School Programs in Speech-Language Pathology

ORGANIZATION AND SERVICE DELIVERY

Fifth Edition

School Programs in Speech-Language Pathology

ORGANIZATION AND SERVICE DELIVERY

Fifth Edition

Jean L. Blosser, Ed.D., CCC-SLP

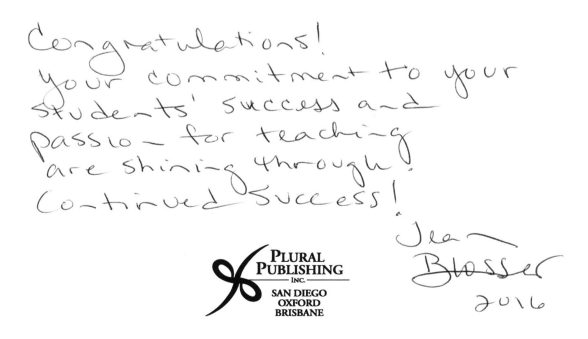

Congratulations!
Your commitment to your
students' success and
passion for teaching
are shining through!
Continued Success!
Jean
Blosser
2016

PLURAL PUBLISHING
INC.
SAN DIEGO
OXFORD
BRISBANE

PLURAL PUBLISHING INC.

5521 Ruffin Road
San Diego, CA 92123

e-mail: info@pluralpublishing.com
Web site: http://www.pluralpublishing.com

Typeset in 10.5/13.5 Palatino by Flanagan's Publishing Services, Inc.
Printed in the United States of America by McNaughton and Gunn
17 16 15 14   5 4 3

Library of Congress Cataloging-in-Publication Data

Blosser, Jean.
School programs in speech-language pathology : organization and service delivery / Jean L. Blosser.—5th ed.
p. ; cm.
Includes bibliographical references and index.
ISBN-13: 978-1-59756-403-8 (alk. paper)
ISBN-10: 1-59756-403-6 (alk. paper)
I. Title.
[DNLM: 1. Speech-Language Pathology—organization & administration—United States. 2. School Health Services—organization & administration—United States. WL 340.2]
LC classification not assigned
371.91'42—dc23

2011031039

Contents

Preface

A look at the early history of the profession of speech-language pathology makes it clear that many changes have occurred since the early 1900s, when the public schools of Detroit and Chicago instituted programs to help children with speech and hearing problems. Some of the most profound changes have occurred in the past several decades, and even more changes are currently underway. Fortunately, the profession has not only weathered the changes but has successfully adapted to them.

This fifth edition of *School Programs in Speech-Language Pathology: Organization and Service Delivery* is written out of passion for the profession and the role speech-language pathologists can play in the school setting, and a desire to inspire others to view schools as the most exciting opportunity to help children achieve their highest potential. I enjoy helping school-based SLPs adapt to, benefit from, and contribute to the many changes in the education and special education landscape that have occurred and are about to unfold. I hope the information serves as a guide to graduate students who are preparing to work in schools, as well as experienced practitioners and clinicians transitioning to schools from other settings.

The major premises and philosophy of this book remain the same as when my former coauthor, Betty Neidecker, originally published it in 1980. The school speech-language pathologist plays a very important role in the schools. Embracing the concept that communication is the foundation of learning and literacy, it is imperative that we strive to provide services and intervention that is educationally relevant in order to help students access the curriculum, participate in their classrooms, and succeed in school. We can only be successful in our role if we collaborate with our education counterparts and our students' families. It is our responsibility to prevent, alleviate, and remove communication barriers that hinder students achieving their full potential and improving their quality of life.

Chapter 1 traces the growth and development of the speech-language pathology profession in the schools, including the philosophy that invited speech-language and hearing programs into the school system, the growth of those programs, and the improvement of quality. An evolution of the speech-language pathology profession is presented. It demonstrates the many changes that have occurred in the SLP's role, focus, and practices. It also shows what changes are on the horizon. The chapter also includes a brief overview of legislation and the emerging role of the school-based SLP.

Chapter 2 includes the role of the *Code of Ethics* of the American Speech-Language-Hearing Association (ASHA), as well as professionalism, certification, and licensing, and professional organizations. It illustrates the breadth and depth of the profession and explores the personal and professional qualifications demonstrated by successful SLPs.

Chapter 3 discusses legislation and important education actions impacting service delivery in the schools. New laws, trends in education, the core curriculum, and national goals and priorities are covered, as well as prevalence and incidence data. The organization of school systems is also presented. Funding for services is discussed, including sources of funding and third-party reimbursement. The SLP's role in inclusion and providing educationally relevant services is introduced. The need for accountability is emphasized. The role of parents as contributing team members is highlighted.

Chapter 4 discusses the SLP's role as a leader and manager and the importance of planning and setting goals. A strategic planning model for developing program change is presented. The chapter also explores time management and planning program, personal, and treatment goals.

Chapter 5 provides a comprehensive description of the facilities for intervention and tools available for use by the SLP. The use of technology for service delivery and record keeping is explored. Suggestions are made for using the Internet to access information or communicate with colleagues and parents. New directions in service delivery via telepractice solutions are explained. Also included is the importance of providing resources to others, including parents, teachers, and specialists.

Chapter 6 explores the importance of documentation and accountability and the driving forces behind the need to include these important elements in speech-language pathology service delivery. Treatment outcomes and the importance of monitoring and documenting changes in students' functional skills as a result of treatment are explained. The essentials of report writing are presented.

Chapter 7 discusses eligibility and decision-making. It explores various methods of assessment including interviewing, observation, functional assessment, curriculum-based assessment, and environmental assessment techniques. Information is included to help understand criteria for determining eligibility, and caseload management is discussed in view of the changing school environment and emerging national educational goals and trends. A section on special populations includes literacy, autism, behavioral disabilities, English as a second language, and transition to work. Highlighted is the SLP's role and strategies for providing service to different groups of students.

Chapter 8 includes the concept and intent of matching students with the most appropriate service delivery options and provides explanations of various models. The concept of considering collaboration as an *essential component* to service delivery rather than a separate service is reinforced. Information on the SLP's workload and caseload is provided. A decision-making framework for matching children to service delivery models is discussed. A range of scheduling and service delivery options, including integrating services within the classroom, are presented.

Chapter 9 reinforces the concept of providing speech-language services that are educationally relevant and designed to help children succeed in school. It explains the SLP's role in developing individualized education programs (IEPs) and individualized family service plans (IFSPs). Also included are methods of providing individualized transition plans

(ITP). Particular emphasis is placed on linking treatment to students' academic needs and working with teachers to facilitate development of communication skills required for classroom success. The importance of identifying and documenting treatment outcomes is stressed.

Chapter 10 focuses on the SLP's role as a collaborative consultant with other professionals and the student's family. The importance of collaborating with others to develop creative solutions to students' communication problems is discussed. The roles and responsibilities of various professionals are included, along with methods of developing and maintaining effective communication and interaction with educators, administrators, family members, and community members.

Chapter 11 explores preservice experiences for students preparing to become school-based speech-language pathologists. It describes the many aspects of the externship experience, as well as providing practical advice. Goals and tasks to be completed during the experience are incorporated. A discussion of ASHA certification requirements is included.

Chapter 12 discusses the importance of lifelong learning and actively engaging in the profession on the national, state, and local levels. Career tracks within the profession, especially in the educational setting, are incorporated in the chapter. Ideas for research within the school setting are also included. Preparation for the job search, interviewing techniques, letters of application, and the resume are covered.

There are discussion questions and projects at the end of each chapter. They are included to help readers consider practical applications of theoretical knowledge and factual information and to stimulate dialogue and discussion with others who are interested in school-based services.

Acknowledgments

Many Thanks

Authoring a text is impossible without the support and contributions of many professional colleagues and associates, coworkers, family, and friends. If this were the Academy Awards, I'd be pulled from the stage for taking such a long time to mention all of the wonderful individuals who contributed to the publication of this book. There are several individuals whose contributions are especially notable. My 90-year-old mother, Mary Prinzo; my sons and their families; and my sister and her family are a constant source of love and support. My son, Trevor, was especially helpful by graphically producing many of the figures and tables. My friends helped me maintain a healthy balance between work, the "book," and enjoying life's adventures. Two of my colleagues in Progressus Therapy, Holly Kaiser and Michael Berthelette, continually provide moral support and positive reinforcement. Many other practicing SLPs reinforce service delivery concepts by implementing them in their schools and providing feedback about practicality and applicability. I feel fortunate to be able to draw from the excellent work of many individuals from within the ASHA community who have led the way in school service delivery. Much of their work is cited throughout the book. I'd also like to thank the members of Special Interest Group 16 (SIG 16) for their lively online discussions about the challenges they face daily while working in schools. Those online discussions often stimulated me to explore new paths. Three passionate SIG 16 members who are exceptionally giving are Les Aungst, Louise Valente, and Shelley Lloyd. I've learned a tremendous amount from each of them. Amazingly, Les continues to enthusiastically provide answers to school-related questions even in his retirement. Finally, I want to thank Jennifer Means, an aspiring young university professor who is dedicated to preparing SLPs to work in the schools in the future. From the moment that I first met Jennifer I knew that she had the energy, commitment, and vision to ensure that SLPs who will practice in schools in the future gain the knowledge and experiences they need to move school service delivery forward. Jennifer and Les willingly reviewed and critiqued the book. Their time, honesty, and recommendations made a difference! Thanks to all.

In Memory

This book is dedicated to Betty Neidecker (1920–2009) in appreciation for her mentoring, commitment, spirit, and vision. Betty authored the first edition of School Programs in Speech-Language Pathology: Organization and Management *in 1980 and subsequently invited me to serve as her coauthor. Betty spent her career nurturing students at Bowling Green State University in Ohio. She was a visionary when it came to school-related services, writing about the roles and responsibilities of SLPs, collaboration, and educationally relevant intervention before the concepts became a trend in our profession. Her philosophy and contributions have shaped the careers of many SLPs and, as a result, impacted the lives of thousands of children.*

1

The Growth and Development of the Profession in the Schools

This chapter provides a historical background of the profession of speech-language pathology and the development of services and programs within the schools of the United States. The philosophy of education that invited speech, language, and hearing programs into the schools is described. Also discussed is the expansion of school speech-language programs, both professionally and geographically. The chapter points out the role of the school-based speech-language pathologist (SLP) in the early days and changes in that role, as well as the factors that influenced those changes. Its also considers the prevailing philosophy and legislation mandating equal educational opportunities for all children with disabilities and its implications for both the programs of the future and the roles and responsibilities of the school speech-language pathologist.

Early History

Although people have experienced speech, language, and hearing problems since the early history of humankind, rehabilitative services for children with communication disabilities were not realized until the early part of the 20th century. The growth of the profession and the establishment of the American Academy of Speech Correction in 1925 reflect the realization of the needs and the special problems of individuals with these disabilities.

According to Moore and Kester (1953), the educational philosophy that invited speech correction into the schools was expressed in the preface to a teacher's manual published in 1897, which contained John Dewey's "My Pedagogic Creed." The preface, written by Samuel T. Dutton, superintendent of schools, Brookline, Massachusetts, stated:

> The isolation of the teacher is a thing of the past. The processes of education have come to be recognized as fundamental and vital in any attempt to improve human conditions and elevate society.
>
> The missionary and the social reformer have long been looking to education for counsel and aid in their most difficult undertakings. They have viewed with interest and pleasure the

> broadening of pedagogy so as to make it include not only experimental physiology and child study, but the problems of motor training, physical culture, hygiene, and the treatment of defectives and delinquents of every class.
>
> The schoolmaster, always conservative, has not found it easy to enter this large field; for he has often failed to realize how rich and fruitful the result of such researches are; but remarkable progress has been made, and a changed attitude on the part of the educators is the result.

Moore and Kester (1953) suggested that child labor laws influenced the growth of speech programs in the schools. Barring children from work forced both the atypical and the typical child to remain in school, and teachers soon asked for help with the exceptional children. A few got help, including assistance with children having speech defects.

According to Moore and Kester (p. 49), it was in 1910 that the Chicago public schools started a program of speech correction. Ella Flagg Young, the superintendent of schools, in her annual report in 1910 said:

> Immediately after my entrance upon the duties of superintendent, letters began to arrive filled with complaints and petitions by parents of stammering children—complaints that the schools did nothing to help children handicapped by stammering to overcome their speech difficulty, but left them to lag behind and finally drop out of the schools: and petitions that something be done for those children. It was somewhat peculiar and also suggestive that these letters were followed by others from people who had given much attention to the study of stammering and wished to undertake the correction of that defect in stammerers attending the public schools. Soon after the schools were opened in the fall, I sent out a note, requesting each principal to report the number of stammerers in the school. It was surprising to find upon receiving the replies that there were recognized as stammerers 1,287 children. A recommendation was made to the committee on the school management to the effect that the head of the department of oral expression in the Chicago Teachers' College be authorized to select ten of the members of the graduating class who showed special ability in the training given at the college in the particular subject and should be further empowered to give additional training of these students preparatory to their undertaking, under the direction of the department, the correction of the speech defects of these 1,287 children. The Board appropriated $3,000.00 toward the payment of these students who should begin their work after graduation at the rate of $65 a month during a period extending from February 1 to June 30.
>
> Instead of gathering the children into one building or into classes to be treated for their troubles, a plan was adopted of assigning to the younger teacher a circuit and having her travel from school to school during the day. The object of this plan was to protect the young teacher from the depression of the spirit and the low physical condition that often ensue from continued confinement in one room for several successive hours at work upon abnormal conditions. It was soon found that the term "stammering" had been assumed to be very general in its application and many children who had been reported as stammerers had not the particular defect reported but some other form of speech defect. (pp. 48–53)

The superintendent of schools in New York in 1909 requested an investigation of the need for speech training in the schools. Two years later the following recommendations were presented to the board of education: First, the number of speech handicapped children was to be ascertained and case histories obtained. Second, speech centers were to be established providing daily lessons of from 30 to 60 minutes. Third, English teachers were to be given further training and utilized as instructors. Fourth, a department for training teachers was to be established. It was not until four years later, however, that a director of speech improvement was appointed to carry out the recommendations (Moore & Kester, 1953).

The Michigan Story

In their fascinating history of the early years of the Michigan Speech-Language-Hearing Association, Costello and Curtis (1989) described the beginnings of the Detroit public school speech correction program.

In 1909, Mrs. Frank Reed, of the Reed School of Stammering in Detroit, contacted the superintendent of the Detroit Public Schools and offered to train two teachers, free of charge, in the Reed Method of the Correction of Stammering, provided the program would be incorporated in the Detroit Schools. A survey was made of the need and 247 cases were found. In May 1910, Mrs. Reed's offer was accepted and during the summer two teachers trained. They were Miss Clara B. Stoddard and Miss Lillian Morley. In September 1910, two centers were opened in Detroit, one on the east side and one on the west side of the city. Wednesday was kept free from classes to call on parents, visit children in the regular classroom and for other activities associated with their work. In 1914, classes for children with other speech defects were begun.

In 1916, Miss Stoddard recommended the establishment of a special clinic at which a thorough physical examination and Binet test be given to children who seemed to have special problems. Regular monthly staff meetings were held and the latest literature on speech was reviewed. The cooperation of teachers and parents was enlisted in the correction of speech. The speech department personnel very early recognized the need for medical care for some of the children. A program for the mentally subnormal in special rooms was inaugurated in 1914 (Costello & Curtis, 1989).

Early Growth

During this same decade there were an increasing number of public school systems employing speech clinicians. Among them were Detroit, Grand Rapids, Cleveland, Boston, Cincinnati, and San Francisco (Paden, 1970). In 1918, Dr. Walter B. Swift of Cleveland wrote an article entitled, "How to Begin Speech Correction in the Public Schools" (reprinted in *Language, Speech and Hearing Services in Schools,* April 1972).

To the state of Wisconsin goes the credit for establishing at the University of Wisconsin the first training program for prospective specialists in the field and for granting the first doctor of philosophy degree in the area of speech disorders to Sara M. Stinchfield in 1921. Wisconsin was also the first state to enact enabling legislation for public school speech services and to appoint in 1923 a state supervisor of speech correction, Pauline Camp. Meanwhile, other universities throughout the United States were developing curricula in the area of speech disorders. Until 1940, however, only eight additional states added similar laws to their statue books (Irwin, 1959). By 1963, a study by Haines (1965) indicated that 45 of the states had passed legislation placing speech and hearing programs in the public schools. These laws provided for financial help to school districts maintaining approved programs, supervision by the state, responsibility for administrating the law, and the establishment of standards. The laws described minimum standards, which the programs were expected to exceed (Haines, 1965).

The first state supervisors, in cooperation with the school clinicians in their respective states, did a remarkably farsighted job in establishing statewide programs in regard to the organizational aspects. With no precedents to follow, they established standards that have retained merit through many years. The Vermont program (Dunn, 1949), providing speech and hearing services to children in rural areas, and the Ohio plan (Irwin, 1949) furnish two such examples. They addressed themselves to such topics as finding children who need the services, diagnostic services, caseloads, the scheduling of group and individual therapy sessions, rooms for the therapist, equipment and supplies, planning time, summer residence programs, in-service training of parents and teachers, and periodic rechecks of children.

A Period of Expansion

The decades of the 1940s and the 1950s were times of growth for all aspects of the profession. In 1943 the American Medical Association requested that a list of ethical speech correction schools and clinics be provided for distribution to physicians. During World War II the entire membership was listed in the National Roster of Scientific Personnel. The organization that started life in 1926 as The American Academy of Speech Correction with 25 dedicated and determined individuals changed its name in 1948 to The American Speech and Hearing Association and in 1979 to The American Speech-Language-Hearing Association (ASHA). Its membership increased from the original 25 persons in 1926 to 330 in 1940, to 1,623 in 1950, and again to 6,249 in 1960. In 1964, the "associate" category was eliminated and there were 11,703 members. By 1975, the membership had climbed to 21,435 with a steady increase until the present time when the membership is approaching 150,000. ASHA is the professional, scientific and credentialing association for its members who are speech-language pathologists and speech, language, and hearing scientists. Several professional journals are published by ASHA and related organizations that are devoted to discussion of the nature and treatment of communication sciences and disorders.

Hearing Handicapped

Initially, programs for children with hearing impairments were designed for children who were deaf. The needs of those with mild to moderate hearing impairments were, for the most part, neglected. Educational programs for the deaf were first established in the United States in 1817 with the founding of the American School for the Deaf at Hartford, Connecticut (Bender, 1960). Children who were deaf received their education in residential schools or institutions until the establishment of classrooms in regular schools. The child in the regular classroom with a mild to moderate or even a severe hearing loss was dealt with by the classroom teacher. In his book, *Speech Correction Methods,* Ainsworth (1948) pointed out that "substitutions and omissions were frequently found in children with hearing loss and may be attacked with articulatory principles employing also visual and kinesthetic avenues of approach." During this era, professionals in the schools were "speech correctionists" and dealt with most communication problems as articulatory problems.

Later the "speech correctionist" became a "speech and hearing therapist" and the public schools therapists included hard-of-hearing children in their caseloads on the same basis as the child with speech handicaps. There were also classroom teachers of the hard-of-hearing in the public schools.

Speech Improvement Programs

School programs designed to help all children develop the ability to communicate effectively in acceptable speech, voice, and language patterns were first called speech improvement programs. The instruction was usually carried out by the classroom teacher, with the speech-language specialist serving as a consultant and doing demonstration teaching in the classroom. Many such programs were initiated in the 1920s, 1930s, and 1940s and were concentrated on the kindergarten and first-grade levels. One of the purposes was to reduce the number of minor speech problems.

The programs were not considered part of the school clinician's regular duties in many states. However, in some cities, speech improvement programs were carried out successfully despite lack of state support.

It was also during these decades that the public school programs increased and expanded, both professionally and geographically. School clinicians found themselves wearing many hats. In addition to selling the idea of such a program to the schools system and the community, the clinician had to:

- Identify the children with speech and hearing handicaps
- Schedule them for therapy at the most convenient time for all concerned
- Provide the diagnosis and therapy
- Keep records and prepare reports
- Work with the school nurse on locating the children with hearing losses
- Counsel the parents
- Answer many questions from teachers who were often totally unfamiliar with therapy services Keep the school administration informed
- Confer with persons in other professional disciplines

- Remain healthy, well groomed, trustworthy, modest, friendly, cheerful, courteous, patient, enthusiastic, tolerant, cooperative, businesslike, dependable, prompt, creative, interesting, and unflappable.

Furthermore, the clinician had to keep one eye on the clock and the calendar and the other eye on state standards.

Language and Speech

Speech-language pathologists have been dealing with children with language problems for many years. Before research and experience sharpened diagnostic tools and awareness, most children were referred to as having "severe articulation disorders," "delayed speech," or "immature language." During the 1940s, 1950s, and early 1960s, there was considerable interest among professionals in articulation and speech sounds.

The focus changed in the late 1960s and early 1970s to an interest in syntactic structures and sentence forms. The past several decades have increased both knowledge and awareness of language problems. Indeed, the title of the professional organization was changed, in recognition of this, from the "American Speech and Hearing Association" to the "American Speech-Language-Hearing Association."

Accompanying the growing awareness of language problems was the realization that the school-based clinician had a commitment to the students whose language is disordered or delayed. Soon school practitioners realized that language was the foundation for learning and that language problems contributed to a student's difficulty in mastering reading or math skills. In addition, language problems were recognized as key characteristics in children who presented hearing impairments, developmental delays, learning disabilities, physical and emotionally impairments, autistic, or environmentally disadvantaged.

Improvement in Quality

The growth in numbers of speech therapists serving the schools was steady during the 1950s and the 1960s. That era concentrated on the improvement of quality as well as quantity by emphasizing increased training for clinicians through advanced certification standards set by professional organizations.

A major project geared toward improving speech and hearing services to children in the schools was undertaken by U.S. Office of Education, Purdue University, and the Research Committee of the American Speech and Hearing Association (Steer et al., 1961). The major objectives were to provide authoritative information about current practices in the public schools and to identify unresolved problems. On the basis of those findings, priorities were established for identification of urgently needed research. Hundreds of clinicians, supervisors, classroom teachers, and university personnel collaborated to develop a list of topics for further study. Research was then distilled by several work groups. The following topics were given the highest priority: the collection of longitudinal data on speech; comparative studies of program organization (with special attention to the frequency, duration, and intensity of therapy); and comparative studies of the use of different speech, voice, and language problems.

Six additional topics were also identified and assigned a high priority: the development of standardized tests of speech, voice, and language; the development criteria for selection of primary-grade children for inclusion in remedial programs; comparative studies of speech improvement and clinical programs; comparative studies of group, individual, and combined group and individual therapy programs; studies of the adjustment of children and their language usage in relation to changes in speech accomplished during participation in therapy programs; and comparative studies of different curricula and clinical training programs for prospective public school speech and hearing personnel.

The study also addressed such topics as the professional role and relationship of the school clinician, the supervision of programs, diagnosis and measurement, and the recruitment of professional personnel to meet the growing needs of children with communication handicaps in the schools. All of these issues continue to be of utmost importance to professionals, ASHA, and school practice today.

The "Quiet Revolution"

School programs changed rapidly in the 1960s and early 1970s. O'Toole and Zaslow (1969) referred to that time period as the "quiet revolution." SLPs became less quiet as they began talking about breaking the cycle of mediocrity, lowering caseloads, giving highest priority to the most severe cases, intensive versus intermittent scheduling, extending programs throughout the summer, utilizing diagnostic teams, and many other issues. The emphasis had shifted, slowly but surely, from quantity to quality.

There were a number of occurrences in the late 1960s and 1970s that attest to the recognition of the public school speech-language specialist as a large and important part the profession. The American Speech and Hearing Association named a full-time staff member to serve as Associate Secretary for School/Clinic Affairs. In 1971, a new journal was initiated, *Language, Speech and Hearing Services in Schools (LSHSS).* In 1999 Special Interest Division 16: Issues in School Service Delivery was initiated and focused on practice in the schools. Subsequently many task forces and committees have worked diligently to foster better understanding of school-based services, children with disabilities, and the role of SLPs in the schools. These steps attest to the importance of school-based practice and have resulted in changes in the qualifications needed to practice in schools, the focus of intervention, improved procedures, and collaboration with our educator colleagues.

Simultaneously, outside influences also asserted pressure on professionals to change the way they provided services to children in schools. Of great significance were changes that occurred in the philosophy and conditions surrounding the American education system. Influences that had the greatest impact included population increases, growing demographic and cultural diversity, limited school budgets, and the importance of literacy, children's right to a fair and appropriate education, attention to special populations, and the adoption of common core standards for education.

Federal Legislation

In 1954, the U.S. Supreme Court's decision in the case of *Brown v. Board of Education* set into motion a new era and struck down the doctrine of segregated education. This decision sparked interest in issues such as women's rights; the right to education and treatment for the handicapped; and the intrinsic rights of individuals, including blacks and minority groups.

Parent organizations have long been a catalyst in bringing about change, and in the case of children with disabilities they were certainly no exception. According to Reynolds and Rosen (1976):

> Parents of handicapped children began to organize about thirty years ago to obtain educational facilities for their offspring and to act as watchdogs of the institutions serving them. At first, the organizations concentrated on political action; since 1970, however, they have turned to the courts. This fact may be more important than any other in accounting for the changes in special education that are occurring now and are likely to occur in the near future.

The PARC Case

An extension of the *Brown v. Board of Education* decision, according to Reynolds and Rosen, was the consent decree established in the case of the Pennsylvania Association for Retarded Children. This decree stated that no matter how serious the handicap, every child has the right to education. The PARC case established the right of parents to become involved in making decisions concerning their child and stipulated that education must be based on problems appropriate to the needs and capacities of each individual child.

Mainstreaming

One of the unexpected aftermaths of the PARC case was to place the stamp of judicial approval on mainstreaming. According to Reynolds and Rosen (p. 558):

> Mainstreaming is a set or general predisposition to arrange for the education of children with handicaps or learning problems within the environment provided for all other children—the regular school and normal home and community environment—whenever feasible.

The intent of mainstreaming was to provide children with disabilities an appropriate educational program in as "normal" or "regular" environment as possible. Thus, depending on the nature and/or severity of the condition, the child may be in a self-contained classroom or a regular classroom for all or part of the educational program. In other words, the child should be taught in the "least restrictive environment allowed by the condition."

Mainstreaming had special implications for the regular classroom teacher as well as other personnel involved in the education of children with handicaps. Reynolds and Rosen (pp. 557–558) said:

Obviously, mainstreaming makes new demands on both regular classroom and special education teachers. In the past, a regular education teacher was expected to know enough about handicapping conditions to be able to identify children with such problems for referral out of the classroom into special education settings. At the same time, special education teachers were trained to work directly with the children with certain specific handicaps (as in the days or residential schools) in separate special settings.

Under mainstreaming, different roles are demanded for both kinds of teachers. The trend for training special education teachers for indirect resource teacher roles rather than narrow specialists is well established in many preparation centers. Concurrently, programs are underway to provide regular education teachers with training in the identification of learning problems. At the local school level, regular and special education teachers in mainstreamed programs are no longer isolated in separate classrooms. They work together in teams to share knowledge, skills, observations, and experiences to enhance the programs for children with special problems, whether the children are permanently or temporarily handicapped. Thus, it has become essential for special teachers to learn the skills of consultation and for both teachers to learn techniques of observation as well as communication.

United States Department of Education

In 1967, Congress created the Bureau of Education for the Handicapped and began a program of grants to speed the development of educational programs. In 1974, Edwin W. Martin, the director of the Bureau of Education for the Handicapped, in an address to the members of the American Speech and Hearing Association, stated that he did not feel we were successfully integrating our roles as speech and hearing specialists in the educational system. He urged that speech-language pathologists and audiologists in schools must be actively involved in interdisciplinary efforts with parents, learning disability specialists, administrators, guidance counselors, classroom teachers, and all educational colleagues.

Over the years, the Bureau has evolved into its present form as the United States Department of Education. The mission of the department is to ensure equal access to education and to promote education success. The Department consists of many divisions and supports numerous programs and initiatives. The most relevant to the field of speech-language pathology services in the schools is the Office of Special Education and Rehabilitation Services (OSERS). The departments within OSERS support programs that assist in providing education to children with special needs, providing for the rehabilitation of youth and adults with disabilities, and supporting research to improve the lives of individuals with disabilities.

To carry out its functions, OSERS consists of three major program-related components. The Office of Special Education Programs (OSEP) is responsible for administrating projects and programs that relate to the free appropriate public education of all children, youth, and adults with disabilities, from birth through age 21. The Rehabilitation Services Administration (RSA) oversees programs that help individuals with physical or mental disabilities to obtain employment through the provision of support services such as counseling, medical, and psychological services, job training, and other individualized services. The National Institute in Disability Rehabilitation Research (NIDRR) supports a comprehensive program of research related to the rehabilitation of individuals with disabilities. One can learn much about the education-related legislation, the goals of education, and support systems in place for professionals by visiting the U.S. Department of Education's Web site https://www.ed.gov. Generally, the United States government defines priorities for education for current time periods. These priorities have impact on the opportunities, findings, and practices for special education including speech-language pathology. We explore some of the priorities that are currently driving education and special education in Chapter 3.

Education Reform and Federal Legislation

Parents, educators, and lawmakers continue to campaign for education reform. Their initiatives inevitably have profound impact on the face of the public education. Each initiative ultimately will also impact the practice of speech-language pathology in schools. The past several decades have seen emphasis on important initiatives including: inclusion of students with disabilities in all facets of the education system; greater focus on increasing graduation rates and preparing students for the world of work; increased involvement of parents in decision making about educational programming; expanding alternative school funding; and the development of programs to deal with students with autism, emotional disorders, and school bullying and violence.

Many key statutes relating to the education of students with disabilities have been implemented over the past several decades. Among the laws that have had the greatest effect on education in America is The Elementary and Secondary Education Act (ESEA) which was originally enacted in 1965 and reauthorized numerous times since then.

The course of special education and speech-language pathology services delivery were most influenced by The Education for All Handicapped Children Act of 1975 (the original Public Law 94-142); an updated version of PL 94-142 called the Education of the Handicapped Act Amendments of 1986 (Public Law 99-457); the most recent version called the Individuals with Disabilities Education Act (IDEA) Amendments of 1997 (Public Law 101-476, later revised as 105-17); and the Rehabilitation Act of 1973 (especially, section 504). The key aspects of these laws are briefly described in the following sections. Although the laws are complex, the intent of supporting positive outcomes for students with disabilities and the mandated guidelines within the laws provide an excellent framework for the provision of quality service delivery programs. Recommendations for developing quality service delivery programs that are responsive to the goals of these laws are discussed throughout the book.

The Elementary and Secondary Education Act (ESEA) and No Child Left Behind (NCLB)

Funding for primary and secondary education was provided through ESEA. Originally funds were to be directed toward professional development, instructional materials, resources to support education programs, and parental involvement. Like other federal legislation, ESEA has been subjected to review and reauthorization every several years. Subsequent reauthorizations include several "Title" programs that focus on specific educational initiatives such as education of children of low income families, supplemental resource centers, educational research and training, improving schools, and providing education to children with limited English proficiency.

The 2001 reauthorization was called the No Child Left Behind Act (NCLB) and has had great impact on educational services, educators and special educators, including SLPs. NCLB (often referred to as "nicklebee") supports standards-based educational reform. This means that setting high standards and establishing measurable goals can improve the quality of educational outcomes. Students' performance in reading and math must be measured annually in third and eighth grades and once in high school. Reading, language arts, science, and mathematics are considered core academic subjects. Schools must demonstrate how students are performing and are judged by their overall performance. Schools with a high number of failing students must make plans for improving their educational practices.

As a result of NCLB, speech-language intervention services have changed dramatically from intervention that is focused on modifying specific speech and language skills to more functionally oriented intervention that is linked to the educational curriculum. Treatment is focused on improving communication skills to help students perform better in learning situations and educational settings.

The next reauthorization of ESEA will most likely respond to ongoing concerns about the effectiveness of our schools. Conversations among interested constituent groups during the pre-reauthorization process in 2010 supported ensuring that students were college ready, empowering teachers and school leaders, and meeting the needs of culturally diverse and English learners, and fostering innovation.

Legislation: PL 94-142

The most sweeping and significant change concerning the education of children with disabilities took place on November 29, 1975, when President Gerald Ford signed into law the Education For All Handicapped Children Act (Public Law 94-142). The major intent of the law was to assure full appropriate education for all children who are disabled between the ages of three and twenty-one. It provided for Individualized Education Programs (IEPs), due process, the use of evaluation procedures for determining eligibility, and education in the least restrictive environment.

The impact of Public Law 94-142 has been beneficial and substantial. It has changed not only the education with handicaps but also has had a wide spread influence on the entire education system. State laws and regulations have been changes, parents have become more involved in the education of their children with handicaps, advocacy groups have influenced education at the local and the state levels, and training institutions and their programs have been affected. Parents and guardians of all children who are disabled are guaranteed legal due process with regard to identification, evaluation, and placement.

Public Law 94-142 has had a pervasive and profound effect on public school speech-language and hearing service delivery. Before the passage of the law, individual states had enacted legislation *permitting* speech and hearing services in the schools, but PL 94-142 *mandated* services for children with speech-language or hearing impairments. In addition, the law established a legal basis for services and provided financial assistance. The scope of speech-language pathology and audiology services are defined in the provisions of the law and mandate the identification and evaluation of children with communication disabilities as well as the development of an Individualized Education Program (IEP) and its implementation. The regulations also cover the provision of appropriate administrative and supervisory activities necessary for programs planning, management, and evaluation.

Legislation: PL 99-457

In 1986, President Ronald Reagan signed into law Public Law 99-457, amendments to the Education for All Handicapped Children Act (PL 94-142). These amendments expanded and strengthened the mandate for providing services to children with handicaps by assisting states to plan, develop, and implement statewide interagency problems for all young children with disabilities from birth through age two. The law included those infants and toddlers who demonstrate developmental delays in the areas of physical development, including vision and hearing, language and speech, psychosocial development, or self-help skills. The law also included infants and toddlers who have a diagnosed physical or mental condition that has a high probability of resulting in developmental delay, or children from birth through age two who may experience developmental delays if early intervention is not provided.

Section 619 of PL 99-457 creates enhanced incentives for states to provide a free and appropriate public education for eligible three- to five-year olds with disabilities. Parent training, family services, and variations in child programming are encouraged by law.

Legislation: PL 101-476 and PL 105-17

In 1990, Public Law 94-142 was further amended. The changed legislation was called IDEA (The Individuals with Disabilities Education Act) or Public Law 101-476. The law resulted in additional major changes. Two new categories of disability (autism and traumatic brain injury) were added. In addition, "person-first" language was introduced changing all references to handicapped children to "children with disabilities." Another change mandated that schools provide transition services to support movement from school to postschool activities.

IDEA was again revised and signed into law by President William Clinton in 1997 (Public Law 105-17). In May, 1999, the final regulations were in effect. IDEA regulations for Part B of the amendment apply to services in school settings. Individual states have the responsibility to establish their own educational requirements. This legislation will have an impact on school programs for the foreseeable future. More revisions will be made as philosophies and knowledge about education for students with disabilities continues to evolve.

Terminology: What's In A Name?

The historical development of school programs in speech and language is interestingly revealed in the titles that have been used over the years. The earliest professionals called themselves "speech correctionists." Some who had previously worked in school systems in this capacity were known as "speech teachers," although they were more concerned with rehabilitation than with elocution. During the 1950s and the 1960s we became "speech and hearing therapists" and "speech and hearing clinicians." All these changes caused no end of trouble, especially in trying to explain the professional's role to others.

During the 1970s we became known as "speech pathologists," and in 1977 the American Speech-Language-Hearing Association in a preference survey found that "speech-language pathologist" was the choice of professionals in the field.

How did we get from "speech correctionist" and speech teacher" to "speech-language pathologist?" The answer is not simple, but perhaps a review of clinical practices may shed some light.

In the 1930s a few universities began programs to train people for clinical roles in public schools and universities. We were "speech correctionists" and "speech teachers." Stuttering problems were the major focus during the earliest days, along with articulation problems. Clinicians were aware of language systems, but problems in that area were treated as speech problems. When faced with students who did not talk, clinicians attempted to stimulate speech by targeting vocal play and babbling. Speech clinicians weren't without their Bryngelson Glaspey Speech Improvement Cards (1941) of Schoolfield's book, *Better Speech and Better Reading* (1937).

Children who did not talk or who had little speech were viewed as having "organic" problems, those related to the brain or neurological systems. Children whose problems in communication yielded to therapy were said to have had "functional" problems. Children who had even minimal vocalization, such as cerebral palsy or hearing impairment, were treated as speech problems. It was at this time the titles of "speech therapists" and "speech and hearing therapists" were used.

Very young children with "delayed speech" and mentally retarded children were excluded from therapy as it was thought they had not reached the proper stage of development to benefit from treatment.

This clinical model was followed for about 30 years, until the late 1950s and early 1960s, when Noam Chomsky's "generative grammar" theories set the stage for the beginning of the profession's understanding of language and language behavior. Although Chomsky offered little help in solving clinical problems, it was at this time that B. F. Skinner's behavioral theories appeared. Speech clinicians still used the functional approach to therapy: however, they did include language-handicapped children on their caseloads for the first time.

One result of these two widely divergent schools of thought was to move the speech clinician's focus away from concentration on problems and articulation.

During the 1960s and the 1970s, the stimulus-response and reinforcement strategies as well as "precision therapy" methods were used to elicit language and speech. These behavior modification methods were widely accepted and speech clinicians freely dispersed rewards and tokens for motivation.

Chomsky's grammar and Skinner's behaviorism prepared the way for the profession's move into semantics and pragmatics and the area of child language. During the 1970s the profession expanded the knowledge base and built on the foundation developed in the 1960s. This had the effect of developing new concepts about language behavior and its component parts.

During the early 1980s children previously excluded form therapy were now included. Children with articulation problems, although still a large part of the speech-language pathologist's caseloads in the public schools, now included individuals with severe language deficiencies, language-learning disabilities, mental retardation, motor handicaps and hearing impairments. Adding impetus to this development was the passage implementation of Public Law 94-142.

Although some may view the trouble with terminology as an identity crisis affecting an entire profession, it might also be constructed as symptomatic of gradual shift in focus from a preoccupation mainly with articulation problems to an interest in language-learning behavior. It also indicates a widening of the scope of services to include prevention as well as remediation, to hone and fine tune our individual professional skills, and to see that these skills are delivered in the most efficient way to the appropriate consumer.

The Emerging Role of the School SLP

Traditionally, in the United States of America, speech, language, and hearing services have been offered as a part of the school program, and a high percentage of the profession has been employed in the schools. Unlike the system in other countries where speech, language, and hearing professionals have follower the "medical model" and have provided services through health and medical facilities such as hospitals, in this country we have followed the "educational model" and provide services in the public schools. Our system is undoubtedly a reflection of our democratic philosophy of education that children have a right to education and that our function in the school is to prevent, remove, and alleviate communication barriers that interfere with the child's ability to profit from the education offered.

Furthermore, the schools constitute an ideal setting in which to provide speech-language intervention services: there is an identified population who are the "consumers" of the services, there are legal mandates for implementation and carrying out the services, and there is local, state, and federal support. Competency in oral and written communication is one of the primary objectives of the school system and today many states, with the encouragement of federal government, have mandated assessment in these areas. Speech, language, and hearing services are the primary support systems in the achievement of these competencies.

Figure 1–1 illustrates the evolution of speech-language pathology service delivery over the past several decades and into the future. For each decade, Column 1

	Focus of Services	SLP Role	Emerging Issues	Treatment Considerations
1970s	• Mechanistic view of language	• Specialist model	• Language use is important	Syntax, Semantics, Phonology
1980s	• Pragmatics	• Expert model	• Language and learning are linked	Content, Form, Use
1990s	• Functional, interactive communication • Preparation for learning, living, and working	• Collaborative-consulting model	• Inclusion • Transition • Efficacy • Accountability • Outcomes	Communication, Learning, Collaboration
2000s	• Social communication	• Facilitator of the service delivery	• Education standards • Alternative schools • Efficacy • Outcomes	Context, Providers, Activities
2010s	• Link therapy to academic performance • Communication for college and work • Cultural diversity and sensitivity	• Education team member/coach • Multiple certification levels • Data oriented	• Common Core Curriculum Standards • Communication for work/college • Integrate technology • Integrate services into classrooms • Evidence based	Evidence, Relevance, Technology

Figure 1–1. Evolution of school-based SLP services.

indicates the areas of communication that were the therapists' focus for treatment. Column 2 shows the roles clinicians have assumed in service delivery. Column 3 lists the emerging issues under professional consideration. This figure shows that changes in service delivery models and the clinicians' role have paralleled the increased understanding of communication disorders and their impact on learning. As issues have emerged and clinical environments changed, clinicians have attempted to modify their practices to adapt to new demands.

The profession is at a new turning point in the evolutionary process. In fact, it appears that the field of speech-language pathology is currently undergoing a metamorphosis in service delivery. Significant changes are taking place in educational settings that are forcing SLPs to reflect on their options for service delivery. In educational forums, public education laws and policies are being rewritten to clarify the meaning and intent of providing services within the classroom setting and in the least restrictive environment. Current perspectives propose an expansion of service delivery options based on communication to serve all children in the learning environment that best fits their individual needs.

At present, speech-language pathologists in school settings are moving toward using inclusive models of service delivery that merge speech and language services with educational programming. Inclusive practices can be described as intervention services that are based on the unique and specific needs of the individual and are provided in a setting that is least restrictive. States are reevaluating services and acceptable service delivery options for all children with special needs. Personnel working in educational settings must demonstrate that their services will support the student so that he or she can participate to the maximum extent possible in social and learning contexts. Based on these directions, the best practice for speech-language pathology services delivery within the school setting would indicate that the general education classroom should be the first step in the continuum of service delivery to students with communication disabilities.

Success is defined in terms of helping students reach measurable, functional outcomes so they can participate in community, family, work, and learning activities. Service delivery has been expanded to include families where possible.

The critical roles of the speech-language pathologist as described in a document entitled, Roles and Responsibilities of Speech-Language Pathologists in Schools (2010, Appendix A) included: working across all levels; serving a broad range of disorders, ensuring educational relevance; providing unique contributions to the curriculum; supporting students' acquisition of language and literacy; and provide culturally competent services. This comprehensive list demonstrates the important contribution the SLPs make in the educational setting.

The school-based SLP plans, directs, and provides diagnostic and intervention services to children and youth with communication disabilities. He or she works with articulation, language, voice, dysfluency, and hearing impairments, as well as speech, language, and hearing problems associated with such conditions as autism spectrum disorders, traumatic brain injury, cerebral palsy, English as a second language, developmental delay, emotional and behavioral disturbances and swallowing disorders.

The speech-language pathologist in the school serves high-risk infants and toddlers from birth to age five in community or school-operated child developmental centers, Head Start programs, special schools, classrooms, or home settings. Also served are children with severe disabilities or multiple impairments in various settings, as well as elementary, middle, and secondary school pupils.

An important aspect of the school speech-language pathologist's duties involve cooperation with other school and health specialists, including audiologists, nurses, social, workers, physicians, dentists, special education teachers, psychologists, and guidance counselors. Cooperative planning with these individuals on a regular basis results in effective diagnostic, facilitative, and educational programs for children with communication problems.

The school speech-language pathologist works with general and special education teachers, administrators and other educators to implement and generalize intervention procedures. Working with parents to help them alleviate and understand problems is also a part of the clinician's function. School administrators are often the key to good educational programming for children, and the school speech-language pathologist works with both principals and program directors toward that end.

The school SLP may also serve as a resource to colleagues and organizations in the community, providing public information about communication disorders and the availability of services for parents and families.

Many school clinicians lead the way in their field by engaging in research to provide evidence of the effectiveness of specific treatment methods. In addition, they initiate best practices for program organization and management and service procedures. The field of speech-language pathology is constantly broadening, and the school SLP must keep abreast of new information by reading professional journals and publications; attending seminars and conventions; enrolling in continuing education programs; and sharing information and ideas with colleagues through state, local, and national professional organizations.

Because the school speech-language pathologist is considered an important part of the total educational program, the size, and structure of the local school district will have much to do with the organizational model used as well as with the nature of the services provided. Often, SLPs travel from school to school throughout the week. Some are assigned to a single school building, whereas others may work in special classes, resource rooms, in classrooms with teachers, or self-contained classrooms. They may be a full-fledged member of the student services team or even work as administrators of speech and language programs.

As the SLP's role as a collaborator or consultant becomes more prevalent, the expectations and responsibilities increase. General education classroom teachers, special teachers, and personnel in other specialized fields may depend on the school speech-language pathologist to provide information on diagnoses, assessment, and treatment of children with communication disorders. As a result, the school-based SLP must be knowledgeable about the school curriculum, the impact of communication disabilities on school performance, and strategies to initiate to ensure that student's performance will improve and they will meet educational standards.

Future Challenges

What is the future role of the speech-language pathologist (SLP) in the schools? Speech-language pathologists working in the schools in the future will need to demonstrate strategies for coping with change. They will need to be well educated, skillful, and flexible. Given the complex American society, they will need to understand and respect the cultural and social backgrounds of their students and communities. They will need to incorporate evidence-based practices for evaluating and treating students. They will need to work with computers for record keeping and incorporate technology into their intervention. Diverse workloads will require them to establish priorities and use better time management skills. Undoubtedly, the federal laws related to special education often serve as a catalyst to programs in the schools and the role of the school speech and language services. It s evident that the laws have enhanced students' access to services and that they have enabled more parental involvement in the educational decision-making process. Some clinicians will implement telepractice to deliver services.

Many of the most significant challenges of working in the school setting have been identified by SLPs during interviews and surveys conducted over the past several years. First and most importantly, SLPs indicate that the changing size and composition of the caseload places new demands on their time, skills, energies, and knowledge base. The type of documentation required to verify compliance with the laws have resulted in increased paperwork, and place great demands on the clinician's time. Perhaps one of the most difficult matters to resolve is the lack of adequate funding necessary to offer quality programs. As America becomes more consumer-oriented, professionals are required to be more and more accountable for their decisions and actions. Administrators and parents are seeking verification of the benefits of speech-language services and treatment outcomes.

Demands such as these can lead to burnout and stress for clinicians. Staying abreast of new trends in treatment, attending professional conferences, working with professionals from other disciplines, and trying new and different strategies in therapy are all positive steps clinicians can take to maintain their interest and energy. To help alleviate the financial constraints, SLPs can work closely with their administration and advocate for change through their professional organizations and political arenas.

Although there are many problems faced by school SLPs and the profession as a whole, there are also exciting and challenging developments. It is difficult to predict how speech-language pathology will be different in the future, but we can make some educated guesses. The makeup of the caseload in schools has already shifted from preponderance of articulation problems to mainly language and learning disabilities. The prevalence and incidence of disabilities such as autism spectrum disorders is skyrocketing. More and more children from diverse backgrounds will be enrolled in the school systems. It will be necessary to develop programs that meet the growing and diverse needs of our multicultural society. There will be an extension of services to preschool children, and, at the other end of the line, services to high school students must focus on preparing them for graduation and employment. Children with severe or multiple disabilities will be placed in general education classrooms and many of these children will have speech and/or language problems.

The role of the SLP as a collaborator and consultant will be greatly expanded, as will the role as a team member in diagnosis, assessment, and placement decisions. There will be increased demand for services designed to help children acquire the skills of reading, writing, and spelling as well as speaking and listening. As has been true in the fields of medicine and dentistry, there will be an emergence of specialists in speech-language pathology. Funding streams for services will be altered greatly. Speech-language pathologists will be expected to use technology for record keeping as well as for diagnosis and intervention. They will be expected to work closely with classroom teachers and health professionals.

SLPs are not alone in their efforts to cope with these trends and changes. The profession as a whole and certainly our professional organizations must focus on these challenges as well. Speech-language pathologists will be expected to be highly educated, flexible, and multiskilled. In addition to consulting, evaluating, or providing intervention, SLPs will have to demonstrate knowledge and competency about social, political, economic, and cultural issues that influence the performance of their roles. Keeping school administrators apprised of their work, the responsibilities, and their program needs will be imperative.

DISCUSSION QUESTIONS AND PROJECTS

1. How does an understanding of the early role of the school speech-language clinician help in understanding the current role?

2. How has the role of the clinician in the schools changed over the years? Do you think this has any relationship to the titles by which we have been and are presently called?

3. Ask 10 of your friends, who are not in the speech-language pathology field, to comment on the titles by which we have called ourselves and what these titles convey to them. Ask the same question of elementary education majors or teachers.

4. Do you think the changes in the profession were brought about by outside pressures or by internal factors?

5. How do you think the role of the SLP in the schools differs from the role of the SLP in private practice? In a community clinic? In a hospital?

2

The Professional School Speech-Language Pathologist

The Code of Ethics of the American Speech-Language-Hearing Association establishes the ground rules for the communication sciences and disorders profession. The principles include conduct toward the client, the public and fellow professionals. Certification is the stamp of approval issued by a responsible agency to individuals who meet specific requirements. It confers the right to practice and the right to be recognized as a professional. It also carries with it the responsibility of exemplary professional behavior.

Organizations are important links facilitating the exchange of new ideas, information, research, recent developments, materials, and professional affairs. School speech-language pathologists must be aware of the various professional organizations and their functions in order to choose the ones with which they will affiliate. Professionalism and professional behavior are discussed in this chapter.

The Code of Ethics

One of the first tasks of the American Academy of Speech Correction, as the professional organization was first called, was the establishment of a Code of Ethics. Mindful of the fact that there were unscrupulous individuals who would take advantage of persons with handicapping conditions by making rash promises of cures and by charging exorbitant fees, the earliest members of the profession felt it necessary to maintain professional integrity and encourage high standards by formulating a Code of Ethics. As may be expected, it was a difficult task, and throughout the history of the organization the code has been periodically updated to meet current problems; however, its purpose and core beliefs have remained substantially the same. The Code outlines the ASHA member's professional responsibilities to the patient, to coworkers, and to society. Thus, it might be said that accountability has always been one of the profession's highest priorities.

Although the Code was adopted for members of the professional association, it serves as the benchmark for the entire profession. In the language of the Code the terms *individuals* refers to all members of the American Speech-Language-Hearing Association and those nonmembers who hold the Certificate of Clinical Competence.

A code of ethics defines a profession's highest standards of integrity and parameters. It should also protect the rights of the consumer. The ASHA Code establishes the fundamental principles and rules considered essential. It addresses confidentiality, the use of persons in research, the supervision of paraprofessionals and of students in training, as well as other matters. The Code has no legal basis except in states where it has been adopted as part of the licensing requirements.

The American Speech-Language-Hearing Association has established an Ethical Practice Board whose major responsibility is the enforcement of the Code of Ethics. A member of ASHA who is a holder of the Certificate of Clinical Competence and who is found guilty of noncompliance may be dropped from membership and have their Certificate revoked. A nonmember who is found guilty of noncompliance would face revocation of the Certificate. The loss of membership status and/or the revocation of the Certificate of Clinical Competence follow procedures of due process set up by the Ethical Practice Board. There is also an appeals procedure. A copy of the Board's practices and procedures as well as the appeals procedures can be found on the American Speech-Language-Hearing Association Web site, http://www.asha.org . It is also reprinted each year in many of ASHA's publications. Examples of cases that have been brought forward for review by the Ethics Board are published and illustrate how the Code of Ethics is interpreted. The ASHA Code of Ethics was last revised in 2010 (ASHA, 2010, Appendix B).

Principles of Ethics

When you read the Code of Ethics you will see that it can serve as a source of the answers to many of the perplexing challenges you may encounter in your day-to-day work. There are four Principles of Ethics and Rules for each of the Principles. The Principles and Rules guide professionals in their responsibility to the individuals they serve, the public, fellow colleagues and the conduct of research and scholarly activities. The Principles are:

> **Principle of Ethics I:** Individuals shall honor their responsibility to hold paramount the welfare of persons they serve professionally or who are participants in research and scholarly activities and they shall treat animals involved in research in a humane manner.
>
> **Principle of Ethics II:** Individuals shall honor their responsibility to achieve and maintain the highest level of professional competence and performance.
>
> **Principle of Ethics III:** Individuals shall honor their responsibility to the public by promoting public

> understanding of the professions, by supporting the development of services designed to fulfill the unmet needs of the public, and by providing accurate information in all communications involving any aspect of the professions, including the dissemination of research findings and scholarly activities, and the promotion, marketing, and advertising of products and services.
>
> **Principle of Ethics IV:** Individuals shall honor their responsibilities to the professions and their relationships with colleagues, students, and members of other professions and disciplines.

Consider the statement in Principle of Ethics I that says, "Individuals shall honor their responsibility to hold paramount the welfare of persons served professionally." There is hardly a professional problem that cannot be solved by asking yourself, "What is best for the client?" versus "What is best for me?" or "What is best for the school?" Your role as a speech-language pathologist puts you in the position of a child advocate. In other words, you are on the side of the child. His or her best interests are your professional responsibility and it is that person for whom you speak.

Deciding what is "best" means that you will have to look at the needs of the whole person. A communication problem cannot be separated from the rest of the individual. The educational, health, psychological, and social aspects must be taken into consideration. Fortunately, you do not have to make decisions by yourself because in a school system SLPs work closely with the family, classroom teacher, school administrator, psychologist, school nurse, physician, social worker, occupational or physical therapists, educational audiologist, and other professionals. The decision concerning what is best for the student is therefore a consensus of those persons in the child's life, who hold paramount the best interests of that individual.

Another important ethical consideration is confidentiality. You will have access to much information about the student with whom you are working and the child's family. This information is given in trust and should be regarded as confidential. The only other persons with whom you might share this information are other professionals in the school who may be working with the child. Within a school system the school policies usually state that pertinent information may be shared among interested professionals, whereas information that may be conveyed to professionals or agencies outside the school system must have the written consent of the parents or guardians. "Shared information" does not mean idle gossip. A conference with other educators should not to be carried on in the hallways, over lunch in the teachers' lunchroom, in front of children or community members, or during social activities.

Ethics Issues in the School Setting

Davis-McFarland (2010) describes the most frequently recurring ethics issues as employer demands, use and supervision of support personnel, cultural competence, reimbursement for services, professional versus business ethics, and clinical fellowship supervision. Practitioners in the school setting can be prepared to respond proactively to ethical issues that confront them if they are familiar with the Code of Ethics and can offer alternative approaches to situations as they arise.

Davis-McFarland illustrates the following ethics issues that have been reported. Some examples of *employer demands* may involve "pressure to provide services without adequate training; adhering to eligibility criteria or program placement recommendations that may be in conflict with clinical judgment; use of old equipment or technology, or providing unwarranted services. Ethics issues regarding *supervision of support personnel* may include, "inadequate supervision; inadequate documentation of supervision; inappropriate delegation of responsibilities; or billing for services by unsupervised students or assistants." Some practices related to *reimbursement for services* that may lead to ethical dilemmas are, "misrepresenting services to obtain reimbursement; billing for services provided by a clinician who is not certified; intentionally misusing incorrect code numbers or diagnostic labels to qualify for payment; billing for services that are not provided or unnecessary." Some common *professional versus business ethics* situations that school-based clinicians may experience are "solicitation of students for private practice from their school caseload; acceptance of gifts or incentives from manufacturers; client abandonment and/or disruption of services; failure to report unethical behavior; or misuse of professional credentials." During the *Clinical Fellowship experience* some ethical issues that may arise for new professionals are "inadequate or inappropriate supervision; inadequate time to meet supervisory responsibilities; inadequate documentation of supervision of the CF's performance; supervisor's failure to maintain their own competence; or misuse of power over the clinical fellow."

Clinicians who are concerned about practices that may be unethical, either theirs or those of another individual, can review the ASHA Code of Ethics for guidance. The ASHA Web site also provides information and reference documents such as the Ethics Q & A for School-Based Speech-Language Pathology Practice (http://www.asha.org) and Ethics and IDEA (ASHA, 2007).

Personal and Professional Qualifications

The communication sciences and disorders profession is multifaceted. Some members teach at the university level, some work in organizations, some supervise in clinics, some administer programs, some provide treatment, some do research, and some are diagnosticians. The SLP who chooses to work in the education setting has the responsibility of preventing, removing, and alleviating communication barriers that may hinder a student from receiving the maximum benefit from the instruction offered in the classroom. In addition, the school clinician is a resource person to others in the school system. Another role of the school-based speech-language pathologist is advisor to the family of the student who has the communication disorder or counselor to that individual. Care should be taken not to provide counsel or advice about issues that are outside the scope of the SLP's role and responsibilities.

In addition to the appropriate education and specialized knowledge and skills, what personality traits are desirable for the school SLP, who must wear so many hats? Among the most frequently mentioned are intelligence, patience, understanding, honesty, adaptability, flexibility, sense of humor, warm and friendly nature, respect for others, acceptance of others, dependability, resourcefulness, and creativity.

Fortunately, many SLPs realize that the skills they acquire will enable them to serve in many interesting roles. SLPs are well prepared to pursue many careers. Examples of alternative career opportunities are provided in Chapter 12. Becoming aware of your unique skills and identifying career and life goals is very important to individuals who wish to function successfully in a complicated school system. In addition to the traditional knowledge base, clinical, and research skills acquired through training and experience, there are many skills that can be applied to the SLP role as well as other professions including:

Leadership

Speech-language pathologists demonstrate leadership skills by serving on committees and participating in activities in their place of employment, in the community, in their state or national association.

Detail/Follow-Through Skills

Speech-language pathologists must present organized and thorough work habits, be detail-oriented, and explicit in communication. These skills are evidenced through daily case management and leadership practices.

Persuasion and Advocacy Skills

Speech-language pathologists influence clients, parents, professionals in related disciplines, physicians, state legislators, and the public about the need of individuals with communication disorders.

Mentoring Skills

Demonstrating intervention techniques to parents, teachers, and related professionals is an integral part of a speech-language pathologist's typical work week regardless of work setting.

Communication Skills

Speech-language pathologists are excellent communicators with clients, on school teams, and with the public.

Human Relations Management

Speech-language pathologists interact with coworkers, employees, students and their families in many different interactive situations.

Coaching and Educational Skills

Speech-language pathologists often teach undergraduate and graduate courses, give lectures at state association meetings and annual conventions, give in-service presentations to parents, teachers, physicians, and other professionals, and provide other continuing education opportunities.

Resource Design and Development

In addition to their other skills, speech-language pathologists frequently design, plan, market, and implement special programs.

Program Review and Author

Many SLPs who are actively engaged in professional associations may evaluate papers for conferences or state association meetings and publish articles in professional journals and newsletters. Some energetic clinicians work with the media to improve public understanding of the profession.

Financial Management

Budget planning and responsible use of funds is a responsibility of many speech-language pathologists, especially in school districts where funding is severely limited.

Fundraising

SLPs raise funds to purchase materials for their program or provide assistance to children in need.

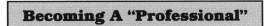

Becoming A "Professional"

Following commencement, graduate students become a professional person with all the rights and privileges as well as all the challenges that go along with being a speech-language pathologist. What does it mean to be a "professional"? For one thing, you earn money for doing the things you did for course credit as a student clinician in the university clinic. During that time, your clinical hours, your intervention plans, and your clinical decisions were subject to review and possible revision by your supervisor. When you turn that corner and become a professional, you become the decision-maker in all these areas. Knowing who you are and your scope of practice as well as where you fit in, together with your values and your attitudes, will provide the basis from which you will make decisions and plans throughout your professional life.

Guidelines for behavior as a professional speech-language pathologist have been set forth in the Code of Ethics. Please note that these are only guidelines. They can only assist you in making ethical, moral, and legal decisions. There are no clear-cut answers to many of the vexing problems that arise.

There are many numerous behaviors that contribute to professionalism. What sort of messages do your mannerisms convey? Are they distracting, annoying, or demeaning? Do you give the appearance of aloofness? Or do you present yourself as being a competent person who shows both friendliness and helpfulness?

Your general appearance also contributes to professionalism. You may be more comfortable in what you wear when relaxing with friends, but on the job this same style of dress may convey an unintended message to parents, coworkers, and to the individuals who are your clients. It goes without saying that cleanliness, careful grooming, appropriate dress, and good hygiene are at the top of the list.

By dressing appropriately you underscore respect for your client and the seriousness of your purpose. No matter what your personal preferences are, you should take into consideration the impression you are making on others. Clothing that is comfortable, clean, and appropriate to your age and setting is another part of your professional image.

Certification, Licensure, and Accreditation

Understanding the various forms of credentials that are required in speech-language pathology as well as other educators and specialists who work in the schools can provide insights about the perspective each individual brings to his or her role. To the neophyte clinician the task may seem formidable; however, some basic information may help clarify the situation.

The Voluntary Agency

Voluntary agencies have developed in countries with a democratic form of government. The voluntary agency is more clearly identified in the United States than in any other nation and usually has evolved out of an unmet need and a concern for one's fellows. The unmet need may be related to social issues, to leisure time and recreation, or to health. Voluntary health agencies may be related to specific diseases or disabling conditions. Usually the membership of voluntary agencies is made up of both lay persons (in many cases, parents) and professionals. Examples of voluntary health agencies are the United Way, the Autism Society, the Brain Injury Association, and the Easter Seal Society. Voluntary agencies are not certifying agencies in the usual sense of the word; however, they perform extremely vital functions for individuals with disabilities and the professionals who serve them. At times members may engage in advocacy or raise awareness about the needs of their constituency.

The Official Agency

The official agency is tax supported and may be on the city, county, regional, state, or federal level. Some agencies bridge two governmental jurisdictions. Official agencies cover myriad categories, including health, education, welfare, vocational, and recreational services. They are interested in the prevention of problems, in research, and in specific disease categories. Examples of official agencies are the city or county health department and the offices that offer vocational rehabilitation services. Some official agencies may be certifying bodies, such as a state department of education.

The Professional Organization

In addition to official and voluntary agencies there are also professional organizations. They, as the name implies, are made up of individuals sharing the same profession. Their goals are to establish and maintain high professional standards, research, recruitment of others into the field, and to share professional information. Examples are the American Speech-Language-Hearing Association, the Council for Exceptional Children, the American Occupational Therapy Association, the American Medical Association, and the National Education Association.

These various types of agencies often work together in a unique fashion, sometimes motivating each other to carry out specific tasks, often supporting each other financially and in other ways, frequently exchanging services and information and preventing duplication of services. The official agencies and the professional organizations also may be accrediting and certifying bodies in addition to the other functions.

Types of Credentials

There are three different types of credentials that directly affect the individual speech-language pathologist, depending on their geographic location and work setting. The type of credential needed to practice in schools varies from state to state and is determined by the state department of education. Obtaining one type of credential does not preclude obtaining another type of credential. In fact, many SLPs hold several credentials and may acquire more throughout their career as they obtain additional professional training or relocated.

In looking at the academic, clinical, and experience requirements of all entities that credential SLPs, you will note that they are almost, if not completely, identical. The academic requirements follow the same pattern. Specific courses can be used to fulfill requirements of several agencies. For example, a course in language development can fulfill the requirements for ASHA's Certificate of Clinical Competence, for public school certification from the state's department of education, and for a license from the state licensure board. There are fees for the original application for a credential and ongoing fees to maintain the credential. It is risky to let a credential lapse because requirements for renewing the credential may change over time. Some states have established reciprocity which means that one state may accept the credentials of another state. Before letting a credential lapse, it is wise to know what steps and verifications will be necessary to reinstate that credential.

Certification by the American Speech-Language-Hearing Association

One type of credential is issued by the American Speech-Language-Hearing Association (ASHA). Unlike licensing and state certification, it has no legal status, but nevertheless it is recognized by various states and by other professions as authenticating the holder as a qualified practitioner or supervisor. ASHA certification is known as the Certificate of Clinical Competence (CCC) and can be obtained by persons who meet specific requirements in academic preparation and supervised clinical experiences and who pass a national comprehensive examination. ASHA grants certification in speech-language pathology. The certificate permits the holder to provide services in the appropriate areas and also to supervise the clinical practice of trainees and clinicians who do not hold certification. Since 1977, persons who are not members of the Association are permitted to obtain the CCC by complying with the requirements.

At least a master's degree is required for certification as a speech-language pathologist (CCC-SLP) by the American Speech-Language-Hearing Association. Furthermore, the graduate coursework and the graduate clinical experience must be obtained at an institution whose program is accredited by the Council on Academic Accreditation (CAA) of the American Speech-Language-Hearing Association (ASHA).

The CCC is held by individuals who provide services in schools, medical settings, universities, speech-language and hearing centers, clinics, private practice, and other programs throughout the United States, Canada, and many foreign countries. Information on how to apply for the CCC may be obtained from the American Speech-Language-Hearing Association Web site http://www.asha.org .

State Credentials and Certification

The speech-language pathologist who wishes to be employed in the public schools of a specific state must obtain a certificate or license issued by that state's department of education. Some states with licensure also grant approval to work in the schools. The qualifying standards are set by each state and include following a prescribed course of study and fulfilling the clinical requirements. Like the CCCs, the state license or certification includes both academic and clinical practice during the university experience. These experiences must be under the supervision of licensed and/or certified qualified professionals.

The recent passage of federal legislation regarding special education service delivery has resulted in activities in many states to improve special education service delivery by upgrading certification standards and requirements. The laws call for personnel standards to be based on the highest requirements in the state applicable to a specific profession or discipline. This is referred to in the law as the highest qualified provider. The majority of states in the United States require a master's degree or master's degree equivalent for state education agency certification. Information on the certification requirements of each state can be obtained by writing to the state department of education or its equivalent. Addresses of the various state departments of education are routinely published in ASHA materials or listed on state government Web sites.

Licensing

A license to practice a business or profession within the geographic bounds of a specific state is issued by that state's legislature, usually through an appointed autonomous board or council. Licensing came about originally to protect the consumer from unqualified and unscrupulous persons. It is also viewed by some as a way to control growth and income of professional interest groups. Obviously, the laws to create licensure are unique to each state.

In the speech, language, and hearing profession, the licensure board may establish rules for obtaining and retaining a license, continuing one's education, and setting standards for ethical conduct. The Board may also administer examinations for applicants and enforce the license law.

Another aspect of licensing is the "sunset law," which means that periodically the legislature may review the licensing agency (and other regulating agencies) and recommend whether or not it should be terminated.

Agency and Program Accreditation

Relevant to the administration of speech-language pathology programs, the American Speech-Language-Hearing Association has established the Council on Academic Accreditation (CAA). Accreditation by CAA assures that institutions offering academic programs in speech-language pathology at the master's level meet minimal standards. ASHA committees and boards continually review the standards to ensure that they reflect the profession's current needs and trends. Complete instructions for fulfilling CAA requirements are available from the national office of the American Speech-Language-Hearing Association. University programs are periodically subjected to review by an external team of CAA reviewers to maintain their accreditation.

Professional Associations

The school SLP has a professional responsibility to keep abreast of new ideas, research, recent developments, materials, publications, and professional affairs. This is a lifelong commitment, and it is part and parcel of what being "professional" means. One way of keeping current and informed is through professional associations. Organizations sponsor meetings with reputable speakers, publish journals and newsletters, and provide an excellent way to get to know fellow colleagues. Speech-language pathologists in schools sometimes feel isolated even though they are in daily contact with children and school personnel. This sense of isolation can be mitigated by being in contact with other speech-language specialists, with whom they can share ideas, information, frustrations, and triumphs.

The most comprehensive and well-established professional organization in the field of speech-language pathology and audiology is the American Speech-Language-Hearing Association. The membership of ASHA is approximately 145,000 members including speech-language pathologists, audiologists, and speech, language, and hearing scientists. This organization has been one of the chief agents for growth and evolution in the profession.

Students are encouraged to affiliate with the National Student Speech-Language-Hearing Association (NSSLHA), which offers many opportunities not otherwise available to individuals in training. It is an affiliate of ASHA, with chapters in colleges and universities. Participation in NSSLHA affords student with the opportunity to engage in learning as well as leadership activities.

Within the ASHA structure there currently are 18 Special Interest Groups. The Groups provide education, leadership and advocacy for members. The divisions focus on specific populations and practice issues including:

Group 1: Language, Learning, and Education

Group 2: Neurophysiology and Neurogenic Speech and Language Disorders

Group 3: Voice and Voice Disorders

Group 4: Fluency and Fluency Disorders

Group 5: Speech Science and Orofacial Disorders

Group 6: Hearing and Hearing Disorders: Research and Diagnostics

Group 7: Aural Rehabilitation and Its Instrumentation

Group 8: Public Issues Related to Hearing and Balance

Group 9: Hearing and Hearing Disorders in Childhood

Group 10: Issues in Higher Education

Group 11: Administration and Supervision

Group 12: Augmentative and Alternative Communication

Group 13: Swallowing and Swallowing Disorders (Dysphagia)

Group 14: Communication Disorders and Sciences in Culturally and Linguistically Diverse Populations

Group 15: Gerontology

Group 16: School-Based Issues

Group 17: Global Issues in Communication Sciences and Related Disorders

Group 18: Telepractice

A number of committees and task forces are formed on an ongoing basis within the Special Interest Group structure as well through the ASHA governance structure to provide information and support for individuals who work in private and public school settings. The Special Interest Groups and many related professional organizations (RPO) hold membership meetings annually at the national convention. They appoint liaisons to keep information and communication flowing between professionals and local or national organizations. Clinicians who are interested in deepening their knowledge or expanding their skills in a specific area or advocating for clients with a particular type of disability can benefit from membership in a special interest group. Being an active participant in association activities enables practitioners to have a voice and shape the direction of the profession and service delivery.

Another organization with which the school speech-language pathologist may want to affiliate is the Division for Children with Communication Disorders (DCCD), a division of the Council for Exceptional Children (CEC). This organization publishes the *Journal of Childhood Communication Disorders*, holds state and national meetings, and is organized as a state group in many states.

Every state has its professional speech-language pathology and audiology association that holds conventions, publishes journals, and sponsors continuing education programs. The state organizations also publish directories of members' names and professional addresses. Many organizations lobby their state legislature for support of professionally related issues.

There may be regional organizations in addition to the state professional organizations. Affiliation with the regional group provides an invaluable opportunity for exchange of information and offers support to individual members. Involvement in such groups is both rewarding and enjoyable. The national as well as state and local speech, language, and hearing professional organizations are concerned with such activities as research, the study of human communication and its disorders, the investigation of intervention and diagnostic procedures, and the maintenance of high standards of performance. The professional organizations are also interested in the dissemination of information among its members and the upholding of high ethical standards to protect the consumer. There are other benefits to be derived from affiliating oneself with a professional organization. Such a group can provide a forum for discussion of issues and can speak with a concerted voice on matters of professional interest and concern. If the professional individual wishes to have a voice in decisions and opinions, the best way to do so is through a professional organization on the state, local, or national level.

There are a number of other related professional organizations with which the school clinician may wish to become affiliated. Membership in other professional groups provides opportunities for valuable exchanges of information and enhances cooperation and understanding. You will learn about other organizational opportunities as you read the professional literature and interact with colleagues throughout your career. Most charge membership dues but the benefits are worth it.

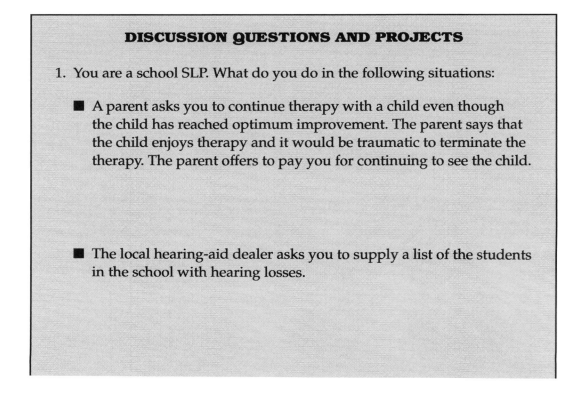

DISCUSSION QUESTIONS AND PROJECTS

1. You are a school SLP. What do you do in the following situations:

    - A parent asks you to continue therapy with a child even though the child has reached optimum improvement. The parent says that the child enjoys therapy and it would be traumatic to terminate the therapy. The parent offers to pay you for continuing to see the child.

    - The local hearing-aid dealer asks you to supply a list of the students in the school with hearing losses.

- An elementary school teacher asks if she may see the records and reports of a middle-school student enrolled in therapy. She asks your opinion concerning whether or not the student is developmentally delayed. (Test results showed that the child isn't delayed.)

- You are asked to do private after-school therapy with a child enrolled in a school in which you are working. The parents are willing to pay for providing the service and you are interested in developing a private practice. The child is already receiving therapy and is on your caseload.

- The parents of a student referred for medical evaluation ask you to recommend a doctor.

- You are asked to do therapy in the school with a student who is currently receiving therapy at a nearby private speech, language, and hearing center. You are aware of this, but the parents did not provide you with this information.

2. Find out the requirements for licensure or certification in your state.

3. Find out what speech, language, and hearing organizations are active in your region. Learn about their membership requirements, purposes, goals, and meeting schedule. Invite an officer of a local organization to speak to your class. Plan to attend one of their meetings. Obtain a copy of their newsletter or journal. Visit their Web site.

4. What are the advantages of joining the National Student Speech-Language-Hearing Association?

5. Investigate ASHA's Special Interest Groups. Join one that interests you.

6. Review the program from a recent state or national convention. Which sessions are of interest to you and why?

7. Contact the president of your state speech-language-hearing association. Ask if they need volunteers for any committees or projects.

3

Foundations of the Program

This chapter provides basic information about the factors that need to be considered in planning and organizing a school speech-language program. As you read, be aware that the information about the structure of the school system is general. Schools are organized in many different ways but have many common features. You, as the school speech-language pathologist, should acquaint yourself with the structure of the educational system in the state in which you live and work. The same is true about the city, county, or district school system in which you are employed. In fact, if you are considering a specific site for future employment, it is a good idea to learn as much as possible before you sign a contract; then continue to increase your knowledge as you go along.

Federal legislation has had tremendous effect on public school special education and speech-language programming. As you read through this book you will find frequent references to several key laws. Your task will be to keep abreast of the changes and requirements of federal and state laws affecting your school speech-language intervention program.

Public schools are supported by state and local taxes as well as by federal flow-through funds. It is important to be knowledgeable about how your program is supported, how budgets are determined, and the process by which funds are allocated. In some cases, the input of the SLP is required or expected and in some instances you may wish to request to have input. Without knowledge of how schools and programs are financed, the SLP is at a serious disadvantage. Another factor in planning a speech and language program is the number of students with whom you will be dealing. It would be nice if these figures were conveniently available, but unfortunately determining prevalence figures is a complex matter. The best we can do is to rely on all the current information at hand and make generalizations that apply to individual school systems. Much more attention is given to determining prevalence figures at the present time than in the past, and the developments in this area are promising.

Organizational Structure of the School System

Program at the State Level

Because of our democratic philosophy of education, we are committed to the concept of education for all. The major responsibility for education rests with each state rather than with the federal government. Through a state board of education, all policies, regulations, rules, and guidelines are set. The laws for education in each state are enacted through the state legislatures, and money is appropriated through this body. A state superintendent of instruction is the chief education officer in each state. A state department of education is responsible for carrying out and developing policies, regulations, and standards related to schools.

State departments of education provide state consultants in various areas of special education. The responsibilities of the consultants in special education and speech-language pathology may vary slightly from state to state, but in general the tasks are similar through the nation. A major task of the professional staff on the state level is to monitor and enforce *minimum* standards of practice in local programs that are partially or fully reimbursed from state money. Along with this, local programs are encouraged to approach optimal goals in serving the needs of students with disabilities. The state staff may provide leadership in assistance with identifying, developing, and maintaining optimal standards.

Following are some examples of ways in which state and local consultants demonstrate their professional leadership to assist school districts, speech-language programs, and clinicians as they try to comply with established standards.

Alerting Districts to Mandates and Requirements

State educational consultants function as the primary source of information for districts regarding legislation, mandates and requirements. They interpret the laws and provide guidelines for implementation.

Providing Access to Relevant Professional Resources and Materials

Busy SLPs sometimes find it difficult to stay abreast of the changing practices and trends in the profession. Consultants often assist by establishing procedures for exchange of resources and materials, providing bibliographies of significant materials, and developing abstracts or summaries of articles that describe important issues.

Organizing and Conducting In-Service Education Programs

In today's climate, the practice of speech-language service delivery is constantly changing. To best serve student needs, the SLP must keep up with changes in diagnostic methods, technology, and intervention procedures. In addition, they must be able to understand and implement new legislation. Consultants assist with this process by organizing and/or conducting meetings and conferences that SLPs can attend to continually improve their skills and qualifications. They also coordinate efforts with professional organizations in the state. Ongoing education such as this will help practitioners in the field develop relationships with other professionals and provides a framework for ensuring effectiveness.

Promoting Professional Relationships with State Agencies and Other Related Professional Disciplines

Speech-language pathology is not practiced in isolation. By working with consultants in other disciplines, the state consultant can help facilitate understanding of how the disciplines can work in collaboration to provide the optimal services for children. In addition, collaboration at that level can help facilitate greater efficiency of effort.

Encouraging Research Studies, Experimental Projects, and Grant Proposals

School-based programs offer excellent opportunities for collecting data and conducting research into the effectiveness of evaluation and treatment methods. In addition, there are numerous opportunities for experimental projects and pilot studies. Consultants can provide direction about the type of data that is needed. They can identify research partners and potential sources of funding. Clinicians who engage in research discover many new perspectives about children with communication disorders and options for treating those disorders. Such efforts can be rewarding and lead to professional growth opportunities. Findings of research efforts often lead to modifications in existing laws and standards.

Identifying Underserved Populations and Unmet Needs

As the demographics of communities continue to change, so will the children who are enrolled in school programs. School-based clinicians sometimes feel frustrated because they experience difficulties fitting new groups of youngsters or different types of communication problems into existing caseloads and service delivery models. Consultants can help identify new needs and broaden the awareness of others so that they begin to understand the types of changes that will enable the program to be more responsive to those who are served.

Conducting Preservice Education Programs

Often, speech-language pathology and special education consultants are asked to contribute to the preparation of future school-based SLPs. They do so by helping universities identify the qualifications SLPs will need to meet the needs of youngsters. They present lectures that help students understand realistic aspects of practice in the school setting. Some individuals are asked to advise university faculty on changes in the federal and state legislation that affect practice in the school setting and assist with review of the professional curriculum to ensure that key aspects are incorporated so that students will be well prepared for their roles.

Serving as a consultant at the regional or state level can be a very rewarding career path to pursue for therapists desire to serve in a leadership role and want to influence how services are provided for students with disabilities.

Compliance with Legislative Mandates

Each state is required to submit annual plans confirming that they are in compliance with the mandates specified by federal legislation. As the laws change at the federal level, states must undergo review of their rules and regulations to determine the types of changes that are necessary so that they can assure the government and citizens that are requirements will be met. One of the responsibilities of the state education agency is to monitor and evaluate the activities of the local education agency (LEA) to ensure compliance with the federal statutes.

Local boards of education are responsible for ensuring proper implementation of mandates at the local level. Funds flow from the federal and state levels to the local level. Districts must verify that they are in compliance with the legislative mandates. There is variation throughout the country on how the mandates are interpreted. This is the result of local philosophy as well as funding availability. There are different rules and regulations for public and private schools. It is incumbent upon the administration and teachers in each school to follow the rules and procedures that are expected. If the rules are not followed, funding can be discontinued, reduced, or withheld.

Regional Resource Centers

Regional resource centers have been established in states as a mechanism for providing the support school districts need in order to develop the programs and processes that are required to ensure that they are in compliance with the federal and state standards. Such centers provide an important link between the state and the local school district. They may be referred to by different names in different states but their goals are fairly common. The centers are generally staffed with special education professionals representing a wide variety of disciplines including speech-language pathology, audiology, occupational therapy, physical therapy, psychology, behavioral management specialists, special education teachers, health care specialists, social workers, and educational administrators, to name a few. Their roles are to provide school systems with the assistance they need to interpret, implement, and comply with legislative mandates, rules, and regulations. Having all of these disciplines work closely with one another permits a truly multidisciplinary and collaborative approach for identifying and planning for the educational needs of children with disabilities. Not all districts can afford to hire such a wide variety of specialists; therefore, the concept of making a central pool of experts available to a region through a central agency has been valuable and cost effective.

Centers provide assistance to school systems in the initiation and expansion of programs and services for children with disabilities. This is accomplished through joint planning and collaboration among school systems within a specific region. As a result, many more youngsters can be served than if each district tried to provide educational and support services on its own.

The centers serve as the mechanism by which school systems can plan, organize, and implement strategies for identifying, evaluating, and teaching children with disabilities. This is the first important step in providing appropriate programs and services for children and their families. In addition, many centers also serve as clearing houses and distribution sources for information pertaining to special education. Speech-language pathologists and other special educators can visit the regional resource center to attend in-service training seminar, learn about newly developed instructional materials and methodologies, or borrow materials. Many centers will even deliver materials to the school system.

By combining resources and personnel, regional resource centers can provide comprehensive services to school districts, education specialists, teachers, and families that might otherwise not be available or accessible.

The Program at the Local Level

On the local level, school systems are organized into school districts. The district is a designated geographical area and may cross county lines. In school terminology, these are referred to as local education agencies (LEAs).

The board of education members are elected by the people of the district and are responsible for governance and for developing and establishing policies. The basic responsibility for each school system rests with the citizens of that community inasmuch as they elect the school board. The school board selects the superintendent, who recommends the needed staff to operate the schools.

The superintendent is the chief administrative officer and chief personnel officer for the school system in that he or she makes recommendations to the board concerning the hiring, promotion, and dismissal of staff members. The superintendent is responsible for the total operation and maintenance of the school system; leadership of the professional staff; and administration of the clerical, secretarial, transportation, and custodial staffs. Most districts have executive level administrators who oversee special services such as curriculum, special education, finance, facilities, and so forth.

The structure of individual school systems may vary from state to state and from community to community. Usually, there are curriculum directors as well as directors of elementary education and of secondary education. There may be directors of pupil personnel service, instructional support services, special education services, child accounting and attendance, guidance and health services, and others.

Building principals are responsible for supervising the professional and support services staff assigned to that building. The role and function of the elementary school principal will differ from that of the middle school and secondary school principal. In addition, roles and functions of principals will vary according to the unique characteristics of the community and will reflect the various cultural backgrounds of the students and their parents. The principal is responsible for managing the school's instructional program, pupil personnel services, support services, and community relations.

An understanding of the structure of the school system is necessary for the speech-language pathologist to function effectively. Obviously there will be variations in organizational structures throughout the country; thus in addition to having a general knowledge of the school system, you, as the SLP, will need to be familiar with the educational facility in which you are employed. Figure 3–1 illustrates a sample partial organizational chart for the special education programs of a school district. Schools are organized in many different ways depending on the size and administrative philosophy of the district.

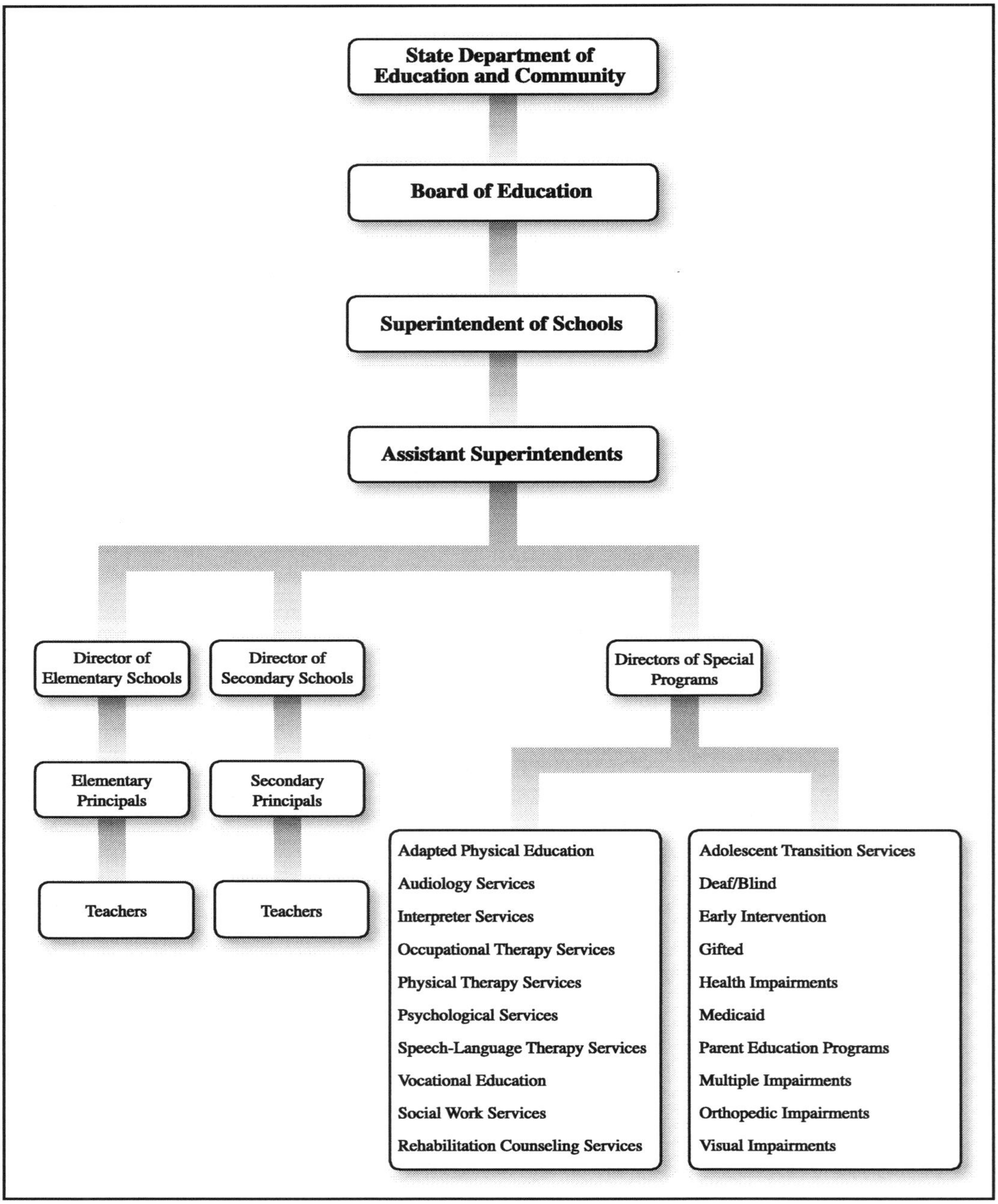

Figure 3–1. School organizational chart.

Public Laws Affecting Speech-Language Service Delivery

Public Law 94-142, The Education for all Handicapped Children Act of 1975, was the original legislation that mandated a free, appropriate public education for all children and youth with disabilities. The dynamics of education, like many other foundational organizations that exist in our country, is continually changing and improving. Therefore, the laws that guide education initiatives and funding are evaluated by our state and federal government. The Education for All Handicapped Children Act of 1975 has been reauthorized multiple times since its inception. The changes made in the reauthorized versions have better reflected changes in education and special education philosophy, children's needs, and parents' wishes. Following is a discussion of the major mandates included in each of the key education laws and the subsequent reauthorizations. Table 3–1 summarizes the federal laws that affect special education and speech-language service delivery. There are several key aspects of the education laws and their reauthorizations that have had remarkable impact on the delivery of all services to children with disabilities, including those with communication impairments. Some of the most significant are:

- Special education and related services must be provided at no cost to the child or parents.
- All children with disabilities and their parents are guaranteed due process with regard to identification, evaluation, and placement.
- A written Individualized Education Program (IEP) must be developed and implemented for each child receiving special services. Individualized Family Service Plans (IFSPs) are required for preschoolers and Individualized Transition Plans (ITPs) are required for students age 14 and over.
- To the greatest extent possible, children with disabilities should be educated with children who are nondisabled. In addition, the education must take place in the least restrictive environment appropriate to the child's needs.
- The laws identify two priority groups among children with disabilities: (1) those not currently receiving any education and (2) those with the most severe handicaps within each disability who are receiving an inadequate education.
- The federal government is committed to assuming a percentage of the costs incurred in providing the programs for children with disabilities. Several types of funding initiatives have been established by various states.
- The local education agencies (LEA) are responsible for providing the appropriate educational programs.
- The local education agencies are responsible for periodic review and monitoring of such programs.

Table 3–1. Federal Legislation and Actions Affecting Special Education

Year	*Law or Action*	*Key Aspects of the Law or Action*
1973	PL 93-112 Section 504 of the Rehabilitation Act	Civil Rights Law. Eliminates discrimination against individuals with disabilities by agencies that receive federal financial assistance. To be eligible for free appropriate public education (FAPE), a child must have a physical or mental impairment. Served as the impetus for the Education for All Handicapped Children Act.
1975	PL 94-142 Education for All Handicapped Children Act (EHA)	Mandated FAPE for students between the ages of 3–21. Provided for Individualized Education Programs (IEPs), due process, protection in evaluation procedures, and education in the least restrictive environment.
1986	PL 99-457 EHA Amendments	Extended protections of PL 94-142 to infants and toddlers (birth to 2). Instituted a formula grant program. Included a mandate for a comprehensive Individualized Family Service Plan (IFSP) as part of the early intervention process. Services provided at states' discretion.
1990	PL 101-476 Americans with Disabilities Act (ADA)	Covered the accessibility of public buildings, transportation, and communication for people with disabilities.
1990	Individuals with Disabilities Education (IDEA)	Expanded the foundations established in Public Laws 94-142 and 99-457. No student can be excluded from public education because of a disability. Procedural due process protections to ensure student and parent rights. Assessment must be fair and unbiased. Students must receive a free and appropriate education in the least restrictive environment. Confidentiality must be maintained. Included the categories of autism and traumatic brain injury as separate disability categories. Defined assistive technology devices and services. Expanded transition requirements.

Table 3–1. *continued*

Year	*Law or Action*	*Key Aspects of the Law or Action*
1993	Goals 2000: Educate America Act of 1993	Described inclusion of children with disabilities in school reform efforts. Developed eight National Education Goals.
1994	PL 103-382 Improving America's Schools Act	Provided for professional development for educators. Lists qualifications and competencies for individuals providing services, including related services and special education.
1997	PL 105-17 Reauthorization of the IDEA	Ensured that children with disabilities had greater access to the general education curriculum. Focused on including aspects of the general education curriculum into IEPs. Stressed the involvement of parents in eligibility and placement decisions. Expanded opportunities for family members, teachers, and other professionals to work collaboratively.
2001	No Child Left Behind	Reauthorization of the Elementary and Secondary Education Act (ESEA). Emphasized accountability for results. Stressed identification of schools in need of improvement and teacher quality. Schools had to include standardized test scores in school performance data. Emphasized using instructional methods based on scientific research (evidence). Provided parents with more information on school performance and expanded options for seeking quality education for children.
2004	PL 108-446 Individuals with Disabilities Education Improvement Act (IDEAIA)	Another reauthorization of IDEA. Aligned IDEA and NCLB. Stressed appropriately identifying students needing special education and provided schools with freedom to exercise reasonable discipline. Identified parameters for highly qualified teachers, reducing paperwork, and fostering more cooperation between parents and schools to reduce litigation.

continues

Table 3–1. *continued*

Year	Law or Action	Key Aspects of the Law or Action
2010	Common Core State Standards for English Language Arts & Literacy in History/Social Studies, Science, and Technical Subjects (the Standards).	Developed by the Council of Chief State School Officers and National Governors Association. Education standards designed to ensure that all students are college and career ready in literacy no later than the end of high school.

- Local education agencies must file a written plan clearly stating the procedures involved in meeting the provisions of the mandatory law. These include: (1) a child-find process; (2) nondiscriminatory testing and evaluation; (3) the goals and timetable of the plans; (4) guarantee of complete due process procedures; and (5) a guarantee to protect the confidentiality of data and information.
- Not only are children with disabilities eligible for appropriate educational programs but they are also eligible for all extracurricular activities such as music, art, and debate. The costs of educating children are borne by the school system. When the child's school cannot provide the appropriate educational placement, the local school system must pay for transportation, tuition, and room and board if the child is enrolled in a residential or tuition-based program.
- The legislation also states that the child with disabilities has the right to a nondiscriminatory evaluation of educational needs. Tests and evaluation materials must not be culturally discriminatory and must be administered in the predominate language spoken in the home. The evaluation is to be administered by a team of professionals and must include the child's parents and/or guardians.

At the center of special education programs for school-age children with disabilities is the Individualized Education Program, or as it is more familiarly known, the IEP. The IEP is the educational roadmap for how we design and implement education for children with disabilities. Essentially the federal law requires that a unique IEP be developed for each child with a disability and reviewed jointly by a qualified school official, the student's teacher or teachers, instructional support personnel including speech-language pathologists, the parents or guardians, and when appropriate, the student. The components of the IEP are explained in Chapter 9.

The special education public laws require each state to submit an annual plan, which is to be approved by the U.S. Department of Education. Each of the components of the act is addressed in the state's plan and the process by which specified requirements will be met is described. One of the responsibilities of the state education agency is to monitor and evaluate the activities of the local education agency to ensure compliance with the federal statutes.

In addition, the state education agency is responsible for the proper use of federal funds in the administration of local programming for children with disabilities. The state education agency is also responsible for the following activities with regard to services for children with special needs: (1) the adoption of complaint procedures; (2) the disbursement of federal funds; (3) an annual report on the number of children served and the criteria for counting them; (4) the establishment of a state advisory committee on the education of children with disabilities; (5) a comprehensive system of personnel development; and (6) records on all activities related to the public law.

Section 504 of the Rehabilitation Act

Individuals with disabilities were assured of participation in and equal access to federally funded program through Section 504 of the Rehabilitation Act in 1973. In order to be eligible, the child must have a physical or mental impairment that substantially limits a major life activity.

Education for Handicapped Act Amendments (Public Law 99-457)

In 1986, Public Law 94-142 was amended to authorize early intervention programs for infants, toddlers, and preschool children who are at either biological or environmental risk for developmental delays. The amendment, known as PL 99-457, expanded the age ranges for receipt of services down to birth and increased the diversity of populations to be served by public school programs. It provided funding incentives for states to facilitate development and implementation of programs and services to children aged 3 to 6 years with handicaps. By the school year 1990 to 1991, states had to implement programs that ensured that the rights and protections of PL 94-142 were available to children ages three to five. State and local education agencies were to supervise the programs. To receive federal funding, school districts needed to include this population in their state education plan submitted annually.

PL 99-457 also established a discretionary program for provision of services to children birth to three years of age. States had to designate "lead agencies" to oversee the implementation of programs for infants and toddlers. In some states, schools accepted the responsibility for these programs. In other states, agencies such as the Department of Health or the Department of Maternal Care accepted the responsibility.

Because PL 99-457 is an amendment to PL 94-142, there are many similarities in the mandates of the two laws. All rights and protections of PL 94-142 are extended to infants, toddlers, preschoolers, and their families. Like PL 94-142, PL 99-457 mandated due process, services provided at no cost to families, interdisciplinary interaction and the team process, a comprehensive system of personnel development, and a comprehensive child-find and child-count system.

PL 99-457, like PL 94-142, had great impact on the role of the SLP practicing in the schools. As the target populations are infants, toddlers, and young preschoolers, the focus of programming necessarily shifted to the family unit. Family services began to play an important role in preschool programs. New partnerships between parents and professionals were forged. Changes were made in service delivery models and intervention procedures employed by speech-language pathologists working in preschool settings. Clinicians searched for infant and family assessment tools and interventions. They began to work with numerous agencies outside of the school system. Services to preschoolers can be provided by private practitioners, community-based programs, local education agencies, or in the family's home because appropriate services are not always available in the child's local school district. To make this happen, public education agencies were required to develop procedures for interfacing with other types of institutions.

The Individuals with Disabilities Act (IDEA) (Public Law 101-476)

As professionals increase their understanding of the needs of persons with disabilities, the federal mandates regulating the provision of education and services continue to change. In 1990, 1997, and 2004, The Education of the Handicapped Act was reauthorized and further amended. Reflecting sensitivity to the negative effects labels often carry for individuals, the title of the law was changed to the "Individuals with Disabilities Act (IDEA)." It reinforced the use of "person first" language, changing all references in the law to handicapped children to "children with disabilities."

IDEA expanded the foundations established by Public laws 94-142 and 99-457. There were six key principles:

- No student can be excluded from public education because of a disability.
- Procedural due process protections ensure student and parent rights.
- Parents are encouraged to participate in their child's education.
- Assessment must be fair and unbiased.
- Students must receive a free and appropriate public education in the least restrictive environment. This is referred to as FAPE.
- Confidentiality must be maintained.

Two new categories of disability were added: "autism" and "traumatic brain injury." Another change mandated that schools provide transition services for students, promoting movement from school to postschool activities. These include postsecondary education, vocational training, integrated employment, continuing and adult education, adult services, independent living, and community participation. The law also ensured that students needing assistive technology services would receive them from trained personnel. The addition of these categories and services influenced the types of students carried on public school clinicians' caseloads. The changes supported developing therapy objectives and procedures that are *functionally based.* IDEA also required the inclusion of a statement of transition services in the IEP for students when they reach the age of 16. Suddenly speech-language pathologists and special educators were expected to collaborate with other educators and agency representatives to plan school-to-work transition services and recommend strategies for meeting transition objectives.

Reauthorization of IDEA (Public Law 105-17)

IDEA was again reauthorized in 1997 (Public Law 105-17). The changes further expanded and changed the role of the school-based speech-language pathologist. The changes were described as the logical next steps in what SLPs had already been doing to assist learners in school settings (Montgomery, 2000). The law stipulated the SLP's connection to the education process. It mandated the use of different service delivery models, the consideration of students' educational performance in the treatment plan and approach, and the SLP's close relationship with other educators. In other words, educators and SLPs have a common purpose—to educate the child. The reauthorized version of IDEA (Public Law 105-17) maintained and refined most of the basic requirements that were in the original Public Law 94-142. IDEA 1997 added new provisions for discipline. A summary of highlights of the reauthorized IDEA law is presented in the following sections and in discussions throughout the book.

- *The definition of disabilities was clarified.* A child with a disability who presents a need for a related service (such as counseling) is not considered to be disabled unless the related service is defined under law as special education. Family counseling, for example, is considered a related service not a special education service.
- *Developmental delays for children age three through nine may be defined as a disability.* This change greatly affected speech-language pathologists' caseloads. Prior to this interpretation, children with developmental delays could not be served unless they were labeled as disabled and eligible to receive special education services.
- *Attention deficit disorder and attention deficit hyperactive disorder may lead to eligibility for special education under the "other health impairment" category.* This is a change from previous versions of the law that limited the other health impairment category to physical conditions. The list of related services was expanded to include orientation and mobility services.
- *Supplementary aids and supports were added to the list of aids, services, and supports that could be provided to children within the context of the general education setting.* This important addition enables more children with special needs to be educated with children without disabilities to the maximum extent possible. Prior to this change, funding that was allocated for children with special needs could not be used in settings where

nondisabled children might also benefit.

- *One of the most complex changes was attention given to the issue of quality of instruction.* The law stated that a child could not be identified as having a disability if the reason for the child's learning difficulty was lack of instruction in reading or math. This ruling has had profound effect on educators. The result is that teachers must obtain appropriate training to ensure that they have the skills necessary to provide quality instruction to students. Thus, the door opened for better collaboration between SLPs and teachers so that teachers could support children with communication disabilities in the classroom. SLPs could feel empowered to train teachers on how to use AAC devices and how to implement communication strategies during their classroom teaching.
- *Evaluations must be comprehensive.* All areas of the suspected disability, including cognitive and behavioral factors, in addition to physical or developmental factors, must be evaluated. A variety of assessment tools and strategies for gathering functional and developmental information must be used. The assessment strategies must also help determine the student's educational needs. The child must be able to be involved and show progress in the general education curriculum. As in previous versions, the parents must consent to the evaluation prior to initiation.
- *States must establish goals for the performance of children with disabilities.* They must develop indicators to evaluate progress. This means that children with disabilities must be included in state and district assessment programs. They may have accommodations as determined by their IEP. If children cannot participate in the assessments, states must develop alternative assignment options. The speech-language clinician can contribute much to the discussion of alternative assessments because many will involve the need to provide alternative methods for communication.
- *The law attempts to help schools develop programming for students with behavioral disorders.* It mandates that a behavioral intervention plan must be developed for students who demonstrate behavioral disability and/or who are removed from school due to situations that occur as a result of poor behavior. Consider the fact that many youngsters who exhibit behavioral disabilities have difficulty understanding communication and being understood.

The 1997 and 2004 changes in the reauthorization of IDEA law led SLPs and special educators to gain a better understanding of the general education curriculum and what students have to learn at various grade levels (Ehren, 2000). SLPs had to reconsider the testing used to determine students' eligibility for speech and language services. Testing should be performance- based. Treatment materials and criteria for success must be based on the requirements for performance in the school setting. The most significant result of the change was that SLPs started to rethink the eligibility criteria for enrollment in services as well as the size and composition of the caseload. They strived to define functional goals. They began to explore and expand alternative services delivery approaches. School systems required teachers to improve their qualifications and skills so they could provide appropriate educational services to children. Perhaps the greatest outcome was that the need for collaboration between general educators, special educators and speech-language pathologists became more critical. The role of the school-based SLP changed significantly.

Elementary and Secondary Education Act (ESEA)

In July of 1999, the United States House of Representatives passed a bill referred to as HR 1995, The Teacher Empowerment Act. Representatives then referred the bill to the Senate Committee on Health, Education, Labor, and Pensions. HR 1995 amends the Elementary and Secondary Education Act of 1965. The bill supports grants to improve the quality of teaching and learning. As a result of the bill, efforts to change teacher training and certification will be inevitable. Schools, universities, and state boards of education will work together to determine ways to promote improvements in teacher preparation including mentoring, measuring educators' performance in the classroom, development of cost-effective and easily accessible professional development opportunities, and changes in tenure and retention of teachers. The Education and Secondary Education Act continues to be reviewed and future iterations likely will focus on literacy and preparing students for higher education and employment.

No Child Left Behind (NCLB)

In 2001, The Elementary and Secondary Education Act (ESEA) was reauthorized and is referred to as No Child Left Behind (NCLB). This act has had great impact on service delivery in the schools. It emphasizes accountability for results. Schools and districts in need of improvement are identified and teacher quality must be ensured. Students' test scores must be considered when evaluating school performance. This is referred to as AYP or Average Yearly Performance. NCLB also expanded parental options for obtaining information about their child's progress and school performance.

In focusing on improving teaching and learning, emphasis was placed on providing instruction that is scientifically or evidence-based. Educators as well as SLPs must use proven (evidence-based) methods of instruction and document that they have used them. Using funds to improve teacher's qualifications and certification was also included.

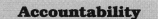

Accountability

The laws that govern education include numerous accountability measures. For example, to receive Title 1 funds, all states have to have in place systematic procedures for measuring student achievement in reading, math and science. This is referred to as standards-based assessments or statewide testing. Students progress toward acquiring appropriate knowledge and skills must be measured in grades 3 through 8.

Not surprisingly, there are many groups of students with disabilities for whom these tests are inappropriate, even with accommodations. Therefore, states must develop plans for alternative assessments. The No Child Left Behind Act (NCLB) requires a statewide accountability system for schools based on standards of adequate yearly progress (AYP). This is aimed at reducing achievement gaps between high-achieving and low-achieving students. Standards are established for each public school, the local education association (LEA) and the state as a whole. The goal for these statewide testing systems is that all students, including children from low income environments and those with disabilities, reach proficient or advanced levels of achievement. The target for accomplishing these goals is 2013 to 2014.

NCLB requires that schools demonstrate adequate yearly progress for all demographic groups. Schools that fail to meet the AYP standard for over two consecutive years are identified as needing improvement. Technical assistance to the school must then be provided to help them improve and students must be offered options for attending another school and/or receiving supplemental services so they can succeed. If the school experiences five consecutive years of failure, corrective actions are warranted. For example, the school may be required to be "restructured." In those situations, the administration and staff may be replaced or the school could be converted to a charter school. Schools that succeed in closing the achievement gap are rewarded for their success.

As part of the school education team, SLPs and services they offer are affected in many ways by these accountability measures. There is much you can do. Take some time to understand your district's performance. Contribute to recommendations of alternative assessment measures. Find out your students' performance on statewide testing. Link your intervention to the curriculum and focus on developing those communication skills that will lead to improved student performance, especially in reading and language arts.

Inclusive Education

Instructing children with disabilities has always been very difficult. The practice of mainstreaming children with disabilities into regular class situations on a full-time or part-time basis was mandated in the original Public Law 94-142. The intent was to provide students with learning opportunities they would not have if they spent their entire day in the special education class setting interacting only with other children who also have disabilities. Mainstreaming worked well in some school systems and not so well in others. Some educators and family members did not feel that mainstreaming went far enough in meeting the full needs to children.

Consequently, leaders in special education advocated meeting the challenge to provide improved programming for children with special needs by embracing the concept of the *inclusive education* (ASHA, 1996). Also, sometimes referred to by some educators as *integration,* the philosophy of inclusion is founded in the belief that children should be educated and completely involved in the activities of their neighborhood schools and within their communities regardless of the severity of their disability. Thus, with the implementation of IDEA, educators began to consider strategies for accomplishing effective inclusion when developing the educational plan. Inclusion involves bringing support services to the student rather than taking the student to the services. Full inclusion means that students will be in regular classrooms full time regardless of their disability and that all services will be brought to them.

Karten (2009a, 2009b) describes the purpose of inclusion as a way of preparing students for adulthood. In order for inclusion to be successful, the student, his or her peers and family, as well as teachers and administrators must all be onboard. Inclusion within the general education classroom is considered the first option on the continuum of services if the student's needs can be met. For inclusion to work, effective strategies for teaching the curriculum must be implemented including modifications, accommodations, and evidence-based instructional delivery. Student's progress and achievements can be verified through ongoing observations and portfolio review.

Inclusion is a very controversial subject. Placing children with special needs into the same classroom as children who do not have special needs makes some people very uncomfortable. The alternative, segregating children with disabilities from those who are not disabled, makes others equally uncomfortable. The concept of inclusion relates to educational values, personal beliefs, and social values. Inclusion implies that all children are valued equally and that everyone is valuable. Accomplishing inclusion presents educators with many difficult challenges. In order for inclusion to work successfully, a great amount of support, communication, and interaction among teaching personnel is needed. Proponents of inclusion favor alternative forms of education service delivery; they are willing to try more creative, flexible methods for educating students.

To effect such wide reaching changes, the entire education system has to rethink its structure and organization. Watching educational programs spring into action and work toward the goal of implementing more effective programs for children with disabilities is very exciting. What you see are regular education and special education teachers forming partnerships and working closely together, *collaborating* to plan the best teaching strategies, materials, and techniques for individual children. The objective is for educators, regardless of their discipline, to combine their knowledge and expertise to jointly develop better solutions to problems than each could have done alone. The classroom teacher maintains the primary responsibility for the student's instructional program. Specialists, including speech-language pathologists, occupational therapists, physical therapists, and other instructional support professionals provide support in designing and implementing special programs to meet the students' needs.

Parents As Team Members

No one cares more about the quality of a child's education than parents or caregivers. The public laws over the past several decades have clearly given parents a major role in making decisions regarding the education and services provided to their children.

The rights and responsibilities of the parents and the school district are described under the *due process* section of the laws for children and disabilities. Due process provides a procedure for reaching resolution when either party is in disagreement regarding the educational program for a child. Both the school district and parents have equal status at meetings. Parents have a right to question why any one procedure is carried out, and whether or not there are alternative procedures. If parents disagree with the recommended procedures they have the right of review with an impartial judge. The purpose of due process is to give parents the right to have the school system explain to them and defend the recommendation procedures. It does not necessarily make the parents adversaries to the system.

On the other side of the coin, the parents have the responsibility of dealing openly and honestly with the school system, accurately describing their child's behavior and reasonably and realistically requesting services. The school district has the right to disagree with the parents. Under due process the parents are entitled to the following procedures:

- A written notice before any action is taken or recommended that may change the child's school program.
- A right to examine all records related to the identification, evaluation, or placement of the child.
- A chance to voice any complaints regarding any matter related to the educational services the child is receiving.
- An impartial hearing before a hearing officer or a judge in the event that the school and the parents cannot agree on the type of school program for the child.
- An adequate procedure for appealing decisions. If parents are not satisfied with the due process procedure, the case may be taken to the state department of education or finally to a court of law.

Public School Reform: Issues and Trends

Public schools are the concern of educators as well as parents, taxpayers, politicians, students, professional organizations, employers, and many other constituent groups. Citizens are concerned about literacy, discipline, drugs, cultural diversity in the curriculum, standardized methods for assessment, and safety in schools. These issues reflect the problems in society. In recent years, calls for education reform have focused on several major issues including: setting higher standards for students; holding schools accountable for students' learning and performance; redefining what type of information is important for learning; gaining consensus about a core curriculum; improving teaching methods and implementing evidence-based instruction and intervention; altering funding streams to permit parents increased choices about how their school-related tax dollars are spent; and responding to calls for changes in the curriculum based on employer needs and/or religious convictions.

Even though problems such as these seem far removed from the therapy room, they do affect how well the clinician does his or her job, which goals are set for the program, the type of students who will receive services, and the funding that is provided for intervention. The national education reform debate is conducted in many arenas and about many topics. The arguments by each side are very compelling. Speech-language pathologists who work within the school setting may be asked to comment about their beliefs and stance on particular issues. Prepare to discuss the pros and cons of national, state, and local issues by following current events in the news media and school district publications.

Goals for Schools

In the past decades there have been increased interest in reforming the way public schools operate and the curriculum that is taught. States and schools strive to rethink and redesign their curriculum, instructional practices, and organizational structure. The driving forces have been to increase student achievement, to prepare students for higher education and the world after graduation, and to keep children safe.

In the Goals 2000 within the Education America Act (1996), eight major goals were set forth by the National Education Goals for America Education Institutions. Goals such as these have had a profound impact on the direction for schools. They brought attention to the challenges that schools face and the potential positive results if the goals are achieved. Unfortunately it is difficult for the goals to be realized because schools continue to lack resources, educators continue to need better preparation for their teaching responsibilities, and viable partnerships have not yet been forged with families.

Goals 2000

Goal 1. By the year 2000, all children in America will start school ready to learn.

Goal 2. By the year 2000, the high school graduation rate will increase to at least 90%.

Goal 3. By the year 2000, all children will leave grades 4, 8, and 12 having demonstrated competency over challenging matter including English, Mathematics, Science, Foreign Languages, Civics and Government, Economics, Arts, History, and Geography, and every school in America will ensure that all students learn to use their minds well, so that they may be prepared for responsible citizenship, further learning, and productive employment in our nation's modern economy.

Goal 4. By the year 2000, the nation's teaching force will have access to programs for the continued improvement of their professional skills and the opportunity to acquire the knowledge and skills needed to instruct and prepare all American students for the next century.

Goal 5. By the year 2000, United States students will be the first in the world in Mathematical and Science Achievement.

Goal 6. By the year 2000, every adult American will be literate and will possess the knowledge and skills necessary to compete in global economy and exercise the rights and responsibilities of citizenship.

Goal 7. By the year 2000, every school in the United States will be free of drugs, violence, and the unauthorized presence of firearms and alcohol and will offer a disciplined environment conducive to learning.

Goal 8. By the year 2000, every school will promote partnerships that will increase parental involvement and participation in promoting the social, emotional, and academic growth of children.

Current Goals for Schools

At this time Goals 2000 have not yet been fully accomplished. However, our education, business, and government leaders continue to make strides for improving education of our youth. Goals and strategies for improving education presented by President Obama in 2010 were to: raise standards for students and teachers; to increase accessibility to early childhood education; to increase graduation rates; and to make college more affordable. Also in 2010, President Obama and our legislators embarked on a broad national effort to turn around America's schools. Schools that fail to make adequate yearly progress (AYP) toward statewide proficiency goals are subject to improvement and corrective action measures. This is referred to as "School Improvement." Turning around the nation's 5,000 lowest-performing schools is part of the Obama administration's overall strategy for dramatically reducing the dropout rate, improving high school graduation rates and increasing the number of students who graduate prepared for success in college and the workplace. The government is making a historic commitment to support state and local education leaders in turning around the nation's lowest-achieving schools.

To accomplish this tremendous task, the U.S. Department of Education is providing $4 billion for this effort. To qualify for this funding under the Title I School Improvement Grant program, states must identify their lowest-performing schools in economically challenged communities and transform those schools using one of the following four intervention models:

1. **Turnaround Model:** Replace the principal and rehire no more than 50% of the staff, and grant the principal sufficient operational flexibility (including in staffing, calendars/time, and budgeting) to fully implement a comprehensive approach to substantially improve student outcomes.
2. **Restart Model:** Convert a school or close and reopen it under a charter school operator, a charter management organization, or an education management organization that has been selected through a rigorous review process.

3. **School Closure:** Close a school and enroll the students who attended that school in other schools in the district that are higher achieving.

4. **Transformation Model:** Implement each of the following strategies: (a) replace the principal and take steps to increase teacher and school leader effectiveness; (b) institute comprehensive instructional reforms; (c) increase learning time and create community-oriented schools; and (d) provide operational flexibility and sustained support.

As you can imagine, these changes can greatly affect the roles and responsibilities of SLPs working within districts that are succeeding or in need of improvement.

Core Standards for Education

Two important organizations that influence the direction of education in the United States are The Council of Chief State School Officers (CCSSO) and The National Governors Association (NGA). In 2010, the CCSSO and NGA set the bar high for improving the quality of education. They established the Common Core State Standards Initiative (Council of Chief State School Officers and National Governors Association, 2010). The driving force in establishing this initiative is the goal to ensure that all students are college ready in literacy no later than the end of high school. Common Core State Standards were developed for English Language Arts and Literacy in History/Social Studies, Science, and Technical Subjects.

The Standards are evidence-based, aligned with college and work expectations, rigorous, and internationally benchmarked. In other words, the standards that are included have been proven to be essential for college and career readiness in the 21st century. The standards will not be static. Like all education initiatives, they will change as better evidence and improved practices emerge. According to explanations provided by the NGA, the standards are an explanation of what students are to learn and provide a guide for understanding for schools, teachers, and parents. They define the knowledge and skills students should gain while in school and the foundation they will need for future success in college and employment. The standards are:

- Aligned with college and work expectations;
- Clear, understandable, and consistent;
- Rigorous content and application of knowledge
- Built upon strengths and lessons of current state standards;
- Informed by other top performing countries; and,
- Evidence-based.

Why Should SLPs Care About Education Goals and Academic Standards?

What do national goals and core standards for education such as these mean for speech-language pathologists and other educators across the country? And, what role can SLPs play in their success? As children enter the school setting, they must present basic communication skills that will enable them to learn to participate in the classroom setting and learn to read and interact with their peers. Competency in specific subject matter depends on their ability to read, comprehend, and respond to materials that are in their texts or presented by their teachers. Speech-language pathologists, like teachers, must maintain their qualifications so they can provide appropriate services to children. To be successful adults and contributors to society, school graduates will have to be able to communicate with their peers and at their jobs. They will have to arrive ready to follow instructions and to participate in complex tasks. Clinicians are expected to involve parents in all aspects of the service delivery program so they can gain a meaningful understanding of their child's communication problems and know how to provide assistance when needed. Professionals cannot do their jobs and students cannot benefit from the school situation when they are afraid for their safety. All will have to demonstrate that violence and other forms of inappropriate behavior will not be tolerated.

Children with speech and language disorders often do not achieve their maximum potential within the classroom setting. They fail because they don't have the speech and language skills needed to be successful within specific aspects of the school curriculum. For example, they cannot be understood, follow the teachers' directions, retain information, ask questions, respond, and so forth. The evolution of our profession has moved from providing remediation therapy to improve the sound and mechanics of students' speech and language skills to collaborating with our educational partners to improve student's communication capabilities so they can succeed in the learning environment and, ultimately, in higher education and life.

Linking our intervention to the core standards for education enables us to ensure that our treatment goals are matched with the demands of students' classrooms and their functional communication needs for success. The standards are the basis of classroom instruction and statewide assessments. Oral and written language skills are stressed throughout the school curriculum. Therefore, the standards that make most sense for linking our intervention are those in the language arts curriculum. There are increasingly difficult expectations for students within the language arts and other content areas in the curriculum from kindergarten through grade 12. Students must master major elements of language and vocabulary for key content areas.

This focus drives several changes in the way special education and speech-language services are provided. First and most importantly, schools must strive to teach students in the general education classroom and to help students access to a standards-based, core curriculum for everyone. Here are some characteristics of this focus for speech-language services:

- Performance goals are based on the state education standards;
- IEP goals must reflect grade level standards;
- Curricular accommodations must be provided to support success;

- Instructional (and intervention) strategies and assistive technology should evidence-based and support access to the standards;
- Placement in special education programs, including speech-language services, should be based on the student's level of need;
- A system for collaborating and consistently delivering interventions should be in place.

High School Exit Tests

The American government and public seek verification that students are prepared to pursue work and postsecondary education after they graduate from high school. A large percentage of the states require that students pass a high school exit test as one mechanism to document that students meet high educational standards. Opponents argue that minority students may have less chance to succeed because of problems that may exist in educational settings that have high numbers of minority students. Similarly, many special educators believe that students with disabilities are at a disadvantage when they take these types of tests. SLPs should be able to discuss the key points surrounding a debate such as this. In addition, they should be able to provide data-based information about problems youngsters with communication disabilities may encounter on high school exit tests. They should be able to pose alternative methods of evaluating the level of learning students have achieved and students' preparation for employment or post-secondary education. If students experience difficulty with the tests, they must receive support and assistance. Tests that are used should be designed to promote success, not failure, for the student.

Prevalence and Incidence: How Many Children Are We Talking About?

The *prevalence* figures of speech, language, and auditory problems, or the *existing* number of persons affected as a *specified* time, are difficult to obtain. *Incidence* figures, the number of *new* cases occurring during a given time period, are usually not available. When reading or interpreting statistical reports, care should be taken not to confuse these two items. Why is it important for prevalence figures to be known? One of the most crucial reasons is that programs and funding for services for children to 21 years of age are based on the number presently being served and those to be served in the future. The infusion of money into states by the federal government is based on prevalence figures. Therefore, these figures should be available and as accurate as possible.

Not only is it important for national and state educational planners to have prevalence information, but it is important on the local level as well. The school speech-language pathologist needs to know approximately how many students in a given school population can be expected to be eligible for speech-language services. The principal needs to know because of space requirements and because it will be important to plan for the coordination of other educational services.

The superintendent needs to know so that an adequate number of speech-language pathologists may be hired and that the budget will accommodate personnel and equipment needs.

Unfortunately, determining the number of individuals with communication impairments is not a matter of simply taking a head count. Reports on incidence and prevalence of speech, language, and hearing problems among preschool and school age pupils have been difficult to obtain, for several reasons. Definitions and terminology regarding disabling conditions may vary from state to state and from person to person so that the reporting of carious conditions is not consistent. There is not yet a universally accepted, comprehensive classification system for speech and language disorders. Sometimes, the data reported are based on too few children, and sometimes survey results are based on reports completed by persons will little or no training in identifying speech, language, or hearing problems. Often, children are not included in survey collection if they are non-verbal, institutionalized, school dropouts, preschool age, or in special classes. Conversely, sometimes children who are English Language Learners are included in counts even though they don't present communication impairments. Many children who might have died at birth or who survived accidents such as traumatic brain injury are now enrolled in public schools with the expectation that services will be available. Years ago children with severe mental retardation were placed in mental health institutions. Due to changes in treatment philosophies and funding mandates, it is not unusual for school systems to be responsible for educating youngsters who may not have been served previously. Factors such as these have led to an increase in the numbers of youngsters reported with communication problems. We do know that communication disorders are one of the most common disabilities in children.

Very few comprehensive prevalence and incidence studies have been completed in recent years. Therefore, a reliable database has not yet been established. Much of the information reported in the literature is still based on studies and surveys that were completed several decades ago. Although this is not ideal, it does provide us with some insights into data available about prevalence and incidence. In addition, some understanding of the prevalence and incidence of communication disorders can be gleaned from data submitted by state departments of education.

Based on research conducted over the past 30 years, it is probably safe to judge that between 8 and 10% of the children now enrolled in school exhibit some kind of oral communications disorder (ASHA, 2011; Hull, 1964; Phillips, 1975).

There may even be indications that the figure of 10 percent is a conservative one. There are possibly reasons for this. In reporting it is often common practice to report the presence of only one disability condition. For example, a child with learning disabilities may also have accompanying speech, language, or hearing problems, but in a survey that child is reported as being learning-disabled only.

The issue of identifying students with language disabilities has become even more complicated as the definition of language disorders has expanded to include pragmatics, literacy (problems related to reading and written language), cognition, emotionally based disorders, and nonverbal communication.

The difficulty in ascertaining the incidence of children with language delay and language deviations continues to be a problem, not only for speech-language clinicians but also for all professionals in the field of special education. The number is actually larger than we suspect Beitchman, Nair, Clegg, and Patel (1986) conducted a study to determine the prevalence of speech and language disorders in 5-year-old kindergarten children in the Ottawa-Carlton region of Canada. Their results indicated that 6.4% of the children exhibited a speech impairment without concomitant language disorder, 8.04% presented language disorders only, and 4.56% showed a combined speech and language disorder. They identified differences between boys and girls in that age group, with the prevalence of disorders being higher among boys than girls. The authors suggested that these results be interpreted cautiously due to the many variables surrounding prevalence research. Their study also did not suggest whether the children identified would benefit from therapy. They recommended further study of these issues.

Recent research in the area of prevalence and incidence remains scant. The American Speech-Language-Hearing Association (ASHA) maintains reports on the prevalence and incidence of communication disorders. In recent years they have increased their efforts to gather and disseminate data due to increased demand for that data for decision-making and reimbursement. ASHA's information is derived from a variety of sources including omnibus surveys, census statistics, the National Center for Health Statistics, National Institute on Deafness and Other Communication Disorders (NIDCD), and annual reports to Congress from the U.S. Department of Education Office of Special Education. Based on sources such as these, staff in the ASHA Research Division reported the following statements that have been made about the prevalence and incidence of communication disorders in children in recent years (ASHA, 2000, 2008; U.S. Department of Education, 1998, 2003):

- Communication disorders are one of the most common disorders in the United States.
- Approximately 46 million individuals in the United States experience or live with some type of communication disorder. Of these, approximately 14 million have a speech, voice, or language disorder.
- The number of children ages 3 to 21 with disabilities receiving services in the 2008 school year was 6,068,802 children. Of these, approximately 1.3% demonstrated hearing loss or deafness. Approximately 24% received services for speech and language disorders.
- More than one of every 25 preschoolers exhibits some type of communication disorder.
- Phonological disorders affect approximately 10% of the preschool and school age population.
- For 80 percent of the children with phonological disorders, the disorders are sufficiently severe to require clinical treatment.
- In addition, children with phonological disorders often require other remedial services.

- Sixty to 70% of the preschool children identified as having disabilities exhibit speech or language impairments. Approximately 1.3% of children ages 3 to 21 served in public schools receive services for hearing.
- Over 3 million Americans stutter, most frequently between the ages of 2 and 6 years when language is developing. Approximately 4 to 5% of children stutter.
- Vocal nodules are responsible for 38 to 78% of chronic hoarseness in children. The reported occurrence of hoarseness ranges from 6 to 23% for children.
- In 1988, over 2 million school-age children received speech-language services; over 57,000 children were classified as hard of hearing or deaf.
- Of the approximately 5.2 million children (ages 6 to 21) with disabilities served in 1996 to 1997, 20% received services for speech and language disorders. Approximately 1.3% (68,766) children received services for hearing impairment.
- Seventy-five percent of children experience at least one episode of otitis media by their third birthday.
- The prevalence of language impairment in preschool children is between 2 and 19%.
- The overall prevalence of specific language impairment in kindergarten children is estimated to be 7.4%. Reading difficulties are associated with specific language impairment.
- It is estimated that the incidence of strokes in children is 2.5 per 100,000 children. Other causes such as brain injury are estimated to be approximately 200 per 1000,000 children.
- Nearly 3 million children ages 3 to 21 have some form of learning disability and receive special education. The percentage of children with a learning disability in the lowest income group is nearly double that of the highest income group. It is estimated that approximately 7 to 10% of children have a learning disability.
- Approximately 28 to 60% of children with speech-language impairments have a family member who does too.

The exact numbers of children who demonstrate communication disorders may be difficult to obtain due to several factors including improved and more discriminating identification procedures, provision of speech and language services outside of the special education delivery system (such as within the regular education classroom), and a current trend to identify students with language disorders as having specific learning disabilities rather than having speech and language impairments.

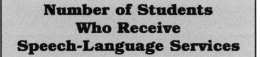

Number of Students Who Receive Speech-Language Services

Each year, the Office of Special Education Programs of the U.S. Office of Special Education and Rehabilitative Services in the Department of Education reports the progress on United States schools are making in the provision of a free appropriate public education for all children with disabilities. The report includes statistical information on the number and percentage of children who received special education and related services in a given time period. It also indicates the implementation of particular sections of the law and the provision of financial assistance to state and local education agencies through formula and grant funding to support the delivery of services.

The system for determining the amount of funds schools receive for providing services for children with disabilities necessitates categorizing and counting children according to the disabilities they present. The data presented in the reports concerning the numbers of children served are referred to as "child count" data. States collect the information annually and these numbers are used as the basis for allocating funds to states in order to provide necessary services. Counts are nonduplicative, representing the number of children served rather than the prevalence of disability conditions. Unfortunately, the statistics are often interpreted as prevalence or incidence data resulting in inadequate funding and limited services. Services provided for the primary disability are referred to as "special education" and are included in the count. Services provided for concomitant conditions are designated as "related services" and are not included in the child count. Thus, only children whose *primary* handicap is speech or language can be counted as receiving speech-language services. Children with other handicaps who receive speech-language services as related services have to be counted in the category that represents their primary disability (specific learning disability, autism, serious emotional disturbance, multiple disabilities, hearing impairment, and so on). Therefore, the numbers reported in the "speech-language impairment" category are not representative of the total number of children actually served by speech-language pathologists in schools. This procedure for counting has made it difficult to determine how many children in the nation have actually been receiving speech-language services and may have resulted in unreasonably low funding for speech-language and hearing services over the past several years.

Caseload Composition

Speech-language pathologists in the schools provide services to students with a wide variety of communication impairments. Results of the 2010 ASHA Omnibus survey showed the following caseload characteristics and trends in the school setting. The findings indicated a median caseload of 50 students. Nearly half (42%) of the caseload of those SLPs who completed the survey were classified as moderately impaired; a third (31%) are mildly impaired, and approximately 22% are severely or profoundly impaired. Another 5% do not have impairments but receive services as a result of a Section 504 plan or Response to Intervention. The survey indicated that the largest portions of speech-language pathologists' caseload are composed of students with language disorders, articulation disorders, and learning disabilities. Informal reports by practitioners indicate that at least 45% of their school caseload was comprised of students who had primary disabilities other than speech-language and were receiving therapy as a related service. Approximately 24% of the SLP's time is spent in direct intervention with the remaining time spent doing other work such as documentation, team meetings, and so forth.

Data collected over the years by the Department of Education reveal that the percentage of children served for communication disorders ranges from 0.9 to 4.1% of the total school-age population. The variance is due to the procedures used for identifying, classifying, and reporting students with speech-language impairments.

The educational placement (environment) for the majority of students with speech and language impairments has been documented as being the general education class versus special education classes. This may change as current trends in education are moving in the direction of greater emphasis on providing prereferral intervention services to children within the general education setting.

Public School Funding

Public education has been the responsibility of government in America for hundreds of years. Education in most states is funded through a combination of local taxes, state funding, and money from other sources such as federal grants, interest on investments, rent, and tuition. Those funds that school districts do receive are allocated to many aspects of the education process including salaries, building maintenance, transportation, educational materials, and special education.

Thomas Jefferson was one of the first proponents of a free, universal education for all children, benefiting not only themselves, but society as a whole. Jefferson believed that education was necessary for democracy to flourish and sustain itself. This was referred to as the "common school movement." Horace Mann, who became known as the "Father of the American School," wrote the following about the philosophy behind the common school movement:

> The cardinal principle, which lies at the foundation of our educational system is, that all children of the State shall be educated by the State. As our republican government was founded upon the virtue and intelligence of the people, it was rightly concluded by the framers, that without a wise educational system, the government itself could not exist, and in ordaining that the expenses of educating the people, should be defrayed by the people at large, without reference to the particular benefit of individuals, it was considered by those, who, perhaps without children of their own, nevertheless would still be compelled to pay a large tax, would receive ample equivalent in the protection of their persons, and the security of their property.

There is a great debate in the United States currently about funding schools. The debate will certainly continue for years to come. Speech-language pathologists must be aware of the key issues and how changes in funding will impact on the types of services they can provide, their salaries, and the environment in which they work. It is not wise to ignore these issues and leave advocacy for better school funding to others. Most school districts and state speech-language pathology professional associations have established committees or employ lobbyists to stay on top of school funding issues.

Funding for School Speech-Language Services

Who pays for speech-language intervention services in the schools? Not surprisingly, the answer is everyone who pays taxes. Our taxes support our schools and their many services. Special education is paid for by local, state, and federal education dollars. Local education agencies are supported in part from local taxes, with reimbursement from state funds. The federal government through the public laws reimburses states for a portion of the expenditures for special education. National statistics show that special education programs claim an increasing share of school budgets. Special education costs include instructors, materials, administrative costs, facilities, meals, and transportation. In 1998, federal regulations took effect that allowed local education agencies (LEAs) to combine IDEA Part B funds with other state, local, and federal funds to carry out schoolwide program activities. The regulations also enabled schools to collect Medicaid funds for serving children who qualify.

States have set minimal standards for special education programs including speech and language services. The standards may cover such areas as personnel qualifications, facilities, equipment, materials, transportation, and caseload type and size. Failure to comply with state standards may result in the loss of significant money to the school district.

There are three basic types of reimbursement to the local education agency: unit reimbursement, per pupil reimbursement, and special. Each state has its unique features in funding patterns, but generally they fall within categories such as these.

In unit funding, states define a specific number of students or a special class as the basis for allocating funds. For example, a unit for a speech-language pathologist may be approved on the basis of 2,000 children in average daily membership. Therefore, a school system with a total population of 5,000 students would be eligible for two and one-half units, which would be two full-time and one half-time SLP. There may be stipulations such as class size, number of children with particular types of disabilities, or number of regular class units.

The per pupil reimbursement model means that the local education agency is compensated for each student receiving special education services. This could be based on average daily attendance (ADA) or average daily membership (ADM). School attendance is generally determined on a given day in the fall and spring of the school year.

A special reimbursement plan usually supplements a unit or per-pupil reimbursement. For example a special unit for speech-language pathology may be approved on the basis of a specific number of children with multiple impairments, hearing impairment, autism, and/or other health impairments in special class or learning center units. Many of these reimbursement formulas encourage high caseloads because the amount of funds generated for a local education agency increases as numbers of students served increases. These reimbursement procedures fail to account for the total number of students with communication disorders or the frequency and intensity of services needed. The special reimbursement model may provide funds for instructional materials and equipment, transportation, facilities, personnel training, pupil assessment, residential care, specific professionals, or ancillary services (physicians, audiologists, psychologists, social workers, physical therapists, occupational therapists, and so on).

The various funding models employed by school districts do not always have a system of accountability built in. Accountability requirements at the national level continue to encourage states to employ systems for funding special education that are linked to standards such as student achievement, student to teacher ratios and types of services. There are also recommendations that funds be allocated specifically for specialized support services such as speech-language intervention services. A similar recommendation supports establishing some means of "equalization" of funding. This means that local and state funds pay equal amounts for special education.

Here is how IDEA funds flow to school districts for special education programs and services (such as speech-language programs):

Funds are appropriated and distributed. Congress appropriates funds to the Department of Education annually based on the federal fiscal year which begins on October 1. The funds are proportioned out to the states in the form of a grant. In addition, funds are reserved for outlying areas and freely associated states and Indian reservations.

Funds are received at the state level. States set aside up to 25% of the federal grant for administration and implementation. The state then allocates funds to the local education agency (LEA) or local school districts.

Use at the local level. Schools then incorporate the IDEA funds into their school's budget. Policy at the local district level dictates how the funds will be distributed and used to support students with disabilities.

How Does the Funding Allocation Work?

Although the intent of the laws that enable government supported education to children with disabilities is noble, the reality is that Congress has never adequately provided the needed level of funding to support services and programs. Congress has authorized that 40% of average student expenditure in the state be covered by these funds. Unfortunately, appropriations have only been at about 20% of total cost. This means that, once states retain the allocation they need and the IDEA funds are distributed to the district, the resulting amount is less than 20 cents on the dollar of per student expenses. The remaining amount needed to support special education costs must come from state and local revenues (State Policy Reports, 2002).

This scenario has created financial difficulty for local school districts. Out of need, schools have had to seek alternative methods of funding programs to help defray expenses for providing education and services to students with disabilities. The regulations that interpret the federal laws indicated that states could use any sources available to pay for services included on the child's Individualized Education Program. The regulations in place for implementing IDEA indicated that "nothing in IDEA relieves an insurer or similar third-party payer from an otherwise valid obligation to provide or pay for services provided to a child receiving special education" (Power-deFur, 1999). That included state, local, federal, and provider funding sources such as insurers or third party payers such as Medicaid (Kreb, 1991; Power-deFur, 1999). As a result, school districts in some states started billing private insurance companies, health maintenance organizations (HMOs), and Medicaid for services provided. Specific terminology must be used to describe the student's disability and recommended treatment protocols in order to be considered for payment by third-party payers. School districts had difficulty trying to collect funds from private and third-party funding sources until Public Law 94-142 was amended in 1986. At that time, Public Law 99-457 required interagency cooperation and coordination of resources. This requirement is still necessary; there must be coordination when a school-age student is receiving services from multiple sources.

Medicaid billing is limited to children eligible for special education and related services under IDEA. This is an important interpretation for speech-language pathology services because it means that students who receive speech-language services but not special education and related services are ineligible for payment for services by Medicaid and other third-party payers (Power-deFur, 1999).

In order to receive Medicaid funding, providers (SLPs and educators) must meet licensing and certification requirements. In addition, they must maintain records and submit documentation according to standards established by the third-party payers. This can lead to additional paperwork and duplication of effort when the district requires one type of paperwork and the payer requires a different type. It is especially frustrating when different entities ask the same questions in different ways and on different forms.

DISCUSSION QUESTIONS AND PROJECTS

1. Why is it necessary for the school speech-language pathologist to know the administrative and organizational structure of the school system on the local level?

2. What questions would you ask about the organizational structure of the school system if you were being interviewed for a position as SLP?

3. What relationship do you see between the prevalence figures for students with speech-language impairments and program planning?

4. Why are most prevalence figures for children with language disabilities difficult to obtain?

5. Public laws state that test and evaluation materials must be nondiscriminatory. Give examples of what this means. How will you know if the tests and evaluation materials you select are discriminatory?

6. Find out the minimum standards for speech-language programs in your state. Who will you call? What paths will you follow on your Web search?

7. Find out if there is a regional resource center in your area. What services does it provide? Visit the center. Interview the provider from the different disciplines.

8. Interview a school SLP to find out to whom this individual is directly responsible in the school structure. What is their role and relationship to you?

9. Invite your state's Department of Education consultant or the Special Education Director from your local school district to speak to your class. Prepare a list of questions to ask.

10. How would you explain the parents' rights and role in program planning to the parents of a child if they do not speak English?

11. Why is it important to use "person first" language when referring to individuals with disabilities? Discuss some of the ramifications of referring to individuals by labels such as "mentally retarded," "learning disabled," "emotionally disturbed," "deaf," and the like.

12. What type of documentation is required in order to receive reimbursement from third-party pay sources?

13. Briefly describe the impact of three key federal laws on the practice of speech-language pathology in the school setting.

4

The Speech-Language Pathologist as a Leader and Manager

When school speech-language clinicians are asked about their programs, services, and day to day work, they are quite likely to make the following responses: "We need more time to plan." "There are too many children on my caseload." "We need more staff members." "I have trouble scheduling students because of all the other school activities." "My budget isn't large enough for me to purchase all of the equipment I need." "It's too hard to keep up with all of the types of disorders I have on my caseload." Interestingly enough, the school SLP generally is pleased with the progress of the children in the program, and the teachers and school administration are pleased with the program. Why, then, the complaints? Very possibly the reason is that each school speech-language pathologist is constantly faced with the challenge of providing the highest caliber of services with the most efficient expenditure of time, money, and resources, including physical, technical, and human resources.

In this chapter we examine how the school SLP, in the role of leader and manager, may utilize time and human resources more efficiently and effectively to provide optimal services to students. A vision of the SLP as a discipline expert and school leader is presented. Topics covered also include proactive planning, establishing goals, managing time and paperwork, utilizing support personnel, obtaining teachers' impressions of and satisfaction with the program, and using technology to carry out administrative functions.

Future Leaders Needed

Leadership in school-based service delivery is a critical need today due to complex challenges clinicians and schools face such as an increasing and diversified population of students with disabilities, reduced funding for special education services, a critical shortage of professionals, and demands for accountability from multiple constituents. In addition, many of the current leaders in the profession are retiring, creating a need and opportunity for new professionals to fill the gaps. School districts seek leaders who have the energy, creativity, and knowledge to resolve problems with innovative solutions. Speech-language pathologists who assume leadership roles in their schools are in a position to influence and change the way things are done.

What makes a good leader? There are many opinions on what it takes to be a good leader. Some authors believe that leaders are born, others believe that leadership skills can be developed. Perhaps it's a combination of the two theories, complimented by experience, nurturing, work context, and a need for leadership that arises at just the right time and place. Susan Moore Johnson explains it this way: "Leadership looks different, and is different, depending on whether it is experienced in literature, on a battlefield, at a rally, on a factory floor, or in a school district" (1996, p. 14). The bottom line is that schools, our profession, and our professionals in schools need good leadership. Delivering speech-language services in schools poses unique realities and demands. There are many stakeholders and each has a different perspective and expectation. Educating children and providing assistance to children with disabilities is an awesome responsibility. Leaders must have interpersonal skills as well as professional expertise. Leaders in the school setting must be many things to many people. They must build networks and connections. And, they must be aware of all aspects of the school organization and people within the organization. To lead successfully, the leader must be connected and engaged at many levels with many constituents.

Many young professionals aspire to leadership roles within their discipline but aren't quite sure how they can accomplish their goals. There are many career paths to lead to positions of leadership. Some are mentored by exceptional leaders, others are recruited to leadership for their expertise and knowledge. Some build a foundation for their future as leaders by observing others lead in their communities and school settings. Many volunteer in professional and community organizations and recognize how important it is to pay attention to local politics. Early leadership experiences may include supervising and mentoring other clinicians, collaborating with education colleagues, organizing a continuing education event, or teaching professional development inservice course.

Leaders can be change agents and change is definitely needed in our schools today. Several leaders in the profession have described their path to leadership and have also offered their insights about the qualities successful leaders possess and their suggestions regarding contributions leaders in our profession can make (Boswell, 2009; Delfosse & Hagge, 2011; Ehren, B. J., 2008; Ehren, T. C., 2005; Estomin, 2010; Flynn, 2010; Golper, 2007; Montgomery & Moore, 2010; Nelson, 2008; Secord, 2007). For example, Tommie Robinson, ASHA President in 2010 wrote that, "Leaders *create* new programs and ideas and expand opportunities for others. Leaders *innovate* and make positive change wherever they are. In addition, the

ASHA Roles and Responsibilities document (Appendix A) describes leadership actions school-based SLPs can take. First and foremost, in the school setting we need leaders who are passionate about providing high quality, evidence-based services to children with disabilities. As discussed by ASHA President, Tommie Robinson (2010), Marshall Loeb and Stephen Kindel define leadership as "the set of qualities that causes people to follow." These qualities might include inspiring and motivating others, listening and acting in a consistent way, and being responsible and accountable. Leaders engage followers in developing vision statements, mission statements, and the strategic plan of an organization.

Following are some important leadership activities that make a difference. SLP leaders advocate for appropriate programs and services for children and adolescents. When leading a team of clinicians, they often focus on developing reasonable workloads and offering professional development opportunities. They strive to increase school administrators' and teachers' understanding of speech-language services. Many also participate in the development and interpretation of laws, regulations, and policies to promote best practice. Leaders play an important role in recruiting and inducting new professionals. In addition through their mentoring and supervision they can facilitate continuity of excellent services. They value the power of data for making decisions and demonstrating results. They have much to offer parents and other educators, including administrators, teachers, and educational specialists. They encourage collaboration as a key pathway to achieving positive outcomes. Many of our professional leaders can be found in universities preparing future professionals or conducting research to generate and support the use of evidence-based assessment and intervention practices. A very rewarding path to leadership is through volunteerism (Delfosse & Hagge, 2011).

Individuals who want to become leaders generally take steps to build their competence and qualifications. Some experiences are planned and others occur when administrators or colleagues detect leadership qualities in individuals. As a result, aspiring leaders develop the knowledge and confidence they need to engage in the critical thinking and problem-solving strategies required in leadership roles in schools, professional organizations, universities, and other professional venues.

Management: Basic Principles

Perhaps the best place to start is to admit to ourselves that to effectively manage our school-based programs we need to acquire new skills, new techniques, and new tools, as well as an understanding of the principles of the management process: planning, organizing, staffing, directing, and controlling. The goal of comprehensive services for all children with disabilities points out the need for appropriate management skills at the local level as well as at the state and national levels.

Presently, there is a trend in health care and educational settings toward implementation of formal systems for program planning, development, management, and evaluation. Strategic planning and continuous quality improvement (CQI) principles have gained acceptance in business, government, and educational settings at the national, state, and local levels. By adhering to the philosophy and processes associated with strategic planning and continuous quality improvement, professionals can identify their program's strengths and weaknesses, determine a vision for the future, and work toward better execution of programmatic goals and objectives. Two basic tenets of CQI are demonstrating outcomes and achieving consumer satisfaction. Speech-language pathology programs serve many different types of consumers including students with communication impairments, teachers and other specialists, parents and family members, school administrators, and the community. Efforts to provide quality services should be supported through all aspects of the program including planning and managing time, developing program goals and objectives, scheduling, implementing assessment and treatment, documentation and reporting, and so on.

It is vitally important to closely examine our school programs. What are they attempting to do? How are they doing it? How effective are they in achieving their goals? The school speech-language clinician today and in the future will need to be acquainted with sophisticated tools and systems for data gathering, evaluation and measurement of programs, personnel, and their effectiveness (outcomes). A "cookbook" approach is not the answer because there is no single "recipe" for a good program.

The SLP's Roles and Responsibilities

The school-based speech-language pathologist wears many hats. The role of the school SLP is a dynamic one with many different areas of responsibility. Recently a team of leaders in the profession worked together on an ASHA task force to define and describe the roles and responsibilities of the school-based SLP. Their knowledge of the goals of education, the demands of practice in the schools, the breadth of disabilities served, and the SLP's relationships with other educators and families served as a basis for describing the roles and responsibilities. The ASHA Roles and Responsibilities (2010) document can serve as a guide for practitioners and their school colleagues. Providing a summary of the document to school administrators would provide a great foundation for building their understanding of the profession and the possibilities of the speech-language program. See highlights of the Roles and Responsibilities document in Appendix B. The full document can be retrieved from the ASHA Web site (http://www.asha.org).

The roles and responsibilities of speech language pathologists have expanded and changed in recent years. The many types of service delivery models employed along with the increasing numbers of children with severe disabling conditions served demand more time and greater expertise of the school clinicians. This means that there must be careful planning and careful allocation of time by the speech-language pathologists in order to get the job done by the end of the day and end of the school year. Although the clinician is responsible for a large number of duties, this doesn't mean that they must "do" each and every one alone.

Organizing and Managing for Success

There was a time when most speech-language pathologists entering the job market had to start from scratch to organize the speech-language therapy program in a school system. Fortunately for you, speech-language pathology programs are already in place in most school systems thanks to federal and state legislation mandating help for children with communication impairments. And thanks, too, for far-sighted school boards and administrators who realized that children need to communicate effectively to benefit from what the educational system had to offer. Last, but not least, thanks to our founding fathers (and mothers) whose foresight and concern established the professions of speech-language pathology and audiology.

Today, however, the picture is different. You, in all probability, will take a position in an already established program. But this situation has its own set of challenges and problems. What are some of the possible roles you may fulfill in a school system?

Following is a list illustrating the many employment situations available for school-based SLPs. This list is by no means complete and it should be pointed out that you could be serving in a combination of these situations simultaneously. You may be:

- The only SLP in a small school district and would be working in several school buildings within the district.
- One of hundreds of SLPs serving a large urban school system.
- One of many SLPs in a rural school district covering a large geographic area.
- Assigned to a special education classroom in one building to serve the needs of a specific population of students.
- Assigned as a specialist in one specialty area of communication disorders (for example, severely disabled) and providing assessment and treatment.
- A consultant in one area of specialization (such as autism) providing consultant services to classroom teachers and other SLPs.
- Serving only preschool and special education classes.
- Providing consultative services through in-class intervention in regular classrooms.
- Offering consultative services through in-class intervention in self-contained special education classrooms (for example, a class for children with autism spectrum disorders).
- Supervising speech-language assistants or paraprofessionals.

- Supervising students in their externship or students completing field experiences.
- Coordinating the speech-language services in a school district or an entire school system.
- Managing a department of pupil personnel services and special education.
- Offering speech-language services in a geographic area encompassing several counties or school districts.

Which of the positions listed above appeals to you most? Regardless of your employment situation or size of your school district, you will quickly learn that organizational and managerial skills are necessary to succeed. Your very first position out of college as an SLP will require that you have a firm grasp of the administrative hierarchy of a public school system and your place within it. You will gain managerial skills as you carry out your own program in concert with others.

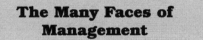

The Many Faces of Management

What is management? Many define management is the art of getting things done through people. The major function of management is to see that people function effectively to accomplish what needs to be done. The skills necessary for good management include the following: communicating effectively; managing time; understanding the job of supervision; understanding leadership and developing a leadership style; and planning, setting goals, and measuring results.

Many colleges and universities offer credit and noncredit courses in management and supervision through their colleges of business, continuing education, or education. Professional organizations such as the American Speech-Language-Hearing Association and the Council for Exceptional Children offer seminars in how to manage programs and supervise others.

The school speech-language pathologist's job is a very complex one consisting of many responsibilities. Let us look at some of the critical tasks the school SLP's job entails:

Program Organization and Management

Much of the therapist's time is spent organizing, planning, implementing, and analyzing various aspects of the school program. SLPs who meet with their administrators on a frequent basis have a greater opportunity to educate them about the goals and purpose of the speech-language pathology program. SLPs who take time to develop and disseminate information about their programs are doing what is necessary to help others learn about communication disorders and see the role they can play in the success of the speech-language pathology program. These communication efforts will pay off in the end.

Screening and Case Finding

In this activity the clinician works with others to identify children with speech, language, and hearing problems who might be eligible to receive speech and language intervention services.

Diagnosis and Assessment

This task includes administering formal and informal instruments to determine the communication characteristics the student presents. Recommendations for treatment are based on the findings of these activities. In most school districts testing is carried on throughout the school year. However, during the first few months and last few months of the school year most SLPs engage in more assessment activities than at other times. Assessment activities may include any or all of the following: administering tests, observing the children in various settings, interviewing parents and teachers, or reviewing portfolios of the students' classroom materials.

Providing Intervention Including Collaborating with Other Professionals

The heart of the speech-language pathologist's role lies in the delivery of intervention services for students with communication disabilities, including direct intervention and collaboration with others to ensure that treatment is carried out in a variety of contexts. When collaborating, the SLP exchanges information and jointly shares responsibility with parents, teachers, psychologists, health care professionals, and others in regard to individual students. Providing intervention does not always mean meeting face-to-face with the student. In service delivery models that employ integrating services into the classroom and collaboration, the SLP may actually provide instructional strategies for others to carry out. School-based speech-language pathologists are a part of the educational organization. Consequently, they must take every opportunity to ensure that their program fits into that organizational structure. This means interacting with all educational colleagues during important school-related activities such as curriculum design, program planning, and social events.

Preparing Materials

SLPs often need to prepare materials for use in their program or for use by others. Materials do not always have to be constructed or designed by the SLP. They must, however, be suited to the students' age, interests, and communication needs. SLPs who work with students with severe disabilities must prepare technologic equipment for students' use in the classroom. They must also train others to use the equipment. This includes setting up computer programs and selecting assistive listening devices.

Documentation and Record Keeping

This task includes all activities involved in maintaining information on the delivery of services to each student and other important programmatic aspects such as the demographics of the caseload, annual activity report, treatment outcome data, program, statistics, and so on. Most school systems have student information systems as well as systems for tracking student's progress on their Individualized Education Programs.

Consultation

Other services, not directly related to students with communication disorders, enable the SLP to maintain, promote, and enhance the speech-language pathology intervention program. These activities are essential to the program. Examples include providing in-service training programs for staff, parents, and colleagues. SLPs must also meet with administrators to discuss program goals and needs and to report outcomes of treatment.

Participating on Curriculum Committees

Speech-language pathologists can make a unique contribution to the decision making process schools utilize to select curricular materials. Many SLPs are not asked to do so because their colleagues in education do not realize the knowledge base that SLPs possess. To really begin articulating the SLP program with the rest of the educational goals for youngsters, SLPs must willingly exchange information with others about how the selected curriculum will positively or negatively impact on a student's performance because of communication requirements and demands within the curriculum.

Other Activities

Many specialists are engaged in research related to the school services. To maintain professional currency, SLPs attend professionals meetings and conferences. Some school specialists spend time supervising university students who are majoring in speech-language pathology. Conservation and prevention programs may be carried out by school-based clinicians. In addition, clinicians participate in public information activities such as making presentations to groups and organizations and interviewing for newspaper articles.

Managing Program Development and Change

Strategic planning is a program planning process that many school districts and organizations use to define their goals and resolve their problems. The strategic planning process incorporates several steps: it involves analyzing the program's strengths, weaknesses, opportunities, and potential problems. After analyzing these factors, reasonable goals and actions are determined that will lead to the fulfillment of the program's mission. This planning method sensitizes you to the school culture and environment. You learn about situations that pose barriers to accomplishing the goals you would like to achieve. The planning process becomes ongoing and never ending. Thus, you stay aware of situations that may change and you can alter your plans accordingly.

Through strategic planning, a staff can be more forward thinking about what they want to do or be in the future. It can be useful as a tool for addressing problems. During the strategic planning process, the expertise of many people is utilized and teamwork is reinforced. The strategic planning process can help an educational staff develop plans for decreasing high caseloads, offering services to a new population, implementing a new intervention program, or acquiring additional resources.

The following sections demonstrate how the strategic planning process can be used to make a change in the program service delivery model.

Determine the Mission

Effective planning requires that an organization very clearly express its mission, or purpose for existing. The mission statement provides direction to program development efforts. When the mission is clear, the decision-making process becomes easier.

Those staff members who will need to embrace and implement the mission must participate directly in its creation. This enables all participants to approach initiation of new goals and actions from the same perspective and with the same philosophical understanding. To develop the mission statement, a multidisciplinary planning group should determine specifically what is to be accomplished. For our example, let's assume that the team wants to implement a collaborative service delivery model in the school building. The mission should be clear and understandable to all individuals who are associated with the program. To increase the chances that this will occur, administrators and educational staff members should participate directly in formulating the program and designing the plan for implementation. The sample mission statement in Figure 4–1 is the type of statement that could be used to guide the planning for a collaborative model. Note that it is stated in general terms.

Scan and Analyze the Environment

In formulating the statement, team members would discuss information obtained from an environment or situational analysis. The team would review those situations that pose problems or barriers to effective collaboration. They would also identify those situations or persons that present opportunities for success. During meeting, the team should identify what has been successful or unsuccessful with regard to current intervention methods or approaches. Following are the types of questions that the team should answer. What kinds of problems can be better solved via a new approach or program model? What resources can be used to solve the problems or eliminate the barriers? Why will such a model be more responsive to meeting the needs of students with communication disorders? A sample environmental scan to determine challenges and opportunities for implementing a collaborative service delivery model is briefly outlined in Figure 4–1.

State the Program Concept

After the mission statement is developed, the team must clearly and accurately describe the type of program they ideally want to establish and what they want it to accomplish. Discussions should lead to descriptions of the population to be served, the type of personnel who will represent the program, equipment to be used, operating procedures to be initiated, tasks and activities to be accomplished, and differences from current practices. Ideas can be generated by viewing model programs, reading professional literature,

Mission Statement for a Collaborative Model

"Our mission is to provide quality, ongoing and comprehensive speech-language assessment and intervention services that interface effectively with the educational program."

Environmental Scan

Strengths

SLPs on staff have expertise in specific areas (integrating technology into therapy, parent training, classroom-based intervention, language foundations necessary for learning and literacy).

Networks have been established among various teachers and clinicians within the school district.

Weaknesses

Personnel and funding for the speech-language program are limited.

School personnel do not understand the impact of communication disorders on academic success.

School district personnel and administrators are resistant to adopting collaborative and/or consultative models.

Parents have expressed a desire for more services provided directly by the SLP.

Opportunities

The school district has just determined that inclusion and Response-to-Intervention strategies should be a priority for the coming school year.

Educators have requested more information about strategies for working with students with communication disorders and struggling learners.

Anticipated Challenges

Administrators believe that direct service by the SLP in the speech-language therapy room is the best mode of delivery for the SLP program.

A principal who was supportive of the SLP program just retired.

Everyone is busy and time to meet is limited.

Funding and resource support is limited.

Evidence supporting the benefits of collaboration and consultative models of service delivery is lacking.

Administrators and education professionals do not understand how SLPs can contribute to the education process.

Target Population to Be Served

Students in grades K–3.

Figure 4–1. Sample strategic plan for developing a collaborative model of service delivery. *continues*

Current Services Provided

Traditional speech-language assessment and intervention services. The SLP tests students, education team members and the family develop the IEP. Speech-language services are provided from September to June in a pull-out service (outside of the classroom) delivery format.

Personnel to Be Involved

SLPs with experience in working with K–3 general and special educators, reading specialist, psychologist, building principal, building special education coordinator, occupational therapist, district curriculum consultant, and the district administrator responsible for speech-language services.

Equipment to Be Used

Standardized or dynamic assessment instruments and teacher/parent training materials (fact sheets, information forms, strategy recommendations).

Objectives to Be Accomplished by the Collaborative Planning Team

Observe and assess the child, formulate expectations and goals, interact with family members, review and select curricular and instructional support objectives and materials, develop lesson plans focusing on identified target skill areas. Provide in-service or education team members.

Benefits of a Collaborative Service Delivery Model for the Population

Language intervention and teaching techniques can be identified and integrated into the child's natural learning environment including home and community. intervention services can be offered to an increased number of children simultaneously. time will be more efficiently used. Professionals' expertise will be shared. Skills that are developed will generalize to multiple learning situations.

Sample Goals for Implementing a Collaborative Service Delivery Model

Conduct a prevalence and incidence study of two school buildings to determine groups of students and types of disorders that would benefit from this type of service delivery model.
Actions: Conduct a screening program. Distribute teacher surveys. Conduct a needs assessment.

Determine two specific content areas of the school curriculum where the SLP program and education program can best be articulated.
Actions: Review courses of study, curriculum objectives, and teaching materials for key target grade levels.

Develop and disseminate written materials explaining the collaborative service delivery model to five key administrators and school personnel.
Actions: Review literature on collaborative programs. Develop simple descriptive materials. Make a presentation at an up-coming administrators and/or teachers meeting.

Figure 4–1. *continues*

Develop resource materials for use when working with classroom teachers.
Actions: Outline the type of materials needed. Review materials currently available commercially and in your resource library. Determine applicable materials. Compile in usable, retrievable, reproducible formats.

Opportunities to Communicate with Others

Conferences	Annual Reports
Progress reports	Newsletters
Parent training programs	Written notes
Observation days	E-mail messages
Budget requests	In-service meetings
Lunch and coffee breaks	Social activities

Figure 4–1. *continued*

and talking with colleagues who have initiated similar (collaborative) programs. Although examples can be drawn from these sources, the mission statement and program concept that are generated should be unique to the specific school district and responsive to its specific needs. It should reflect the resources and expertise available in the district. Figure 4–1 shows a sample program concept for a collaborative model.

The implementation of a new program does not need to be an all-or-nothing approach. After reviewing your environment, present situation, and resources, you may realize that a collaborative model might be most effective in only a few aspects of the SLP program. For example, you might decide to launch the new model with only high risk infants and toddlers, with students needing augmentative communication systems, or with students from diverse cultural populations. You may decide to implement a particular model in one school building rather than another because the teachers are more willing to work with you. In such a case, you would determine one or two specific areas of concentration on which to focus the collaborative services for the first year. You would then make a plan for the second and later years. Team members should decide how to phase in the mew model so resistance to change is reduced. A key factor in the successful initiation of any new program will be the way it is introduced and explained to others in the building or school district.

Formulate Goals or Objectives

Goals, objectives, and an action plan are developed after the challenges are identified, the mission statement is written, and the program concept is developed. The goals and strategies for achieving those goals need to be formulated using "operational terms." This means the goals should be *feasible, acceptable to colleagues and administrators, valuable,* and *achievable.* They should be either *quantifiable* or *observable.* Goals should be designed to take you in the direction of your mission. Write goals that tell administrators and colleagues what they can expect from the new model and how they will benefit from it. A goal statement such as "to increase accuracy of teacher referrals by 15%" indicates clearly what is to be accomplished by adopting the new service delivery model. Care should be taken to be realistic when developing goals. If they are not realistic, the chances are slight they will be realized or that you will yield the results you want. Sample goals are illustrated in Figure 4–1.

Your mission and strategic goals are achievable only when they are based on accurate information and developed in a systematic manner with input from a variety of sources, including those professionals who will be charged with implementing them. There are a number of interactive planning techniques that can be used when formulating your mission and goals, including developing storyboards, creating scenarios, brainstorming, and using consensus-building techniques. You may want to invite a consultant in to work with the staff by facilitating an open discussion about what they want and what would work for them.

Develop and Action Plan for Accomplishing Goals

Through discussion with the team, prioritize your goals and then develop an action plan indicating major activities for accomplishing each goal. A number of activities will be required for accomplishment of each goal. This is where the team effort is important. Encouraging participation in the planning process will engender teamwork and ownership in the program when it is up and running. Work with people to identify tasks they wish to pursue and skills they can bring to the project. To keep participants on task, list deadlines, persons to be involved, individuals responsible for overseeing each action step, potential obstacles to completion, and enabling steps. Be realistic in establishing deadlines. You want these activities to be an enjoyable, doable task. Monitor progress by reviewing actions taken on each objective periodically. Take corrective action when it appears that efforts are off-track. Figure 4–1 provides examples of actions that can be taken. Of course there will be objectives, steps timelines, and assigned responsibilities for completing each of the actions.

Evaluate the Organizational Structure to Determine Support for Implementation

The organizational structure has to be conducive to adopting a new model if implementation is to be successful. Therefore, during the planning process, the organizational structure should be examined. The organization needs to be designed so the mission and goals can be accomplished. For example, in order to collaborate with educators about ways to improve students' academic abilities, a professional must be available who understands what specific needs are important for classroom success, the subject content that is taught at various grade levels, and what classroom techniques need to be enhanced or adapted. Administrators must be supportive of the change.

Administrators will need to be convinced with concrete data and evidence that the new program or model is going to have a positive impact on the treatment practices and educational methods used with students. Only then will they provide the support that is needed and create a school environment that is conducive to ensuring success. The potential for this occurring is increased in districts where organizational management is participatory, where there are well-developed communication systems, where administration is responsive to staff members' ideas, and where there is a willingness to be creative and innovative. Recognize that it may be impossible to change the organizational structure of the school or district. However, analyzing the existing structure with respect to the model you want to implement will give you the advantage of knowing the forces you will confront.

If top-level management embraces the program change and goals, top-down changes can be initiated to support it. School building and caseload assignments can also be adjusted accordingly. Financial resources can be allocated to support its development.

Develop Systems for Sharing Information

To implement your program effectively, there must be an organized flow of information to professionals involved in the program and to consumers of the services. With clear exchanges of information, individuals can function responsibly to carry out goals, understand priorities, and form effective relationships. Examine the communication style, needs and opportunities in your organization (school district). Ask yourself and your team, "Who in this school district needs to know and understand what we are trying to do?" In order to create an information-based system, there needs to be mutual understanding, shared values, and mutual respect. As part of your strategic plan, develop a plan for communicating with your various colleagues and consumers to make them aware of your new program and get them involved in it. Figure 4–1 lists numerous methods for communicating with colleagues and consumers about our sample case. Communication strategies are discussed more thoroughly throughout the book.

Conduct Ongoing Planning and Evaluation

If the new model was given life by a small group of individuals, efforts need to be made to integrate the new program into the comprehensive plan of the whole organization (e.g., special education program, related services division, pupil personnel department). Duplication of services and efforts must be avoided or eliminated. Already scarce resources will need to be shared. For example, for a new service delivery model to work, there will need to be frequent and systematic interactions with individuals involved and periodic review to see if modifications are needed.

After the planning team has taken a good look at what actions the strategic plan entails, he or she must determine priorities. Inexperienced clinicians in a new situation sometimes try to do everything the first year. This is not only unreasonable, but also unwise to attempt. The result may be that of spreading oneself too thin and not accomplishing anything satisfactorily. For example, the team may have to decide whether a teacher in-service program or parent in-service program is more important during the first year. The clinician may then rationalize that the teachers are more readily available and need to understand the program more immediately than do the parents, so the in-service program for teachers would take precedence. During the following year, however, the therapist may decide to devote more time and energy to the parent in-service program, and that program would be given top priority.

The goals for the year should indicate the time (or times) of the year that the goals would be implemented and accomplished as well as the amount of time involved. Goals may be written for an entire school year or for one semester at a time.

Monitoring and evaluating the evolution and development of the program are important aspects of the strategic planning process. There are many mechanisms for evaluating and maintaining control over the program. Evaluation can be achieved by means of periodic staff meetings, reports of activities, periodic progress reports, and feedback from colleagues. As planning is a cyclical process, results should be reviewed on an ongoing basis and corrective actions are taken in light of new situations. The program change should be evaluated periodically to determine if modifications are needed. During each review period, strengths, weaknesses, opportunities, and potential problems ought to be reconsidered. The following questions could guide a discussion of changes that might affect the program. Have there been major changes in personnel or school policies that will impact the program? Has anything new emerged? Future direction and ideas for expanding the program to other grade levels, school buildings, and disorder populations should be reviewed and/or approved by administration.

Program goals should not be confused with goals that individual SLPs establish for themselves. These clinician's goals and the program goals may not necessarily be at odds, but it should be kept in mind that although clinicians may come and go, programs, it is hoped, go on forever. Setting goals for the program, with the clinicians as the implementers, will allow smooth, continuous functioning of a program despite changes in personnel. There is probably nothing more frustrating for a school clinician who is stepping into a job than to learn that the previous clinician left no records concerning what was planned, what was accomplished, when it was accomplished, how long it took, and what remains to be done.

In addition to establishing yearly or semester program goals based on a priority list of the tasks involved in the speech-language pathologist's job, other information would have to be available, including:

- Number of speech-language pathologists on the staff
- Number of schools to be served
- Amount of travel time between schools

- Enrollment figures for each school building (enrollment by grade level and enrolment of special education classes, including hearing impaired, physically impaired, developmentally delayed, emotionally disturbed, and so on)
- Number of preschool children in the school district
- Number of students with IEPs, types of impairments, functional communication status, and so forth.

The school clinician can use this information to decide on the appropriate methods of delivery-of-service and scheduling systems.

More About Writing Program Goals and Objectives

The school SLP, although responsible to another person in the hierarchy of the administration, is responsible for the management of the school's speech-language pathology program. The school system may be a large urban system, a small community system, or a sprawling countywide system, and the school SLP must assess the needs in light of the local situation and plan accordingly.

If the school system employs more than one SLP, there must be coordination of their activities. If it is a large or moderately large system, one SLP may be designated as the coordinator of the program. But even the school SLP who is working alone in a small school system needs to have a plan of action.

Planning ahead is the key to a successful program. Setting goals and objectives is one of the most critical elements of the planning process. Once the goals and objectives have been determined, the next step is writing them down in such a form that they clearly communicate their intent to all the persons concerned and involved in the program.

The utilization of written goals and objectives has many potential advantages in the school speech-language program. First, it allows for change, because through the system of periodic review, objectives will need to be revised and rewritten. Also, it creates a positive pressure to get things done. Communication among professionals will be improved. There will be more precise definitions of the roles and responsibilities of the school speech-language clinician. A system for evaluating and assessing the overall program is inherent in the written goals and objectives. Better utilization of each staff member's time and capabilities will be encouraged. And, finally, there will be a better basis for understanding the program both within the school system and in the community.

When trying to determine goals and objectives, it is helpful to view the program and your responsibilities in terms of a problem that needs to be solved. First, there is a need to establish major goals, objectives, and policies that guide decision-making. In the larger context, it is helpful to ask yourself some questions:

1. What is the purpose of the (speech-language pathology or education) program?
2. What are the major goals, objectives, and policies that guide the program's decision making?
3. What is the structure that is in place to assign responsibilities for the various

tasks that must be achieved in order for accomplishing the objectives?

4. What resources (space, equipment, furniture, staff, and supporting services, to mention only a few) are available to support the program so the purpose can be accomplished?

Goals are long-term and short-term, tangible, measurable, and verifiable. They are not nebulous statements but specific statements of a desired future condition. Ideally, goals should be set by all persons involved in the structure so there is a commitment on their part. Once the goals have been determined it is crucial to get them down in writing. The language must be clear and concise and must communicate the intent to all relevant parties. Let us look at some examples of goals and objectives. We first consider writing long-range program goals, assuming that you have already evaluated the existing situation and have determined the overall needs of the program. Keep in mind that although these are long range and broad in focus, they still need to be stated specifically and concretely. Examples are listed below:

- One year from (date) the SLP will have developed and written a language curriculum guide for special education teachers in the county.
- By (date) the SLP will have completed a research project related to determining criteria for case selection at the kindergarten level.
- By (date) 90% of the pupils in Conrad Elementary School identified as having communication problems and needing intervention will be receiving the appropriate service delivery model.

Some goals and objectives may be narrower in focus and have a shorter time frame.

- By (date) the SLP will have obtained referrals from 75% of the K to 6 teachers.
- By (date) the clinician will have conducted group parent meetings for parents of all children enrolled at Pelland School.
- During the second week of school in September, the SLP will acquaint teachers at Lennox School with referral procedures through an in-service meeting.
- By (date) the SLP will write an article for the local newspaper and prepare items for the local radio and television stations announcing the prekindergarten communication evaluation program to be held during the first week in May.

A *criterion*, or *standard of performance*, is the description of the results of a job well done. It represents the desired outcome or benchmark for success. Using numbers or another indication of quantity such as *how much* and by *when* provides a framework for determining if the goal has been achieved. The outcome should be realistic and high quality enough so that when the task is completed it will have been of value to the program. Some examples follow:

- Dismiss 30% of the pupils enrolled as functionally corrected by April.
- By (date) the SLP will provide three demonstration

language-development sessions in 50% of the first grade classrooms of Coleman School, and receive written positive feedback from 90% of the teachers involved.

The *evaluation* is the method used to determine if the goal or objective has been accomplished. An indication of the evaluation may be a report sent to the coordinator of speech language and hearing services. Or it may be a list of post-test scores, a list of referrals made, or a chart indicating that change has occurred as the following example shows:

- By (date) the SLP will have completed speech-language screening tests of 95% of the first-grade pupils in St. Xzavier School, and a report will be submitted to the school principal and the director of speech-language and hearing services.

Occasionally, objectives are difficult to measure or confirm, even though they are activities or events that when accomplished lead to the overall improvement of a situation or condition. The following example demonstrates this:

- The SLP will attempt to improve communication with the classroom teachers by eating lunch with the teachers at least two times per week; inviting teachers to observe therapy sessions and attending as many school meetings and social functions as time permits.

School SLPs are familiar with the process of writing goals and objectives for the students with whom they work. Program goals are also important so that there is a clear understanding of *where* the program is going, *how* it will get there, and *how* to know when the objectives and goals are achieved. The manager of the program should be sure everyone understands the goals and, ideally, each participant should have a part in formulating them.

Managing the Workload and Time

The management of the workload and time to accomplish important tasks and responsibilities are important aspects of the role of the school SLP. Due to mandates within the state and federal laws, SLPs are confronted with great amounts of paperwork in the implementation of procedures. Although this undoubtedly has accounted for an increased expenditure of time, there are ways of managing time that can lead to increased productivity. It is extremely important to create a system for setting up your workload, caseload, and schedule. Some people create their own scheduling systems. However, there are tools that make the scheduling process more efficient. One such tool, Caselite Scheduling Software, provides a computer-based solution and relevant suggestions for designing a schedule plan (http://www.CaseliteSoftware.com).

Planning for the Week

In planning for the week the key word is *flexibility*. The school clinician will have to decide how much time during the week will be spent working directly with students, providing guidance to teachers, supervising assistants, or traveling from school to school. Specific blocks of time can be allocated for each of these categories of activities. An activity such as parent training may be carried out in a block of time. The school clinician may want to reserve blocks of time at certain times of the year or the semester for various aspects of the program.

Such activities as diagnosis and assessment, staffing and placement, and consultation are necessary parts of the program, and time for these activities may be set aside in daily or weekly blocks. For example, the staffing and placement team may not meet every week, so the block of time set aside weekly could be used on alternate weeks for meetings to discuss placement recommendations or for conducting diagnostics or providing consultation.

Record keeping and time spent in organizing, planning, implementing, analyzing, and evaluating the program could be scheduled at times of the day when staff members are in the school but children are not present. For example, mornings before children arrive at school and afternoons after they are dismissed could be utilized for these activities. Many school systems set aside a time usually referred to as *coordination time* for tasks of this nature.

Two very important activities are consulting and collaborating with the classroom teacher and other educators. This may be done on an informal one-to-one basis or as part of an in-service training presentation for teachers, school administrators, other school personnel, and parents. Because communication is the keystone of the education process and because even the most skilled classroom teacher cannot teach a child who has not developed adequate communication skills, the school speech-language pathologist has much to offer in helping to improve communication abilities. The school SLP needs to plan for time for consulting and collaborating with others.

Over the last decade, an increasing number of SLPs began to expand the types of service delivery models they use to meet the needs of youngsters on their caseload. For example, it has become commonplace to provide intervention within youngsters' classrooms or to teach critical communication skills alongside of the classroom teacher. Each of these service delivery models requires time to plan and execute. Other clinicians have hired assistants to work side by side with them. If assistants and aides are assigned to the program, time must be planned to train them and time must be allocated for the supervision of such personnel.

For many of the activities mentioned, time is not planned on a regularly scheduled basis but certainly must be set aside to include these important facets of the program.

Planning for the Day

In planning time for the day, the school clinician will have to know how many hours per day the children are in school. What is their arrival time and what is their dismissal time? How much time is allowed for lunch and recess?

The time that the teachers are required to be in school and the time they may leave in the afternoon is set by school policy, and school clinicians should follow the same rules that teachers are required to follow. This sometimes poses a problem for the school clinicians who is scheduled in School A in the morning and School B in the afternoon, but who must return to School A for a parent conference or staff meeting after school is dismissed. The problem arises when the teachers in School B think the clinician is leaving school early. Difficult situations such as these can usually be alleviated by following the rule of always informing the principals of School A and School B of any deviation from the regular schedule.

The school SLP will have to decide the length of the therapy sessions and amount of time devoted to diagnostics and other services. There does not have to be a predetermined length of time. Sessions may range from 15 minutes to an hour or more. The length of treatment depends on a number of factors including the student's unique needs, the composition of the caseload and resulting demands, and the school schedule for classes, recess, lunch, dismissal time, and so on.

Future chapters will include an in-depth discussion of factors that must be considered when constructing a workload, caseload, and schedule. Among the considerations are the total number of children to be seen, range of disorders to be served, extent of services to be provided, composition of caseload, and structure of therapy sessions (group versus individualized sessions versus classroom-based intervention). Also, children will inevitably progress at different rates. Some may be in the final phase of therapy and won't require as much time as children who are just beginning. The caseload and schedule should be "fluid" to accommodate children moving into and out of treatment as their communication skills and needs change.

It is wise to schedule the sessions a few minutes apart to allow for children to arrive on time or to allow time for the clinician to locate a child whose teacher has forgotten to send a child to therapy. In planning the daily schedule the school clinician will need to retain as much flexibility as possible. Children change and their needs change. The child who once required 30 minutes of individual therapy per day may later need only 15 minutes twice a week. Or the child who once needed individual therapy may need the experience of a group or in-class activity to continue making progress. The principal and the teachers must also understand the benefits of offering a flexible program. It is the responsibility of the clinician to interpret the rationale involved in making changes in schedules.

As a result of inclusion and the influx of more children with serious disabilities into the public schools, the school clinician must allow time for working with classroom teachers of youngsters who are developmentally delayed, dysfluent, emotionally disturbed, hearing impaired, learning disabled, autistic, and multihandicapped. In fact, any child with communication disabilities may require direct as well as indirect intervention by the speech-language pathologist.

Allocate Time for Planning

In most school systems, the SLP sets aside a specific time which is allotted to the numerous activities that must be carried on in addition to the time spent in therapy. This is usually referred to as "planning time" or "coordination time." This may be a block of time allocated during the week or it may be several periods of time during the week that are not scheduled for therapy. Or it may be a combination of the two. Planning time is not a "right" and should be used wisely or others may interpret that it is not needed.

SLPs spend their planning time accomplishing a broad range of tasks and activities. These might include conducting screening programs, administering diagnostic tests, completing re-evaluations, participating in teacher conferences, attending administrative conferences, contacting parent, making phone calls, writing individualized education plans, completing summary reports, attending professional meetings, making referrals, observing youngsters in class or other settings, volunteering for state professional associations, attending in-service meetings, reviewing and ordering materials, organizing resources, gathering data, and reading professional literature.

Successful service delivery requires administrative support. You will quickly lose that support if others perceive that you are wasting time and not meeting the goals and objectives of the educational organization. The best way to gain the support you need is to demonstrate that you are engaged in your program and accomplishing what you are expected to do.

Personal Time Management

The school clinician who is the sole speech-language specialist will have much greater responsibility than a person stepping into a job where there is an ongoing program with other school clinicians already involved. In the latter situation, the new clinician fits into the program that has already been set up. In the former, the clinician may be the key planner and organizer. The school clinician must take into consideration two factors in overall time and workload management. The first is the need to plan time on a long-term, yearly, semester, weekly, and daily basis; the second is the need for the clinician to manage his or her time within the larger framework. With respect to both factors, planning is an essential first step. The next important step is setting priorities and sticking with them.

Use of time is a matter of personal preference but time efficiency experts make some useful recommendations. Time-saving techniques are not necessarily new. Most people think they are too busy to implement them or perhaps do not know how to implement them. One technique is to make a list of things to be done today, then to set priorities on that list and follow them. Long "To Do" lists become more manageable if you first prepare a list and work from your list throughout the time period, checking off tasks as they are accomplished. Group similar tasks. For example, make all phone calls, prepare written reports, administer tests to children, or conduct conferences within given time periods. If possible, delegate tasks to others. Organize materials so they are easily retrieved and accessed.

Keep a file containing alphabetized names and telephone numbers of persons and agencies necessary to the work. A record of incoming and outgoing telephone calls might be recorded in a notebook or computer file, providing a record and synopsis of those conversations.

Another important factor in personal time management is not to let paper work or E-mail messages pile up. One efficiency suggestion often heard is, "Handle each piece of paper (or E-mail message) only once." A period of time each day or each week should be devoted entirely to this task. It is also important to look at habits or practices that may be wasting time, for example, attending too many meetings, spending too much time on phone calls, allowing too many interruptions, or attempting to do multiple tasks in a short time. Most school clinicians would like to add an extra hour to a day now and then or think in terms of an occasional 8-day week. Because time is scarce it must be managed with maximum effectiveness. Experts in time management tell us that selecting the best task from all the possibilities available and then doing it in the best way is more important than doing efficiently whatever job happens to be around.

No matter how one looks at it, we are dealing with that precious and fleeting commodity—time. It is scarce, inelastic, does not have a two-way stretch, cannot be stored or frozen for future use, and cannot be retrieved. It can, however, be managed effectively.

Professional Development Plans

Administrators in some school districts require educators, including speech-language pathologists, to submit a Professional Development Plan (or Professional Growth Plan). There are important reasons for such a document. First, it enables administrators and practitioners to mutually agree upon issues such as the workload, responsibilities, and duties. Second, the plan makes a statement of competencies and skills the clinician needs to have to effectively provide services to youngsters. To ensure accountability, the Professional Development Plan often specifies how training for those competencies and skills will be accomplished, including when, where, and who will pay for the training. This is especially necessary when new competencies are needed to serve a child with a particular type of disorder or to implement a new service delivery model. The use of professional development plans demonstrates the necessary and expected link between treatment outcomes for the student, competencies needed by the SLP, program development goals, and accountability.

Many districts and some state boards of education require educators to have a Professional Growth Plan tied to student learning. For example, they might require that the plan be educator directed and focused on acquisition of knowledge and skills related to the state education standards, subject content, instruction methods, technology, assessment and data analysis, classroom management, and school safety. Staff development efforts are generally aligned with student and instructional personnel needs. If the school principal identifies a teacher's performance as deficient, then a Professional Development Plan is generally constructed. Different needs assessment instruments can be used to determine the skills and competencies the educator must learn including inventories, classroom observations, interviews, self-assessments, student achievement data, and the like. Educators may engage in a wide range of learning activities as part of their Professional Growth (or Development) Plan including: study groups, action research, journal reading groups, in-service training programs, self-guided study, peer coaching, workshops, college courses, and independent studies. Figure 4–2 shows excerpts of key elements from the professional development plans of a speech-language pathologist.

Rationale for Professional Development Plans

Demonstrate the necessary and expected link between treatment outcomes for students, competencies needed by the SLP, the speech-language program goals, and accountability.

Make a statement of the competencies and skills the therapist needs to effectively provide services to students.

Facilitate agreement upon issues such as responsibility, workload, and duties.

How to Establish a Professional Development Plan

Identify your professional strengths, skills in need of improvement, career goals and aspirations. Consider changes that have occurred in your workload, caseload, responsibilities, and duties. Think about the five major areas of service delivery: evaluation, intervention, program management, collaboration, professional relationships.

Specify competencies and skills you would like to acquire. These may be competencies and skills that your supervisor has identified as in need of improvement or new skills you need in order to provide services to a new population or advance your career.

List 3 learning outcomes that will result from execution of your Professional Development Plan.

Formulate a Professional Development Plan for the year (calendar year or school year) based on your self-evaluation.

> Determine how these competencies and skills can be achieved. Consider a wide range of learning and continuing education activities including: in-service training, seminars, workshops, self-guided study, journal reading, university courses, peer coaching, mentoring, web exploration etc.
>
> Specifiy methods you will use to determine if you have acquired the competencies and skills or accomplished your goals and learning outcomes. Methods for determining may include observations, interviews, self- assessment, caseload or student performance data.
>
> Establish a time line for accomplishing each task on your annual Professional Development Plan.
>
> Evaluate your progress *quarterly* within the one-year time period. Make adjustments where necessary.
>
> Implement your new competencies and skills in your program and career.
>
> Reward your success with by sharing your accomplishment with peers, supervisors, and administrators.

Figure 4–2. Establishing a professional development plan.

Quality Improvement

Another aspect of the management of school speech-language pathology programs must be taken into consideration. This aspect is *quality*. The profession's commitment to quality began as early as 1959 when the American Speech-Language-Hearing Association established its accreditation program with the founding of the American Boards of Examiners in Speech Pathology and Audiology (ABESPA). Later, the name of the accrediting body was changed to the Professional Services Board (PSB). At the present time, standards and guidelines are established by ASHA for the accreditation of educational programs, certification standards for professionals, and standards for professional services. These standards and guidelines are continually reviewed and, when necessary, changed to meet current needs.

Quality Improvement of Professional Practices

The communication disorders profession is continually evolving. Our understanding of the nature and impact of disorders is improving as are our techniques and approaches to diagnosis and treatment. Consequently, it is important to monitor and review professional practices on an ongoing basis to assess the quality of service delivery and to determine adjustments needed to make improvements.

Speech-language pathologists in various settings have begun to develop and use continuous quality improvement (CQI) approaches to improve performance and service delivery in order to better meet consumer expectations and needs (Frattali, 1990). State and local education agencies, third party payers, government regulators, and accreditation agencies have supported these efforts. School clinicians should establish a comprehensive quality improvement plan which is appropriate to the school setting. The plan should reflect a commitment to ongoing program assessment and continual improvement. It should focus on all activities of the program. It should include a process for monitoring, assessing, and evaluating various aspects of the program's work process and service delivery such as the program *structure* (facility and staff characteristics), the *process* (methods of treatment and care), and the *outcome* (end result) (Frattali, 1999). The plan should also state the specific elements (e.g., criteria, indicators, standards, or protocols) against which aspects of quality are compared. The intent is to use performance-based and outcome-oriented measures to identify areas in service delivery in need of improvement. If deficiencies are noted then actions or steps must be taken to make improvements.

It is important that staff members work as a team in developing and implementing the quality improvement plan. This means jointly assuming responsibility for identifying problem areas and implementing change. Therefore, to be effective, the plan should incorporate procedures for peer interaction and review. In this way, problems can be discovered and resolved before they interfere with the quality of services. It should encourage collaboration among staff and administration in joint planning efforts to improve areas where problems are noted. The concept of continuous quality improvement crosses all health and education settings. It is a professional and ethical responsibility. Frattali (1990) recommends the following 10 steps for designing a quality assurance process:

1. Select a structure, process and/or outcome approach (e.g., *structure* [clinician qualifications, condition of test equipment, adequacy of test environment], *process* [treatment methods, selection of diagnostic measures, appropriateness of goals], *outcome* [client satisfaction, functional communication, goal attainment]).
2. Define a target client population (e.g., age group, diagnosis, disorder severity).
3. Choose a method of assessment (e.g., retrospective, concurrent, prospective).
4. Select a data source (e.g., clinical records, interview, observation, survey questions).
5. Select or develop standards against which to measure the quality of care provided.
6. Set the level of compliance.
7. Specify expectations.
8. Collect and analyze data. Evaluate the quality of services.
9. Formulate corrective action if deficiencies are found.
10. Monitor the service until deficiencies are corrected.

Lastohkein, Moon, and Blosser (1992) developed a sample quality improvement plan appropriate for the school setting. As a process for review, they selected the implementation of a collaborative service delivery model within a local school district. Following is an explanation illustrating how each of the ten steps described by Frattali would be applied to evaluate and improve collaborative efforts (Table 4–1, Quality Improvement Plan).

Step One (Assign Responsibility)

The first step in Frattali's model is to determine who will be responsible for monitoring the speech-language pathology program's collaborative efforts. The following individuals will most likely be involved in collaboration: the speech-language pathologist, audiologist, parents/caregivers, special education director, principal, superintendent, classroom teacher, social worker, school nurse, psychologist, and other professionals in special education.

Any of these professionals could function as the quality improvement coordinator responsible for assigning each individual with specific responsibilities and establishing a formal reporting mechanism. For the purpose of this discussion, the SLP on the team is designated as the quality improvement coordinator.

In order to determine the effectiveness of collaborative efforts and areas where improvement is needed, it was necessary to narrow the focus of the quality improvement plan by delineating the scope of care in the following ways.

Step Two (Delineate Scope of Care)

The second step, delineating the scope of care, determines the who, what, when, where, and how aspects of the QI process.

Table 4–1. Quality Improvement Plan

Aspect of Care	*Quality Indicator and Threshold Evaluation (TE)*	*Data Source*	*Collection Method*	*Time Frame*
Administrative Issues: Time Constraints and Scheduling Conflicts	Establish regular meeting times.			
	A) Full Team TE: 90% attendance at scheduled meetings	Records of meeting dates and attendance at meetings	100% review; Concurrent	Quarterly
	B) 2–3 Person Collaborative Partner Teams TE: 90% attendance at scheduled meetings	Records of meeting dates and attendance at meetings	100% review; Concurrent	Monthly
Long-Term Plan	All team members (as listed in Step 1) will participate in setting long term goals (e.g., goals to be met in 5 years). TE: 90% actual participation	Staff minutes and reports	100% review; Concurrent	March
	All team members will participate in setting short-term goals used to achieve above long-term goals. TE: 90% actual participation	Staff minutes and reports	100% review; Concurrent	June
Participants' Responsibilities	Specific responsibilities will be assigned to each team member for completion during a specific period of time (e.g., 3-month increments over a 2-year period). TE: 85% completion of all task assigned	List of assigned tasks, activity reports, summary reports	100% review; Concurrent	Quarterly

Aspect of Care	*Quality Indicator and Threshold Evaluation (TE)*	*Data Source*	*Collection Method*	*Time Frame*
Team Members' Expertise and Competence	Team members identify areas of knowledge necessary for collaborative model to be successful (e.g., knowledge of each others' disciplines, knowledge of speech and language development, impact of communication on academic success, school curriculum, process of collaborative model). TE: 85% agreement on topics selected	Topics for discussion identified by team members at staff meetings or via questionnaire	100% review; Concurrent	Ongoing
	Team members obtain information on specified topics necessary for the collaborative model to be successful. TE: 80% participate in learning activities	Agendas and brochures from in-service programs, continuing education credits, academic records, summaries of literature reviews, information received from other professionals	Periodic review; Retrospective	Ongoing
Case Selection Criterion	Accurate identification of students with language-learning disabilities to be served under the collaborative model TE: 90% agreement of team members regarding eligibility criteria and case selection	Test scores of students placed in learning disability classes	50% of caseload; Concurrent	Semiannually

In our school collaborative program the following guidelines are specified.

- *Who*—Individuals needing services in schools who may be served under a collaborative model include elementary children who have language-learning disabilities with class placement in a program designated for children with learning disabilities.
- *What*—Services provided under a collaborative model include but are not limited to the following: consulting with other professionals, in-servicing the caregivers and other professionals, establishing goals and treatment plans, co-treating, maintaining and exchanging reports, teaching other individuals to implement intervention strategies, and counseling caregivers/individuals regarding student's communication disorders and the impact on education.
- *When*—Collaboration should continuously be occurring among professionals. This may take place throughout the school day, at weekly staff meetings, or at IEP meetings.
- *Where*—Collaboration can occur in the students' learning environment, at staff meetings, at IEP meetings, or via other forms of communication exchange.
- *How*—Collaboration can be achieved by communicating face to face (e.g., at staff meetings, IEP meetings, in the classroom), via written communication (e.g., exchange written reports, memos, newsletters), or via telephone.

Steps Three Through Six (Identify important aspects of care, identify quality indicators, establish thresholds for evaluation and collect and organize data, respectively)

Important aspects of care must be identified to provide a focus for the quality improvement efforts. Aspects of care required for effective collaboration include: long-term planning, assigning responsibilities, improving participant's competence in specified areas, identifying case selection criteria, and addressing administrative issues such as scheduling conflicts and time constraints. For each aspect of care identified, a quality indicator, threshold evaluation, data source, collection method, and time frame are established. To complete the process, Frattali indicates that the following four steps are necessary.

Step Seven (Evaluation of Care)

If a predetermined threshold is not met, the data should be analyzed to determine if opportunities for improvement exist.

Step Eight (Action Plan to Improve Care)

If improvements can be made, an action plan to improve care should be established. Because this steps provides an opportunity to make revisions (i.e., review plan, change indicators, identify new indicators), this is a critical step in the model.

Step Nine (Assess the Actions and Document Improvement)

Procedures should be established for continuous monitoring, evaluation, and documentation of revisions specified in step eight.

Step Ten (Communicate Findings)

Finally, a report to communicate findings is distributed to all team members involved.

This chapter has focused on the management and planning aspects of the speech-language pathologist's role. Most new professionals never anticipate that they will find themselves in the position of working on a district-wide planning team or thinking of ways to solve problems such as school violence, curriculum selection, or service delivery models. Yet, this is the nature of the job in today's school environment. The most important benefit for professionals who use this planning process is that the result will be a systematic process for making serious, important decisions that affect children's lives. One hopes it will inhibit the urge to just jump in to implement a new service delivery or approach without careful review and advance planning. Without such efforts, new programs are likely to fail or have less impact than is possible.

DISCUSSION QUESTIONS AND PROJECTS

1. Describe the mission of the program in which you are currently participating at a university, a local hospital, or school district. Is the mission in writing in any of the marketing materials?

2. Obtain a copy of the strategic plan for your local school district. Request to meet with administrators who oversee implementation of the strategic plan.

3. What are some yearly program goals you, as the SLP, might develop?

4. What are the advantages of written program plans and goals?

5. What are various ways of quantifying or measuring the success of a speech-language pathology program?

6. Develop a quality improvement plan for initiating a parent or teacher training program in your local school district.

7. Identify three program goals that will improve service delivery to children in your school districts.

8. Write a personal professional development plan that includes statements of how to improve your clinical skills in a particular area.

5

Tools of the Trade: Space, Facilities, Equipment, and Materials

Adequate facilities and equipment are necessary to enable school speech-language pathologists to appropriately serve students. Additionally, comprehensive accountability procedures and efficient record keeping practices can assist the clinician in documenting responsible service delivery. Space, facilities, equipment, materials and reports may be considered representative tools of the trade. Just as a carpenter needs good tools, so does the SLP. In this chapter, we consider the basic needs and how they can be met.

Physical Facilities

At the present time there is a wide variation in the quality of workspace and work environment available to school-based SLPs. The reasons for discrepancies from school site to school are not always clear. Some schools are overcrowded and the school clinician is in competition with other school personnel for the available space. Many school districts are financially strapped and can't provide the space. School buildings, new as well as old, may not have been planned with the speech-language services taken into account. In some cases the school administration is either unaware or apathetic about the issue of adequate working space. On the other hand, increasing numbers of school systems provide excellent facilities.

Minimal Standards for Facilities and Space

Appropriate facilities are necessary to provide an adequate atmosphere for performing responsibilities and implementing program goals. State and federal guidelines stipulate that the workspace for the delivery of speech language intervention services be suitable and appropriate. Several committees within ASHA have recommended minimal standards of operation for programs offering speech-language and hearing services. As a general guideline, the standards suggest that the physical facility should be barrier-free, in compliance with all applicable safety and health codes, and suitable for the conduct of those activities required to meet the objectives of the program.

In many states, minimal standards for facilities are established by the state department of education. These do not necessarily describe superior facilities, but they do provide a standard below which schools may not go. There sometimes is confusion about this issue, and the school clinician needs to be aware of exactly how the standards are worded. Some local school districts and professional organizations have also developed recommendations for physical facilities and equipment necessary for operating programs effectively. This can be determined by visiting the organization's Web site, reviewing operational manuals, or interviewing program administrators.

The beginning school clinician needs some sort of "yardstick" by which to evaluate and define adequate facilities. The checklist presented in Table 5–1 can be used as a reference when observing a school speech-language pathology program, selecting a site for your school externship experience, or interviewing for a job. If several elements are inadequate, don't be afraid to discuss them with program administrators. Although it is not advisable to engage in confrontations, questioning an administrator based on sound information and a desire to provide the best services possible can result in improved understanding of the speech-language program and an improved environment for service delivery.

Pleasant, Comfortable, and Functional Space

In establishing criteria for evaluating physical facilities, the factors of "realism" and "idealism" must be taken into account. Although it might be ideal for the speech-language clinician to have a room used exclusively for the speech language intervention program, it may not be realistic. The speech-language pathologist may be following an itinerant schedule. Other educators could utilize the space on the alternate days.

Another factor to consider is the existing facilities (things as they are today) and the potential facilities (things as they might be with some modifications), particularly in setting up a new program. It is important to establish a set of criteria that indicates how the existing facilities could and should be modified in the future. In assessing this aspect of the program the policies of the school must be known. For example, is the supervisor of the speech-language pathology program involved in the planning of new facilities or the modification of existing ones? Will staff members be included in future planning? Are alternative plans considered, such as the use of mobile units, remodeling of areas of buildings, or rental of additional space? What are the budgetary allowances and constraints?

Table 5–1. Program Environment Checklist

Room

Location

______ Quiet, private enough to permit confidentiality; free from distractions

______ Easy to locate; accessible for individuals who are nonambulatory or exhibit severe learning disabilities

______ Near students' classrooms and restrooms

______ Designated for exclusive use by the SLP program during all times when the speech-language pathologist is on site

______ Easy access to emergency exits

______ Secured for storage of equipment and materials

Lighting

______ Suitable for reading and manipulating pictures and objects

Power

______ Adequate number of electrical outlets for operating program equipment (e.g., recorders, computers, amplification systems, augmentative devices, printers, telephones, etc.

Size

______ Adequate to meet safety standards for the maximum number of persons who will be in the room at a given time

Temperature

______ Adequate ventilation, heating, and cooling; thermostatic control available

Safety Devices

______ Audible as well as visual safety devices (fire and smoke alarms)

Furniture

Chairs

______ Appropriate size and number to accommodate clinician, students, and observers; matched to the table size and space

Desk

______ Adult size, office style with lockable drawers

File Cabinet

______ Lockable

______ Appropriate size for number and type of files used for the program

Tables

______ Appropriate height and number to accommodate a broad range of students' sizes and ages

______ Adequate support for equipment (computers, printers)

Shelves

______ Adequate number and structure for storage of books, therapy and testing materials

Assessment and Instruction Materials

______ Most recent version

______ Age appropriate

______ All parts and pieces available and in working order

______ Sanitary and in good condition

______ Appropriate mix of standardized and nonstandardized instruments

______ Ample number of protocols

Equipment and Materials

Audiometers

______ Appropriate for testing pure-tones and immittance

______ Properly calibrated

continues

Table 5–1. *continued*

Amplification Devices	*Recording Device*
______ Appropriate to meet individual and group needs	______ Designated for exclusive use by the speech-language program
Augmentative Communication Systems	______ Appropriate for recording and playback
______ Appropriate for various age and functional communication levels	*Telecommunications Display Device*
Computers and Other Technology	______ Available if needed to meet the needs of students who are hearing impaired
______ Available according to need	*Telephone*
______ Suitable for word processing and data storage	______ Available when needed
______ Appropriate software for program management and intervention	______ Located in a private area
______ Accessories necessary to operate uniquely designed programs	*Video-Recording and Playback Equipment*
Expendable Materials	______ Available and easily accessed
______ Conveniently located	______ Appropriate for recording and playback
______ Easily accessed	______ Designated for exclusive use by the speech-language program
Mirror	
______ Appropriate size for viewing faces and bodies	
______ Constructed of safety glass	

In addition to evaluating the room itself, there are other considerations. First, the room must be accessible to pupils who are disabled and located in an area of the building convenient to others who use it. Perhaps it should be located near the youngest students in the building because these children sometimes have difficulty finding their way to and from the room.

Space is often at a premium in school buildings, and many buildings are old and not well planned for present-day needs. With a little imagination and resourcefulness, however, some simple remodeling and rejuvenation can transform unused space into completely adequate facilities for the school pathologist. In buildings where space is limited, SLPs can work with administrators, teachers, and plant maintenance personnel to identify space that could be partitioned and utilized for the SLP program.

If a new building is being contemplated, the speech-language clinician potentially can be in on the planning stages to insure adequate space allotment. School architects are not always well informed about the space and facility needs of the program, and the school pathologist can be of invaluable assistance by providing recommendations and useful information.

The policies of the school in regard to space also must be known when planning physical facilities. For example, the school pathologist should know how space is assigned in a building and whether or not staff members are consulted when the assignments are made. The school SLP should also know whether or not there are provisions for modifying the room. If space is to be shared, staff members should obtain input from all the persons sharing the room.

Most people feel better and do better in surroundings that are attractive, comfortable, and pleasant. Children are no exception. Color, adequate lighting, and comfortable furniture are conducive to good results in therapy. A child who is seated on a chair that is too big for him or her is going to be very uncomfortable. In a short time the child will begin to squirm and wriggle and will be unable to focus on whatever the clinician is presenting. The child may seem like a discipline problem to the unaware clinician, but in reality the little boy or girl may simply be attempting to find a comfortable position.

One of the most attractive therapy rooms I have seen was in an old school building in a rural area. The whole building sparkled with cleanliness. Wooden floors were polished, walls were painted in soft colors, and furniture was in good repair and arranged harmoniously. The therapy room was pleasant, with a carpeted floor and colorful draperies. A bulletin board served both a useful and decorative purpose. The obvious pride in the surroundings was reflected by the way that the children treated the therapy room and its furnishings. The clinician reported that everyone in the school, including the custodian, the principal, the teachers, and the children were proud of their attractive building and worked to keep it that way.

Space Allocations

The space allocations in schools have improved over the years. Perhaps this is because SLPs now spend more time in each school and more schools have full time or nearly full-time speech-language intervention programs. Also, school administrators are becoming more aware of the importance of speech-language pathology programs, and the needs of the programs are receiving more attention. Nonetheless, it is of vital importance that the school SLP assumes the responsibility of making the needs of the program known to the principal, director of special services, and superintendent. The school SLP must be assertive and forthright in this endeavor. The student with a hearing loss, language-learning disability, fluency problem, voice disorder, or phonological problem cannot benefit from therapy in a room where there are constant interruptions, exposure to illnesses, noise from band practice, or a storage room that is inadequately lighted, ventilated, and heated or cooled.

Overcrowded schools and substandard space within school buildings have prompted some speech-language pathologists to look elsewhere for the solution to the facility problem. Mobile units and stationary trailers located on the school grounds have provided solutions for many clinicians. There may be a number of advantages in using mobile units. They contain everything necessary for the program, thus eliminating gathering up and storing items every day. Equipment will not be broken when it remains stationary and doesn't have to be transported in the trunk of a car. Mobile units provide quiet facilities for testing. They may also represent a savings in tax dollars in comparison to the cost of building permanent facilities.

Special Considerations for Special Populations

Careful thought and planning should go into designing, organizing and decorating your therapy room. Keep your students' special needs, ages, learning capabilities, and interest levels in mind. Decor should be attractive and motivating. Care should be taken to avoid arranging the room in a way that is distracting or condescending to students' ages or intelligence. Certain groups require special considerations.

Infants, Toddlers, and Preschoolers

As a result of federal legislation, school districts are responsible for providing services to a younger group of children than they had accommodated previously. Many school buildings are not designed for such a young group. Room location, furniture size, and equipment selection is of utmost importance. The environment must be bright and stimulating. Children in this age group do not learn by sitting quietly at a table and taking turns talking. Learning quite often takes place on the floor or while the child is in motion during play. Therefore, the atmosphere and materials should invite manipulation, creativity, movement, and interaction. Toys are appropriate, especially if they can be used to encourage investigation, experimentation, imitation, and questioning. Because of the way in which children play with toys, they will need to be cleansed frequently and maintained in proper working order.

Adolescents

Obviously, facilities for intermediate and high school students will be different than those for elementary and preschool students. The size and type of furniture as well as the arrangement of the classroom and decorations should facilitate group discussions and lessons. The typical classroom or rows of desks is not conducive to the type of learning that takes place in a typical situation. The use of carrels and learning centers provides the opportunity for independent work. Activity centers related to specific learning skills could incorporate vocabulary cards, work sheets, and learning games. Learning centers might include tape recorders, objects that can be manipulated, and computers. A library center might have reading materials, books used for book reports, story wheels, and writing materials. A career education center might contain materials related to various occupations, job application requirements, and forms.

Children with Severe and Multiple Impairments

There is likely to be wide variation in skill levels, capabilities, mobility, sizes, and intervention needs for children with severe and multiple impairments. Consequently, facilities for this group of children should be designed so that easy adaptation is permitted throughout the day. Furniture should be of sturdy construction, adjustable, and easily moved to meet positioning requirements. Treatment materials should be selected to permit teaching important concepts and skills while still being motivating. Augmentative and alternative communication systems are valuable assets to children whose communication skills are severely restricted.

Some children with severe and multiple impairments become easily distracted by auditory or visual stimuli. Children with sensory problems, brain dysfunction, or developmental delays may have difficulty functioning in a room that is too stimulating or distracting because of garish colors or busy patterns. To accommodate these youngsters' needs while still providing a bright, stimulating environment for other children on the caseload, the clinician may wish to arrange one section of the therapy room in such a way that all potentially distracting materials are out of the child's range of vision.

Facilities for Observation

The school clinician may want to invite parents, educators, and school administrators to observe diagnostic and intervention services. This would provide opportunities for involving valuable members of the child's world in the therapy program, teaching others about the profession, and promoting collaboration.

One way to facilitate observation is to invite persons to join you during the session. If the presence of others would distract the students, one-way mirrors and intercom systems can be used to enable observation without interruption. Through observational experiences such as these, parents and teachers can learn important speech and language stimulation and correction techniques. Team members such as school psychologists can observe the child's communication skills under optimum conditions to obtain valuable diagnostic information. Administrators can learn about the scope and services of the speech-language program.

Often, school clinicians hear the comment from others, "But what do you actually do in a therapy session?" Having people observe would take some of the mystery out of therapy and would make vividly clear the role they can play in the therapy process in the home or classroom. This ultimately would help the child generalize what he or she has learned. Observers will be able to follow the flow of the session better if they are provided with a brief explanation of the goals of the session and the intent of activities they are about to observe. One effective method is to write those goals on a blackboard or sheet of paper.

Demonstration Centers

Some large school districts and regional resource centers house demonstration centers where parents, students, and teachers may go to learn about communication devices including assistive listening devices and alternative/augmentative communication systems. By displaying devices, potential users are able to gain an understanding of assistive technology that is available. They can learn about how the technology works or how the device might help in adapting the classroom environment. In addition, visitors can gain a sense of the possibilities that are available for enhancing the communication experience. Children with hearing impairments can be exposed to alerting, listening and telephone devices. Youngsters with limited verbal skills can sample various types of voice synthesizers and response options.

Equipment and Materials

In addition to the therapy room and its furnishings, several types of equipment, materials, and supplies are needed for a successful program. Equipment and materials should be appropriately selected to meet the needs of the students and types of disorders being served. Appropriate schedules of maintenance and calibration should be followed to ensure that equipment remains in proper working order.

Equipment is an item that is not expendable; retains its original shape, appearance, and use; usually costs a substantial amount of money; and is more feasible to repair than to replace when damaged or worn out. Materials and supplies, on the other hand, are considered expendable. They are used up, usually inexpensive, and are more feasible to replace than to repair when damaged or worn out.

Integrating Technology into All Aspects of the Program

The growing use of computers and other types of technology in instruction, business, and everyday life has become a reality on the American education scene. School SLPs who use computers have discovered that they are able to save time, conserve energy, increase benefits to students, and cut down on that greatest of all time-thieves, paperwork. School clinicians have discovered that computers can be invaluable tools for managing program information and as an integral adjunct to intervention. SLPs use computers to record students' screening and test results, track case management information; create their schedules; develop and catalogue therapy materials; maintain therapy logs; and compile statistical data for accountability to school administrators, boards of education, and state departments of education.

Much of the SLP's workload involves paperwork and reporting tasks. Computers can provide a number of advantages by helping the SLP save time, conserve energy, and increase benefits to clients. Software programs that permit word processing, data management, and spreadsheet functions enable SLPs to communicate with other professionals, and store and efficiently manage important information and reports.

School systems use computer-based information systems to track student information including demographic information, present levels of performance, IEPs, goals, attendance, services provided, and progress. Clinicians must learn to use the systems and allocate time in their schedules to enter data on a routine basis. School systems provide training in entering and maintaining data.

Data can be stored for administrative, research, and budgetary purposes. Decisions are made and funding is allocated based on the student information systems so accuracy is required and expected. An analysis of data can help identify trends such as increases in the caseload size, disorder type, or a population shift within the school district. Accurate caseload figures, demographic figures, and disorder and severity data can promote more efficient use of school personnel and program development. Required reports can be compiled more quickly, efficiently, and accurately. Computerization now permits clinicians to prepare reports that are comprehensive, easier to read, and more professional in appearance. In addition, the time saved can be used for an extension of direct therapy time.

A centralized information management system can store a large number of data. Test results, pertinent medical information, referral sources, treatment outcome data, and follow-up information unique to each student can be added at any time. Sorting options for producing printed reports are numerous. For example, a report that alphabetically lists student enrollment data by grade and room number for a given school can be printed for the school principal. Results also may be sorted according to those students enrolled in a special education program or as a compilation of students with a particular type of disorder. This flexibility for storage and maintenance of records eliminates time-consuming, cross-checking tasks and provides accurate records for studying screening, testing, and intervention data.

Software programs have been developed that can save SLPs considerable time and effort in dealing with the deluge of paperwork involved in developing Individualized Education Programs. Computers can be used in the generation of IEPs and for documenting completion of steps necessary for compliance with due process. The memory capacity of the computer allows storage of a virtually unlimited number of items in the goal and objective bank. In addition, items may be added to the bank for students who are not adequately described by existing statements or whose team members request additional objectives.

The stumbling blocks to computer usage in the schools include lack of familiarity with computers, financial restraints, limited connectivity, constantly changing technology and applications, lack of understanding about how to best use technology, and a dearth of speech-language professionals who understand its potential applications. Computers may be purchased by a school system for use by the speech-language pathology staff. Before purchasing a computer system and software programs, identify your needs and the applications you plan to use. Take into account the goals you are trying to achieve and service delivery models employed.

There are many issues to be decided prior to investing in technology. Prior to spending valuable funds to purchase a computer, an iPad, applications or software, clinicians should determine how they plan to use the technology. The school SLP contemplating the purchase of computer software is faced with a bewildering array of information and material. Many professionals review currently available computer software and accessories. Care should be taken before spending limited school funds on computers and software. They should offer broad use and flexibility.

Here are some questions to guide decision making about the purchase of technology and software. The responses to these questions can help formulate a proposal to administrators that includes an explanation of the type of technology being requested, the rationale, and the costs.

- Will it be used for program management and administration or for intervention?
- Who will be the primary user—the speech-language pathologist, a staff person, an assistant, or the students?
- What are the skill levels of the users?
- Will additional training be necessary?
- Where will the computer be located?
- Who will have access?
- Will security measure be necessary to protect data and equipment?
- Will Internet connectivity be necessary?
- Are specific software programs required?
- Will the computer be networked with others to permit exchange of information and integration of school district records and information?

Technology in Service Delivery

In the past, speech-language pathologists' equipment use was limited to audiometers, recorders, and simple amplification devices. They used word processors only for preparing reports or organizing data. Many clinicians are now routinely integrating more advanced technology into their service delivery programs. They are also recommending the incorporation of technology into the classroom setting to improve conditions for communication exchanges within that environment. It is not unusual to see students with communication disorders wearing assistive listening devices or the teacher speaking through a microphone. Children can be observed sitting at computers practicing language exercises or using a voice synthesizer to express their needs. Today's clinicians are using technology to manage program information as well as develop their students' communication skills.

Computer technology presents a window of opportunity for people with disabilities. If applications and software are selected properly, they can be used to facilitate drill practice, encourage transfer and generalization of learned skills, and permit individualized practice and self-correction. For example, treatment for students who are severely impaired can be enhanced through computer programs that use interactive learning and synthesized speech. The computer is also valuable to students as a means of access to information and visually oriented training and instruction. Computers won't replace competent clinicians but the use of computers by SLPs and audiologists in the schools can make a positive difference in the delivery of services to students with communication impairments.

Telepractice as a Service Delivery Option

In recent years many SLPs and school districts have explored the option of delivering speech-language services from a remote setting. We discuss this mode of service delivery further in Chapter 8. If therapists engage in service delivery using telepractice, they should make sure that the equipment meets recommended specifications. Those specifications will vary depending on the nature of the client and desired outcomes. Telepractice can be accomplished using telephones, the Internet, Web-based programs, through teleconferencing, and a variety of other technology solutions. It is important to make sure that the sound and image quality are sufficient for clinical applications. ASHA's Division 18 has provided guidelines and recommendations for all aspects of telepractice.

Augmentative and Alternative Communication Systems (AAC)

Perhaps the most exciting result of advanced technology is the increased opportunity for persons with severe impairments to communicate with others in their world. Speech-language pathologists are teaching persons with disorders such as dysarthria, verbal apraxia, aphasia, glossectomy, dysphonia, developmental delays, autism, brain injury, tracheostomy, and deafness to interact with their families, peers, and teachers via augmented and assisted-communication systems. Augumentative communication refers to communication systems that supplement speech. This can be accomplished through common techniques such as writing, gestures, and pictures or via more specialized techniques including electronic aids (Vanderheiden & Yoder, 1986).

Experts in augmentative communication believe that trying to "fix" the speech of a person with a severe motor disorder so that it is intelligible results in a sense of failure for the student as well as the SLP. One cannot fix a severely impaired neurological system, but you can offer the student alternative modes of communication. Even very young children become frustrated when they are unable to communicate. Early exposure to augmentative communication systems helps them understand how to communicate.

Today's clinician needs to know how to work with students' families and professionals representing a broad range of educational, medical, and technological disciplines to help select augmentative and alternative communication systems which will be optimally suited to the student's needs (Silverman, 1989; Yorkston & Karlan, 1986). Vanderheiden and Lloyd (1986) describe several dimensions professionals can use to determine the usefulness or advantages of particular augmentative communication system components for meeting functional communication requirements. They group these dimensions into three broad categories that include: functionality/ability to meet needs; availability/usability; and acceptability/compatibility with the environment.

When selecting and implementing augmentative and alternative communication systems, it is necessary to match the student's physical and cognitive skills with the devices that are to be used. This is not an easy goal to accomplish. Many experts who confront such decisions on a frequent basis generally base their selection on the knowledge they have about devices and the knowledge they gain about the student through comprehensive assessment. The student's potential ability to use the device to communicate should be the driving issue. Other aspects to consider when making a selection include: ease of use, growth potential, keyboard layout, rate of communication output, voice output, visual output, auditory output, structure for positioning and mobility, adaptability for rapidly changing needs, client response capabilities, funding resources, and the like.

Experts in the field of alternative and augmentative communication believe that AAC-based intervention should be implemented as early as possible to help students effectively participate in their home and school activities. The benefit of increased understanding of interactive and pragmatic communication can make a great difference in the student's ultimate success in home, school, community and work. Children must be able to proceed at their own pace. The clinician must be sensitive to frustrations and make the learning experience fun and rewarding.

Clinicians who are interested in learning more about alternative and augmentative communication intervention would benefit participating in ASHA's Special Interest Group 12: Augmentative and Alternative Communication. The manufacturers of augmentative and alternative communication products participate in a national not-for-profit organization, The Communication Aid Manufacturers Association (CAMA) in Evanston, IL. They conduct educational outreach projects such as workshops and in-service training. In addition, they provide helpful guidelines and suggestions to SLPs who provide AAC intervention. Efforts such as these help clinicians stay abreast of rapidly changing technologies.

After selecting the device, the clinician is then involved in instructing the student and facilitating the incorporation of the communication system into classroom and social communication activities. The school clinician interested in incorporating augmentative and alternative systems into the speech-language program is faced with an important decision-making task. There is great variability in capability and complexity in the devices available on the market. Cost can be high. Sometimes, it is necessary to help the student's family seek financial assistance. The Prentke Romich Company (a company that develops, manufactures, and distributes augmentative communication systems) suggests that there are numerous sources that can be sought for funding the purchase of devices including:

- insurance companies and Medicaid programs;
- vocational rehabilitation programs;
- school system equipment funds;
- private corporations;
- trust funds;
- service clubs;
- fundraising agencies; and
- organizations that grant wishes to people with specific disabilities.

Working with Teachers to Maximize the Potential of AAC

Training must be provided for teachers of students who use augmentative and alternative communication systems. Student success will be greater if teachers contribute to the discussion of the type of device to use and learn to integrate educational and functional activities with AAC intervention. This will help to merge the speech-language and classroom goals. Training is most effective if the SLP and teacher interact with one another frequently. This helps to facilitate a team approach; encouraging both to collaborate in the selection and structuring of activities. Planning must first begin with identification of the students' needs and competencies. Teachers and others who engage in communication interactions with the student must learn to prompt use of the communication device and engage in conversation with the student.

Gillette, DePompei, and Goetz (2009) developed a tool to focus collaborative discussions between teachers and SLPs regarding the potential use, benefits, and selection of personal digital assistance devices (PDAs). The guide helps teachers and SLPs jointly explore key aspects that can lead to the selection of appropriate devices for helping students with memory and organization (Figure 5–1). Using the guide, team members can assess the need for electronic memory/organization intervention, develop an intervention plan, and monitor progress through evaluation forms. Students can develop functional skills using features such as address books, alarms, calendars, E-mails, cell phone use, and more.

As technology development continues to progress, it is essential that school-based SLPs gain the expertise they need to match students with the appropriate technology and devices so they can develop communicative competence. One device cannot possibly meet the needs of the broad range of students in a school district. There are numerous device options that should be considered such as the type of voice output and accessories such as optical pointers. E-mail continues to offer students with severe disabilities opportunities to connect with others in their school, community, or the world at large. Most regional resource centers make augmentative communication devices available on loan to parents. They also offer regional training workshops and in-service programs.

Intervention Materials

During recent years, there has been an increase in the amount of commercial materials available for testing and intervention. Some of them are excellent and some of them are not useful for the purposes they claim to accomplish. On the other hand, there are many excellent homemade materials. These have the advantage of being inexpensive, and because many of them are designed for a specific purpose, they are useful. Without decrying the use of materials, homemade or commercial, the clinician would do well to evaluate them from another point of view. Do they accomplish a goal in therapy for the child, or do they serve as a prop or a "security blanket" for the clinician? This letter from a student clinician who completed an externship in an early intervention camp for children with communication disabilities, illustrates the point:

> Before I went to the summer camp in Maryland, they sent me a list of things to bring along. I didn't notice any mention

PDA Intervention Plan

Implementing Electronic Memory and Organization Aids

Using this Guide

Use this guide to provide assistance for intervention team members to assess the need for electronic memory/organization intervention, develop an intervention plan, and monitor progress through evaluation forms.

Electronic Memory Organization Aids

PDAs, Smartphones, and cell phones all include personal assistance functions. Cell phones are included since many feature the same functions as PDAs.

PDA stands for personal digital assistant and is the most complex and computer-like of all the devices. In fact, PDAs are often referred to as pocket computers or palmtops. Functions include address books, alarm, calendar, internet, e-mail, and word processing software.

- Examples: Palm Zire™, Dell Axim™

Smartphones combine a full-featured mobile phone with handheld computer functions such as touchscreens, miniature QWERTY keyboards, calendar, address book, and notepad.

- Examples: Blackberry™, Nokia™

Cell phones are portable electronic devices used for mobile communication. Memory aids on cell phones include alarms, calendars, and e-mail access.

- Examples: Motorola™, Nokia™, Samsung™, etc.

Key Concepts

- Increase independence for your client
- Assist with organization and memory
- Provide a means of planning
- Promote increased socialization with peers and family

Tips for Interventionists

- Acquire knowledge and experience about devices to better assist your client.
- Work on your client's responses using the device and then move to teaching entry if possible.
- Involve the intervention team in the use of device.
- Begin with frequent intervention and gradually increase sessions over time.
- Encourage your client to wear the device, for example on a lanyard, to prevent loss or theft.
- Get feedback from team and your client on a regular basis.
- Encourage exploration of device through use of various functions, including games.
- Remember that the use of device is not limited to work-tasks and can be used for fun.

The University of Akron

Yvonne Gillette, Ph.D. yg@uakron.edu
Roberta DePompei, Ph.D. rdepom1@uakron.edu
Elaine Goetz, B.A.
The School of Speech-Language Pathology and Audiology, The University of Akron, Akron, Ohio 44325-3001

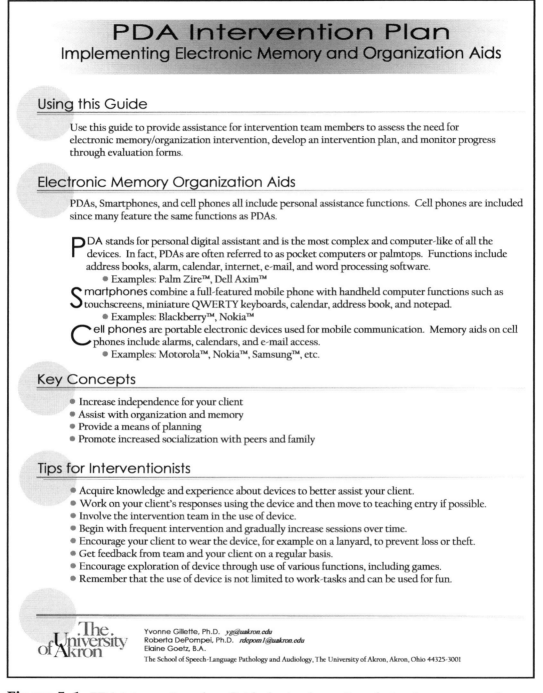

Figure 5–1. PDA intervention plan: Guide for implementing electronic memory and organization aids. Teams can use this tool to assess the need for electronic memory/organization intervention, develop plans, and monitor progress. *Source:* Gillette, Y., DePompei, R., & Goetz, E. Project funded by the National Institute on Disabilities and Rehabilitation Research. Project Number H13A030810. *continues*

Memory and Organization Assessment

Answer the following questions in relation to your client to assess for memory/organization intervention.

Name of Client: Date:

Appointments (day, time, event)

How well does your client keep track of appointments?*   1 2 3 4 5 6 7
Could a device assist with this issue? Currently__ In 1 year__ In 5 years__ Never__
What is your client's current organization method? (PDA, cell phone, Smartphone, planner, other)
Would a device help for keeping track of appointments? YES NO

Contacts (name, address, phone, other)

How well does your client keep track of contacts?*   1 2 3 4 5 6 7
Could a device assist with this issue? Currently__ In 1 year__ In 5 years__ Never__
What is your client's current organization method? (PDA, cell phone, Smartphone, planner, other)
Would a device help for keeping track of contacts? YES NO

To Do list (daily, weekly, long-term)

How well does your client plan or follow to do lists?*   1 2 3 4 5 6 7
Could a device assist with this issue? Currently__ In 1 year__ In 5 years__ Never__
What is your client's current organization method? (PDA, cell phone, Smartphone, planner, other)
Would a device help for planning and following to do lists? YES NO

Calculator, Expense List

How well does your client keep track of finances or use a calculator?*   1 2 3 4 5 6 7
Could a device assist with this issue? Currently__ In 1 year__ In 5 years__ Never__
What is your client's current organization method? (PDA, cell phone, Smartphone, planner, other)
Would a device help for use of a calculator or expense list? YES NO

Self-reminders (voice or written memos)

How well does your client keep track of reminders/memos?*   1 2 3 4 5 6 7
Could a device assist with this issue? Currently__ In 1 year__ In 5 years__ Never__
What is your client's current organization method? (PDA, cell phone, Smartphone, planner, other)
Would a device help for self-reminders? YES NO

Camera

How well does your client keep track of personal events?*   1 2 3 4 5 6 7
Could a device assist with this issue? Currently__ In 1 year__ In 5 years__ Never__
What is your client's current organization method? (PDA, cell phone, Smartphone, planner, other)
Would a device help for a record of personal events? YES NO

*Independence Rating Scale:

- **7** = independent (no prompts needed)
- **6** = modified independence (independent with certain partners/opportunities)
- **5** = low assistance (prompts needed in 2/10 attempts)
- **4** = moderate assistance (prompts needed in 4/10 attempts)
- **3** = moderate/high assistance (prompts needed in 6/10 attempts)
- **2** = high assistance (prompts needed in 8/10 attempts)
- **1** = total prompting & assistance

Figure 5–1. *continues*

Memory and Organization Plan

This is a guide to create a projected plan of intervention for a memory/organization device aid. Review the guidelines on the left and create a plan on the right.

Name of Client:

	Plan Guidelines		Plan Date:
Environments & Partners	*In what environments could your client potentially use a memory/organization aid?* ○ school ○ work ○ home ○ community/social	*Who are potential partners?* ○ teacher ○ classroom aide ○ parent ○ spouse ○ sibling	
Opportunities	*According to environment, which opportunities might be aided by the use of a device?* ○ reminders for taking medicine, appointments, meetings, tests/assigments, shopping/shopping lists ○ keeping contacts organized and accessible ○ to-do/task list at work or school ○ planning the day and keeping to that schedule (calendar) ○ financial management ○ healthcare management and maintenance ○ interacting with peers/co-workers ○ easy access to e-mail, computer funcitons, Microsoft Office™		
Functions	*What functions might be helpful for your client?* ○ calendar ○ contact list (address/phone) ○ task list ○ notes/memos: ○ written ○ oral ○ calculator	○ camera ○ games ○ computer functions ○ Microsoft Office™	
Skill Outcomes	*What outcomes are initially pertinent for your client?* ● You may want to start with recognition of alarms and move to outcomes specific to your client's needs. Examples: ✎ Appointments: responds to one task in a timely manner each day. ✎ Contacts: Finds and calls 1-2 people when indicated. ✎ To Do List: Completes a job after alarm reminds to do so. ✎ Calculator: Adds simple amounts to determine total charge for lunch. ✎ Self-reminder: Follows through with taking medications on time. ✎ Camera: Takes pictures to use as a focus for discussion with family members. *What is the present level and projected level of this skill?* ● Refer back to the independence scales on page 2 for present level functioning.		
Schedule	*When would your client be using the aid?* ● *What activities?* ● *What days?* ● *What times?*		

Customizations Possible:

The following features allow for personalization of the device. Some may be important to your client.

● ring tones, font changes, screen sizes, backgrounds, & color schemes

Figure 5–1. *continues*

Memory and Organization Intervention Note

Name of Client:
Environmental Support Person:

Device:
Date:

Today's Plan:
- Skills established:
  Rate skill outcomes on the independence scale of 1-7.
- Skills to continue:
- Skills to develop:

Instruction
- What was the most effective method of instruction (verbal, visual, modeling)?
- Did the client require multiple repetitions (if so, how many)?
- Was there a need for additional cueing, prompting in addition to directions?
- Additional comments:

Device
- What features seemed to help/hinder?
- Any missing features that could have helped?
- Additional comments:

1. How often does your client use his or her device?
   a. daily: ___ times per day
   b. couple times per week
   c. once a week
   d. less than once per week
   e. never
2. If your client never uses his or her device, why is that?
   a. forgot how to use it
   b. no one helps me with it
   c. I don't like it
   d. I need more help with it
   e. technical problems
   f. other: (explain)
3. If your client does use the device, what is he or she using it for?
   a. taking photos
   b. playing games
   c. contact lists
   d. calendar for reminders
   e. memo pad
   f. calculator
   g. to-do list
   h. "synching to computer"
   i. voice recording
   j. other: (explain)
4. Where is your client using the device?
   a. home
   b. school
   c. work
   d. community
5. Who helps your client the most with the device?
   a. self
   b. family member
   c. teacher/staff member
   d. peer
   e. other: (explain)
6. What other functions would you like to see your client learn to use?
   a. camera
   b. calendar for reminders
   c. calculator
   d. create contact list
   e. task lists
   f. create memos
   g. games
   h. Microsoft Office (if applicable)
   i. note-taking
   j. other: (explain)
7. Is there anything you would like to share or ask?

Client Self-Assessment

1. How often do you use your device?
   a. daily: ___ times per day
   b. couple times per week
   c. once a week
   d. less than once per week
   e. never
2. If you never use your device, why is that?
   a. forgot how to use it
   b. no one helps me with it
   c. I don't like it
   d. I need more help with it
   e. technical problems
   f. other: (explain)
3. If you do use your device, what are you using it for?
   a. taking photos
   b. playing games
   c. contact lists
   d. calendar for reminders
   e. memo pad
   f. calculator
   g. to-do list
   h. "synching to computer"
   i. voice recording
   j. other: (explain)
4. Where are you using your device?
   a. home
   b. school
   c. work
   d. community
5. Who helps you the most with your device?
   a. self
   b. family member
   c. teacher/staff member
   d. peer
   e. other: (explain)
6. What other functions would you like to learn to use?
   a. camera
   b. calendar for reminders
   c. calculator
   d. create contact list
   e. task lists
   f. create memos
   g. games
   h. Microsoft Office (if applicable)
   i. note-taking
   j. other: (explain)
7. Is there anything you would like to share or ask?

NIDRR

This work is produced in partnership with the Assistive Technology Collaboration on Cognitive Disabilities (University of Akron, Temple University, Spaulding Rehabilitation Hospital, and the Brain Injury Association of America) and was funded by the National Institute on Disabilities and Rehabilitation Research (NIDRR) Project Number H13A030810.

Figure 5–1. *continued*

of therapy materials. Should I take some along? I had been working as student clinician in the university clinic and either used their therapy materials or created my own. What should I do? Well, if they didn't tell me to bring any, perhaps they furnished staff with them after you got there. When I got to camp, no materials in sght! What was I expected to do for therapy! I panicked. Within a very short time we were plunged into the camp program and things moved along at a fast clip. Suddenly, in the middle of the summer, I realized I had been doing therapy for several weeks and hadn't even missed my therapy materials. How could this be! In analyzing the situation I realized we had been using the life experience situations at camp, the activities, the surroundings, the educational programs and the other people in the camp as our "materials." The therapy grew naturally out of the environment.

Educational Materials

We often overlook the most obvious source of materials: the school and people with in the school. If therapy in the schools is to be meaningful to the child it must be a part of the school program. The school clinician needs to know what is going on at various grade levels in the way of instruction and should then tie the therapy to the classroom activities. Looking at the books children read, talking with the teacher about the instructional program, becoming familiar with the school curriculum, and looking around the classroom itself will help the school clinician become more familiar with classroom instruction and will suggest ideas for intervention techniques and motivational devices. School districts develop curriculum guides that outline the objectives of the curriculum and activities that should be a part of the educational program. Appendix D is a representative curriculum for Language Arts.

Most districts and regional resources provide some resources designed to improve the quality of instruction for children with disabilities. Instructional and diagnostic materials are available on a loan basis to school clinicians. The instructional resource centers provide other services with which the school clinician will want to become familiar. Visiting the resource center gives the clinician an opportunity to examine a large number of tests, materials, and books before making a decision on which ones to purchase for the school. Personnel at the resource centers are also helpful in discussing the use of various items of material and equipment.

Regional, state, and national meetings of speech-language pathologists usually include displays by commercial companies of equipment, materials, and books. Company representatives provide demonstrations of equipment. This is also a good opportunity to get on the mailing lists of commercial companies. The school clinician may want to maintain a file of company brochures and current prices.

Integrating Multimedia into Treatment

There are many multimedia computer systems and CD-ROM technology programs that feature language learning activities. These offer motivating and effective intervention tools for children. Creative speech-language pathologists may want to consider incorporating software for music, artwork, and other creative forms into treatment sessions. Research has shown that youngsters can progress at a rate comparable to what they achieved in traditional therapy if properly administered by qualified clinicians. The graphics, sound, text and animation capabilities incorporated into computer programs may help to keep students focused on activities. Remember, however, the computer is an intervention tool. To be effective, a qualified professional must develop the goals and plans for use.

Computer applications and programs can be located in catalogues from publishers of clinical materials. In addition, some commercial software programs that involve language use can be adapted for speech-language therapy. Care and attention should be given to the selection of computer-based products. As with other clinical materials, the programs should be relevant for the students' academic curriculum and communication needs. The cautious clinician will review articles in the professional literature to determine the potential efficacy of using various devices including software programs.

Surfing the Net

The World Wide Web (www) offers university students and practitioners many avenues for exploration. Speech-language pathologists can find information about a wide range of topics such as treatment protocols for specific disorders or interesting resource materials to suggest to parents by accessing the many commercial and free Web sites offered by businesses and organizations. Judith Maginnis Kuster (2010) has been a leading influence in the discipline by cataloguing hundreds of the most useful speech-language pathology websites and links. Her columns have appeared in the *ASHA Leader* for several years and are archived so that they can be accessed (http://www.mnsu.edu/comdis/kuster4/leader.html). The site features a communication disorders library, a speech and language disorders section, an annotated bibliography of references; global links; an extensive list of interactive discussion forums, guidelines for designing and presenting research and much more. ASHA's Web site is also a good launching pad for professionals and consumers who want to investigate communication disorders.

Assistive Listening Devices

Students' success in the classroom and in therapy is often limited by their in ability to monitor their own speech or hear, attend to, and discriminate others' speech during conversations and classroom discussions (Flexer, 1999). The acoustics in many school buildings is so noisy that it interferes with students' and teachers' abilities to communicate effectively. Noises come from heating, ventilation, and air conditioning equipment, noise from outside and adjacent rooms and hallway activity. Although some gains have been made in efforts to establish standards for classroom acoustics, there still are not uniform standards that are applied nationally (Nelson & Blaeser, 2010).

Audiologists and speech-language pathologists have found assistive listening devices (ALDs) to be very useful tools for working with students who have hearing impairments as well as students with other types of communication and learning impairments, including second language learners, or auditory or attention problems (Flexer, 1989; Nelson & Blaeser, 2010; Nelson, Kohnert, Sabur, & Shaw, 2005). Assistive listening devices include various FM or infrared amplification systems and products that provide solutions to problems created by noise, distance from the speaker, or room reverberation or echo. ALDs offer effective means for sound amplification by improving the intelligibility of the speech signal by enhancing the signal-to-noise ratio (Flexer, 1991, 1992; Nelson & Blaeser, 2010).

Two types of devices, personal FM units and hardwire assistive listening devices (ALDs), can be beneficial to individual children in the therapy situation or groups of children in the class room setting (Flexer, 1989). To use these units, the teacher/clinician wears a microphone transmitter and the student wears a receiver unit equipped with insert earphones. The cost and design of this equipment varies, but inexpensive portable devices can be assembled without much difficulty. The amount of amplification needed is dependent on a number of factors and individual needs for amplification vary greatly. The advice of an educational audiologist familiar with the performance potential and benefits of various types of assistive listening devices should be sought when recommending units for particular children or classroom situations.

Evaluating Materials to Determine Quality and Applicability

At the present time there are numerous speech and language assessment and intervention products on the market. Unfortunately many of them have not been field tested on a variety of populations. The clinician that purchases them may have no information concerning their effectiveness, applicability, validity, or reliability. Clinicians should not purchase communication intervention products unless the information necessary to evaluate their usefulness is available from the company publishing them. New tests in particular should be evaluated carefully before they are purchased. Advertising brochures should not be the only criterion for selection, and the clinician should seek the pertinent information by querying the publishing company directly. Some school districts that are experiencing financial constraints limit the funds that can be spent on materials. Publishers will often provide free use of materials if SLPs offer to conduct and report field test data.

Prior to purchasing programs, tests, or equipment, clinicians should request to use the materials on a trial basis. This will provide opportunity for clearly determining the applicability to specific populations, the capability for meeting your program objectives, and to predict the durability, frequency of use, and maintenance requirements.

Shared purchasing of equipment. Another way to become familiar with materials and equipment is to discuss them with other clinicians in the area or with university staff members, if there is a university training program nearby. School clinicians in a geographic area may want to consider joint purchase of expensive pieces of equipment that could be shared. Or one school district may purchase one item which could be loaned to a neighboring district, whereas that district may purchase another item with the idea of setting up a reciprocal loan system. Time sharing policies and insurance considerations would have to be worked out in advance.

Portability. The portability of materials should also be taken into consideration. The clinician on an itinerant schedule should keep in mind the bulk and the weight of the materials. Lugging materials and equipment in and out of buildings, not to mention up and down long flights of stairs, several times a day requires the stamina of a packhorse and has caused more than one school clinician to trim down the amount of materials used.

Organizing Materials and Intervention Activities

Graduate students start to collect therapy materials and ideas during their clinical experiences, and the habit continues throughout their careers. It is useful to create files of various intervention and motivational ideas. If the file is well organized it can be expanded and ideas can be added for years to come. The file should be organized in such a way that material can be easily retrieved and replaced after sessions or at the end of the day. It is suggested that information consistently be placed in uniform size files or on uniform size file cards.

Some clinicians find it convenient to color code the file, whereas others prefer to alphabetize the information under topical headings. Computers and technology offer a very dynamic way of producing, storing, and organizing resources, treatment materials, and motivational activities.

Here are the ingredients for a dynamic, practical filing system:

- Various ways to teach a child to produce a consonant or a vowel
- Lists of words containing specific phonemes in different positions within words
- Words taken from the student's spelling, reading, mathematics, and science books.
- Sentences loaded with specific sounds
- Ideas for auditory discrimination and bombardment
- Poems, riddles, finger plays, and stories
- Flannel board ideas
- Barrier games
- Worksheets for home practice
- Exercises for tongue and lip mobility
- Unit topics (cultures, holidays, sports, good nutrition)
- Role-playing ideas
- Experiential activities for parents to try at home
- Progress sheets or charting methods

- Bulletin board idea (holidays, seasons other topics of general interest.)
- Word lists and pictures related to holidays
- Puppets for use in therapy and diagnostics
- Laminated picture cards illustrating nouns or verbs
- Lists of music and books for children
- Lists of suggestions for mentoring parents and teachers
- Movement activities
- Ideas for speech development and speech improvement lessons in the classroom
- Teacher study guides and work books
- Careers and vocational information

The file can serve a number of useful purposes. It can be an inventory of available materials and publications; it can aid in lesson planning; and the materials can be easily removed from the file and used during the sessions. In addition, it can serve as an aid when consulting with classroom teachers in speech and language development and improvement and serve as a source of ideas when working with parents. Plus, it is concise, easy to construct, convenient to use, and inexpensive.

Expendable Materials

Supplies, such as paper, crayons, chalk, and some materials that can be used only one time, are usually supplied by the school; however, it does not necessarily follow that the school clinician has access to an unlimited supply. These items may be rationed or budgeted to the clinician on a yearly or semester basis. The clinician should be aware of the school's policy in regard to supplies. It should also be pointed out that because clinicians may function in several different schools within the same system, each school may have its own policy in regard to the availability of supplies.

Sometimes budget allowances are made on the basis of pupil enrollment. Both money and supplies may be determined in accordance with the total number of children enrolled or the number enrolled at any given time. Because budgets must be made in advance, the figures may be dependent on last year's enrollment or the estimated enrollment for the next year.

Budgeting for Materials, Equipment, Supplies, and Professional Development

Speech-language pathologists need tools in order to do their job. Schools are aware of this but budgets are tight. Funds are used to purchase materials, supplies, and equipment. In addition, they set aside funds each year for the staff's professional training so that clinicians can continue to build their expertise and maintain their credentials.

There are many ways to get the funds needed. However, you may have to draw from several sources and be very creative to access the funds. Therapists who are skilled at expressing their need and rationale for funds can be highly successful Most districts establish a departmental fund to be used to provide clinicians the tools they need to deliver services. They establish processes for requesting the funds and justifying how they will be used. In addition to the department funds, many school districts use funds generated through their Medicaid services to purchase equipment and materials or to sponsor national speakers for conferences. Often, school districts and employment companies provide a professional development allowance to each therapist. Funds from that allowance can be used at the clinician's discretion for preapproved items such as testing and therapy materials, registration at conferences, and equipment. There generally is a fixed sum and should be spent carefully by setting priorities regarding how to spend the funds, spreading the funds over the school year, and evaluating the quality of the product or training course to determine its value for enhancing the services you are providing. Generally there is a fixed amount and you must seek approval of a supervisor to spend the funds. Some districts and counties also have grant funds that can be accessed through application.

When considering the purchase of equipment, keep in mind that although the initial expenditure may be great, the equipment should not have to be replaced for many years. There is, however, the matter of repair, maintenance, and general upkeep to be considered. For example, an audiometer needs yearly calibration; computers need to be upgraded. Take these factors into consideration before purchasing expensive equipment.

Commercial therapy materials are subject to wear and tear if they are used frequently and may have to be budgeted periodically. Considerations in the purchase of therapy materials might be whether or not they can be adapted for a variety of uses and occasions and whether or not they serve the purpose for which they are being purchased. They must be appropriate to the age, maturity, and interest of children.

Another matter to be considered is insurance on audiometers, computers, assistive devices, augmentative systems, and other items of electronic equipment-a figure that should be in the budget. Also, if equipment is to be leased, the rental costs will have to be included in the budget. When budgeting for a program, don't forget to account for ongoing material needs such as office supplies (DVDs, paper, pens, paper clips, and the like).

Budgeting for Professional Materials

Professional books may also be included as part of the school clinician's equipment and therefore would be justifiable budget items. The clinician may want to add to his or her own library of professional books, and these, of course, would not be a part of the school budget. The same is true for dues for professional organizations.

Budgeting for Travel

Some school systems allow travel money and expenses for employees who attend professional meetings. It is wise for the new clinician to check the policy in regard to this matter. If a clinician must travel between schools as part of the job, a travel allowance is available. Some school clinicians are paid a flat amount for a specified period of time, whereas others receive reimbursement on a per mile basis. Some school systems make up for this difference by paying the clinician a higher salary that the person whose job does not entail travel between schools during the working day, for example, the classroom teacher.

Accessing Funds

Creative clinicians can accomplish their goals by submitting an explanation of their pet project to local, state, and national businesses and organizations that offer grant programs. Many organizations that support education and special education list grant opportunities on their Web sites. Although competitive, the guidelines for application are relatively straightforward. Many clinicians have accessed these grant opportunities to obtain funds for training or purchase augmentative and assistive devices or to support a team charged with developing a literacy-based language curriculum. Large department store chains, insurance companies, social organizations, and county education associations are all possibilities.

Inventory Records

It is a good idea to maintain a systematic record or inventory of materials and equipment purchased for the program. This will facilitate sharing materials between several clinicians, locating articles when needed, and replacing articles should they become misplaced or damaged. The inventory record should include the name of the article, the manufacturer's name, address and phone number, the date purchased, the cost, serial numbers if applicable, the intended use, the storage location, and dates equipment was repaired or calibrated. Computerized data management systems often include software programs which can be used for developing inventory records and reports. The storage of equipment during the months when school is not in session, or equipment is not in use, is a matter to be determined by the SLP and the administration.

DISCUSSION QUESTIONS AND PROJECTS

1. Visit several school speech-language programs and rate their facilities using the Program Environment Observation Checklist in Table 5–1.

2. Are mobile units used in your state? What are their advantages and disadvantages? Under what conditions would you use one?

3. You are the school SLP. The principal has assigned you to a small former storage room with no windows but a convenient location. You are not satisfied with the room. Would you try to have another room assigned or would you modify the assigned room? Outline the steps you would follow, using either alternative.

4. Collect five advertisements from publishing companies of speech-language assessment and intervention materials and equipment. They can be brochures or advertisements in professional journals. Determine the strengths and weaknesses of the materials.

5. Start an activity file. Justify the method you have chosen to organize it.

6. Interview a SLP to find out how he or she budgets for equipment and materials and how the materials are procured through the school system. How are maintenance and insurance handled?

7. Draw a design plan for your ideal therapy room: (a) for an elementary school and (b) for a high school.

8. Start a collection of record and report forms used in the schools. How would you organize report forms for a school system?

9. Technologic assistance is needed to select appropriate iPad apps and augmentative communication devices for intervention. Make a list of 10 questions you might ask of persons who have technologic expertise with these devices.

6

Documentation and Accountability

The American public is demanding that school systems be accountable for the educational results of their students. This has come about because there are a number of problems in the schools that are troubling to the public. Problems that are most distressing with regard to students with disabilities are differential educational opportunities based on type of disability and geographic location; disruptive behaviors in classrooms; high drop out rates; low graduation rates; high unemployment rates; lack of preparedness for work and advance education, and limited community integration of adults with disabilities. Research on effective schools and effective teaching has repeatedly proved that student achievement is not at the expected level. The achievement gap is noticeable in grades, standardized test scores, dropout rates, and limited pursuit of higher education (Education Week, 2004). In addition, teachers are not adequately prepared for the challenges they face in the classroom. Models of special education programs that pull children away from the regular education classroom may actually compound problems by interrupting the time students spend in class or interrupting the presentation of critical information.

Observations such as these have led to increased calls for accountability, proof that services are effective, and ways to measure student outcomes. Schools have initiated various options for documenting the performance of students with disabilities. Options include alternative assessments, progress monitoring, diplomas, certificates of attendance, or certificates of competency. Changes in methods of assessing performance have also evolved to include the use of performance-based assessments such as portfolios. Speech-language pathologists have a responsibility to document and report their results as well. Comprehensive accountability procedures and efficient record keeping practices can assist the clinician in documenting responsible service delivery. The scope of practice and responsibilities of speech-language pathologists continue to broaden and change. In addition to changes in the educational world, speech-language pathologists now may provide more complex procedures than in the past such as treatment of swallowing disorders. This raises the potential risk for liability. Problems can be decreased or avoided when SLPs document services properly.

Documenting Treatment Effectiveness

School-based SLPs continue to seek valid methods that can be used for describing students' communication skills, monitoring progress, and measuring change in communication status following intervention in a school-based program. A uniform methodology is needed to describe the populations served, verify that students are eligible for services, report intervention models used, measure treatment outcomes and benefit, and ultimately make caseload and treatment decisions that are cost effective. Our public is seeking verification of the outcomes of our intervention. To respond, we need to describe what constitutes a learning outcome for each or our students and develop mechanisms to assess how well students achieve the outcomes. Simply explained, one of the primary indicators of the positive outcome of speech-language intervention is increased communication independence (understanding others and them understanding the student) and reduced dependence on the support of others for communication (reduction in the amount of assistance needed to understand and be understood). Positive outcomes indicators for students enrolled in therapy would include: no longer classifying the student as eligible for therapy, reducing the frequency and intensity of services, dismissal from therapy, and improved performance in the classroom and other home, school, and community activities.

The evidence should:

- be comprehensive covering all of the skill areas addressed in therapy;
- include multiple judgments from more than one source;
- include use of skills in multiple contexts not just performance in the speech-language program; and,
- be derived from multiple types of formative and summative measures including direct observation, evaluation, and demonstration of student's abilities.

Increasingly SLPs are faced with complex challenges in the current school environment. These include: high caseloads diverse student needs, inconsistent scheduling patterns among clinicians, financial constraints, limited personnel, and increasing demands for accountability, efficiency, and cost effectiveness. Recent trends in special education and speech-language service delivery encourage greater consistency and evidence to support service delivery decisions. Practitioners seek better methods of describing the populations they serve, selecting service delivery models for intervention, and determining the effectiveness of treatment.

The Rationale For Better Record-Keeping Procedures

Typically, speech-language pathologists across the country do not have access to data collection methods and tools that promote or permit the following practices:

- Consistent service delivery practices among all SLPs within the district;
- Consistent descriptions of students' communication status at the time of admission and discharge;
- Adherence to eligibility criteria or guidelines by all team members;
- Consistent documentation of treatment interventions provided;
- Documentation of educators' perceptions of students' functional communication skills based on classroom performance;
- Results of treatment (outcomes); and,
- Documentation and comparison of clinical decision-making and service.

Consequently, SLPs continue to express concerns about caseload and workload management issues that occur due to inconsistent procedures for:

- Referring children for SLP services;
- Describing communication skills and impairments;
- Identifying the impact of the impairment on school performance;
- Confirming eligibility for services;
- Verifying that the expertise of an SLP is required;
- Specifying appropriate intervention approaches;
- Communicating meaningfully with education colleagues about students;
- Collaborating with educators to ensure that therapy strategies are integrated into the classroom;
- Determining progress in treatment;
- Measuring and comparing treatment effectiveness of various intervention models; and,
- Making decisions regarding referral for additional services or dismissal.

This type of information has broad implications beyond the speech-language pathology program. The diversity of the population and number of students with communication disorders creates several service delivery challenges for SLPs and educators. SLPs struggle to accurately identify students who are most in need of speech-language pathology services. They try to determine the effect of students' communication disabilities on school performance and participation in other home and community activities. They strive to establish priorities for treatment and to select appropriate service delivery models to accomplish goals. They seek methods for documenting progress and effectiveness. In addition, SLPs want to provide quality services to students with diverse needs in spite of complex barriers such as competing priorities, lack of time, fiscal constraints, a shortage of qualified professionals, increasing demands for accountability, efficiency, and cost effectiveness.

Records and Record Keeping

School-based SLPs often remark that documentation and record keeping in the school setting is overwhelming. However, documentation and record keeping are necessary for all types of settings where people receive health care or educational services. There are ethical, legal, reimbursement, and fiscal reasons (Johnson, 2003, 2004; Swigert, 2002). Therefore, SLPs must become masters of proper documentation, regardless of setting. To prepare and maintain excellent documentation and records, SLPs must be aware of national, state, and local regulations and requirements including IDEA, Medicaid, and district policies. There are legal and professional reasons for maintaining a comprehensive record and report system on the speech and language program.

Federal and state laws place tremendous emphasis on accountability in the school system. Accountability has made it urgent that special services in the schools develop methods for reliably and accurately reporting data on children with disabilities. Historically, the school clinician has maintained written records for many reasons:

- To verify the needs for and benefits of clinical services;
- To inform others about the program and specific services;
- To keep track of the services provided;
- To provide continuity both to the program and to the child's progress in therapy;
- To serve as a basis for research;
- To coordinate the child's therapy with the child's school program; and,
- To serve as a basis for program needs and development.

Parents often question the nature and quality of the educational program or special education services their child is receiving. Their concerns may include instructional support service programs such as speech and language intervention. As a result, they may request detailed information about the goals of therapy and techniques used. On rare occasions, there may be enough disagreement with placement decisions and the educational professional's practices to pursue due process or legal recourse in order to implement changes.

Several court decisions in the past few decades have ruled in favor of the parents' concerns about the school's failure to provide appropriate education or services. Some examples include: *Greer v. Rome City School District*, 950 F.2d 688 (11th Circuit Court, 1991); *Oberti v. Board of Education of the Borough of Clementon School District* (3rd Circuit Court, 1993); *Sacramento City Unified School District v. Holland* (9th Circuit Court, 1994). In these cases, the school districts have incurred large financial obligations. This can be financially detrimental to a school district and professionally damaging to the practitioner. The clinician that keeps detailed records of diagnostic findings, treatment procedures, and outcome of therapy will be in a better position to explain and defend the clinical decisions he or she has made. Another legal issue relates to professional qualifications. Many states require licenses or credentials for speech-language pathologists. Districts specify the qualification and credentials that they require to serve particular student populations or educational settings. This implies a legal responsibility for service delivery and the need for accountability. Professionals are at risk for losing their license or being reported for unethical practices if they provide services without the required credentials or training. It is the professional's responsibility to know the state and district requirements.

Laws have been passed which enable school districts to seek reimbursement for services from third-party payers such as Medicaid and private insurers. The 1999 final regulations of 1997 IDEA (34 CFR 300.142) stated that if a child is eligible for services through a noneducational public agency and receives the services in an educational setting, the noneducational public agency is financially responsible. In order to obtain third-party funds, documentation of services must be provided including the diagnosis, rationale for therapy, treatment procedures, short- and long-term goals, amount, duration, and frequency of treatment.

There is increasing competition for scarce tax dollars among educational, health care, and social organizations. As a result, many government agencies require statements of accountability prior to awarding funds to create new programs or sustain existing programs. Local, federal, and state agencies want to know what results are being obtained for the tax money spent. Schools and administrators must provide evidence that demonstrates compliance with federal and state department of education rules and regulations. Appropriate speech-language records and documentation can provide the proof needed that the speech-language program is being managed efficiently, that it is meeting goals, that professionals possess the required credentials, and that students are making progress. Documenting success in these ways can result in new or continued funding from government or grant agencies.

There are a number of important questions that SLPs should ask themselves frequently throughout the school year in order to be accountable for their program services, the composition of their caseload, and clinical decisions. Asking the following questions will help make programs more manageable and may reduce the challenges of a high caseload that often cause stress for many SLPs:

- Is the decision to enroll a student for therapy based on specific eligibility criteria?
- Does the student's communication impairment adversely affect school performance?
- Is the expertise of a speech-language pathologist required to meet the student's needs or could he or she be served via the school curriculum or by another type of education professional or specialist?
- Have you identified the most appropriate intervention protocol to meet each student's needs?

- How appropriate is speech-language intervention for each student in your program?
- Have therapy goals been established that, if accomplished, will make a difference such as enabling the student to better access the curriculum or perform school tasks?
- Is the time spent in therapy used in an effective way so that taking students away from their academic subjects is justified?
- How much progress is each student making?
- Is progress documented and recorded?
- Is there a documented rate or level of change in each student's functional skills and academic performance?
- If progress is slow or nonexistent, are changes made in the type of services provided or the intervention approach implemented?
- How many cases have been followed through either to complete habilitation or rehabilitation or to the greatest degree of compensatory skills that can be expected? If not many, why not?
- Is treatment time used as effectively as possible?
- Can all time be accounted for by describing workload activities?
- Is time that is not scheduled with students justifiable?
- Are available knowledge and resources utilized?
- Are children progressing at an appropriate rate or are factors related to the way the program is organized influencing a reduced rate of progress?
- Are adaptations made to meet unique personalities and needs?
- Do school supervisors and administrators understand what the SLP does each day and the support that is necessary to ensure a quality program?

In addition, the federal mandates add impetus for appropriate record and report keeping. It makes good sense for the clinician to keep a running account of a child's progress in therapy simply because the clinician is dealing with a large number of children and it would be impossible to remember all the facts and details pertinent to each of them. Good records about the nature and needs for services, the services provided, and the student's progress provides a means of communication between professionals, billing documentation, proof of compliance, and legal evidence.

Management of Student Records

In order to be useful, record and report systems should permit quick retrieval of information regarding the status, disposition, and intervention of individual students as well as the collective data that must be recorded to report program statistics. There is increasing demand for accurate record keeping, case management reporting, and statistical data for accountability to school administrators, boards of education, and state departments of education.

The majority of school clinicians will find a computer or Web-based student information system already operational in the district. Most districts have linked their student information systems, their special education documentation systems, and their IEP tracking systems. The systems generally establish special coding systems. In order to maintain excellent records of services, it is necessary to be familiar with the coding system and to be diligent about the codes used to describe each student's impairment and services that are provided. If systems are not in place, clinicians will need to create their own methods for capturing and tracking data. In both instances it will be necessary to evaluate and monitor the system continually and make the necessary changes in the procedures and forms to be in compliance with state and federal regulations.

Written information about students must remain confidential. Therefore, school districts have procedures in place for sharing and storing records and reports. The policies regarding security measures should be established and in writing. The same is true of the availability of such records and reports to other personnel, administrators, referral sources, other clinicians on the staff, and parents. Policies and procedures for sharing information must be adhered to. For example, parents must provide written permission for release of records or information about their child.

Time should be reserved on the SLP's weekly schedule to prepare and manage the abundance of required records and reports. Some of the most time-consuming tasks are filling out reports, keeping information up to date, and filing and retrieving material. These tasks must be completed daily. When weekly, monthly, or yearly reports are involved, a large chunk of time is needed. Many school systems provide a central office or Web-based repository for the school district clinicians and in this way a uniform filing, retrieval, recording, and security system can be utilized.

School SLPs have to abide by the polices of the school system with regard to how long records and reports on individual children should be retained, which records should be retained, and how records are transferred from school to school as well as from school system to school system. Policies of some districts require storage for five to seven years. It is essential for clinicians to ask what type of information should be in the student's official record. Statistical information with relation to program management and incidence figures can be very useful to clinicians in planning future programs and serving as a basis for research. The school clinical staff might make decisions about retaining of this type of information. Provisions for where information is stored, how it is retrieved and who can access information is generally described in district-level speech-language program handbooks.

Records and Reports

While the exact content and format of reports may vary from district to district, there are some common features that are generally included in the documentation of program and student records. Table 6–1,

Table 6–1. Overview: District Organization and the Speech-Language Program and Services

Speech-Language Program Information
School district organization and leadership
Policies and Procedures
Schools within the district and locations
Special education and speech-language services
Organization
Reporting structure
Speech-language services team
Number of SLPs
Qualifications and special expertise
Student demographic information—Composition of student body
Average daily membership (number of students in district)
Number of students with special education needs
Number of students classified needing speech-language services
Grades and special education programs
Economic/cultural status
Travel time between buildings
Schedule for servicing each building
School schedule—important dates and events
Therapy facilities
Budget
Individual Speech-Language Pathologist Information
Names of individuals providing speech-language services to students
License and/or certification documents
School designated as home-base or office location
Schools assigned to serve
Area of specialization and/or interest
Projected Need for Services
Caseload size and composition
Types of disabilities served
Ages
Functional status and severity levels
Numbers of students served
Number of continuing cases; number of new cases

Table 6–1. *continued*

Services Provided
Range (continuum) of services provided
Prevention
Prereferral (including Response-to-Intervention)
Screening
Assessment
Intervention — range of intervention approaches
Professional development / In-service programming
Criteria of Case Selection
Eligibility criteria
Functional status rating criteria
Severity rating criteria
Prioritization criteria

Overview: District Organization and the Speech-Language Program and Services, characterizes the school district organization, special education programs, speech-language caseload and services. Efficiently capturing this information can serve as a foundation for discussing your program with constituents and planning appropriate services. The information also demonstrates where the speech-language program fits within the realm of the entire school organization and would enable you to analyze program data to effect changes in program design and practices.

Table 6–2, Outline of Key Components of Student Reports, illustrates an overview of the type of documentation required for meaningful clinical record keeping. This outline is an excellent resource for school clinicians' interested in reviewing and/or improving their clinic record-keeping procedures. Understanding what and how to document is critical to the provision of high quality services. Basically, documentation and record keeping can be very time consuming, but it can be done efficiently if the SLP is organized and works from a template or outline. Using technology as much as possible helps. It is expected that the challenges and burden of documentation that clinicians experienced in the past will be reduced by the wonderful applications that are emerging every day.

Many individuals are likely to review the speech-language pathology records including parents, school administrators, teachers, attorneys, advocates, and fellow speech-language pathologists. Therefore, records should be written so that they are understandable and contain the type of information others will be able to use better understand the student and determine the services that are required. Care must be

Table 6–2. Outline of Key Components of Student Records

Identifying Information
Student's identifying information
Name
Caregiver's name
Address, phone number, E-mail address
Chronologic age
Social security number or school student ID number
School district, building, grade or placement, homeroom, teacher
Referral source, date of referral (if new referral)
Student History (documentation of function, abilities, previous interventions)
Medical history and/or diagnosis
Educational history
Communication disorder diagnosis (behaviors observed)
Prior functional communication status
Prior treatment for speech, language, hearing problems, and outcomes of that treatment
Frequency, length, duration of treatment during the reporting time period or in prior settings
Description of Current Functional Status and Abilities (communicative and educational)
Date of multifactored evaluation
Current level of functioning (level of independence and amount of support and assistance needed)
Baseline testing (standardized, nonstandardized procedure)
Observations
Interpretations of test scores and results
Other relevant clinical and educational findings (contributed by other educators and specialists)
Impact of impairment on educational performance (adverse effect on education and participation in the educational context)
Rationale for needing the expertise of a speech-language pathologist in order to improve
Statement of potential for improvement and response to intervention—estimate student's abilities based on findings

Table 6–2. *continued*

Treatment (Intervention) Plan
Date treatment plan is established
Long- and-short-term functional communication goals
Functional and measureable goals and objectives based on impairment and function level
Recommended intervention approach based on the impairment or disability
Recommended service delivery option including location, amount, frequency, and anticipated duration of treatment
Expectation that treatment will improve the student's condition
Documentation of Treatment
Date treatment is initiated
Number of times treatment was provided to date
Objective measures of communicative performance (use functional terminology; compare performance against original measures)
Significant developments that might influence rehabilitation potential
Documentation of collaboration with educators and caregivers
Changes in treatment plan
Recommendations for follow-up treatment, continued service, or discharge
Record of consultation and/or collaboration with other individuals and outcomes
Documentation of Clinician and Qualifications
Signatures (including credentials on all reports and records)

taken to make sure that the content of reports and student files is at all times professional. Written comments should not be made that could be construed as hurtful or slanderous.

Critical information is generally incorporated into the student's master file held in a central record-keeping system or location in the school district. The SLP, teachers, and other educators working with the student also help keep pertinent materials in their offices or work stations. These are sometimes referred to as "work folders." Materials might include physician reports, test results, work samples, observation notes, attendance logs, and much more. Much care should be placed in the development of written documents including the Individualized Education Program (IEP), the Individualized Family Services Plan (IFSP), and Individualized Transition Plan (ITP). They should be securely located, yet accessible since they should be referred to often to verify goals, document progress, and determine future steps.

There are numerous questions that school speech-language pathologists should consider as they develop and store records. First and most importantly, the records should be available to provide the type of accountability others seek about the speech-language program. Soon after receiving an inquiry, the SLP should be able to provide responses to questions about the caseload, treatment goals, kinds of disabilities served, goals for treatment, impact on education, intervention schedule, and students' progress. School administrators and program supervisors may visit periodically and must understand the SLP's role and the type of students served in the program.

HIPAA and FERPA

We have a responsibility to our students and their families to adhere to the highest standards of practice. In 2006 a set of rules referred to as HIPAA was established. HIPAA stands for the American Health Insurance Portability and Accountability Act of 1996. HIPAA ensures that all medical records, medical billing, and patient accounts meet consistent standards with regard to documentation, handling, and privacy. Patients (or students' families) must be able to access their own medical records, correct errors or omissions and be informed regarding how personal information is to be shared and used. Schools, like health care organizations, must follow these rules as well. Care should be taken not to share information with unauthorized individuals.

The Family Educational Rights and Privacy Rights Act (FERPA) is another legal protection that schools and educators must keep in mind. FERPA provides parents of student and students who are 18 years or older with privacy protections and rights regarding student records. The records covered by FERPA regulations include information that is directly related to a student and retained by an educational agency or institution.

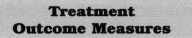

Treatment Outcome Measures

There is great pressure for speech-language pathologists, health care professionals, and other educators to demonstrate the efficiency and effectiveness of their services (Blosser, 1997, 2010; Eger, 1998). *Treatment efficiency* addresses the efficiency of treatment and the time and cost it takes to achieve optimal outcomes. It requires controlled conditions. *Treatment efficacy (effectiveness)* and *treatment outcomes* are important elements for determining quality of services. Information can be gathered in a number of ways and results are used for multiple purposes. Treatment outcomes assess the broad value of treatment. They include the clinician's and client's perceptions of change that has occurred. Outcomes are measured at the time of discharge from a program. They are based on the student's functional ability. Spady (1994) defines outcome as, "clear learning results that we want students to demonstrate at the end of significant learning experiences" (p. 2). This means that educators at every level within the school district, including SLPs, must establish what it is that students will be able to master at given points in time as they progress through school. To accomplish the goals Spady outlines in his work, schools must establish systems for ensuring that students are equipped with the knowledge, competence, and qualities needed to be successful. Schools must be structured and operated in ways that enable the outcomes to be achieved and maximized for all students (1994). Outcomes must be measured and managed so that students can learn and succeed. To summarize, consumers are asking what they are getting for students' efforts in school and therapy and what they are getting for their education dollar. There is a shift of focus from process (what we do) to results (what we produce).

Outcome results can help clinicians demonstrate the effectiveness of services. They can also provide some insights about the prognosis for successful treatment. Parents, teachers, and students with communication disabilities often ask how long intervention will take. Administrators want to find out how much the services will cost. Clinicians can use the information to determine if others perceive that the approaches they are using are effective. This information is especially valuable for planning budgets and resources, demonstrating accountability to administrators, and verifying that standards are being met. When results show that treatment efficiency and effectiveness are not quite as expected, the information can be used to identify program or staff needs and to plan staff development opportunities.

Schools must redefine how IEPs are written and used. The days of writing IEPs that target improvement in only speech-language skills are gone. Rather, the IEP must be jointly prepared by the education team, including the SLP. The speech and language segments of the IEP and goals should clearly describe how intervention will enable the student to function and perform better in the school environment. Professional jargon must be eliminated so that others have the benefit of understanding the student's problems and needs as well as the role they can play in the treatment. Blosser (2010), Eger (1998), and Ehren (1999) suggest writing speech and language outcomes in the context of learning instead of writing speech and language goals that are directed toward improving the sound and flow of communication alone. As a beginning, education teams should determine what one communication skill, if improved, will have the most impact on the student's performance in the educational environments.

Goals should be measurable. *Measurable is observable.* Significant communicators in the student's life can learn to make observations of the student's communication in order to determine if changes are occurring as a result of treatment. *Measurable is repeatable.* The target behavior should be repeated in a variety of contexts. Evaluations of performance can be made over a regular period of time. *Measurable is functional.* The behavior should be observed in a variety of settings and authentic conditions. *Measurable is understandable.* Teachers and parents who are asked to be involved in observations and monitoring activities should understand the reason for collecting information. *Measurable is achievable.* Treatment should be altered on an as-needed basis to meet the student's current needs. Following are a few examples based on these principles:

- The student will apply problem-solving and decision-making skills in math and English class as measured by the teacher's observations of the accuracy of the student's responses during classroom discussions.
- The student will follow written instructions on objective tests as measured by review of the student's responses on social studies tests.
- The student will employ effective fluency strategies when confronted with a stuttering episode during a classroom presentation as measured by observation made by two peers using a checklist.
- The student's interview skills will be increased by recalling specific information when questioned as measured by an interview rubric completed by the job coach.
- The student will increase his or her ability to use complex sentences to tell about experiences as measured by a transcribed language sample collected by the speech-language pathologist.

Another indicator of learning outcome is service completion (sometimes referred to as dismissal, exit, or discharge criteria). National standards for dismissal criteria have not yet been developed. Clinicians continue to wrestle with this issue. We must determine dismissal criteria for each communication disorder. However, there are some guidelines that SLPs and their school teammates can follow for recommending that students should be dismissed and services completed. Examples are as follows:

Mastery of speech-language goals. Provide evidence that the student has achieved the speech-language goals that were on the IEP and that he or she no longer meets the criteria for enrollment in services. Students who can appropriately use compensatory skills or assistive technology would also be described as having mastered their goals. Provide evidence that the impairment no longer effects participation in the classroom situation or educational performance.

Goals can be addressed within the curriculum. Students are not eligible for services if they no longer require special expertise of a speech-language pathologist or specialized intervention approaches.

Inadequate progress. Students who make minimal or no progress towards achieving their goals can be discharged. This recommendation should only be taken after trying a varied of potential solutions and alternative interventions. Of course, it is necessary to document attempts to try different approaches and how the student responded.

Lack of motivation or participation in service. One of the keys to success in therapy and other learning situations is engagement and participation. Students who are not participating and engaged in their therapy program no longer will benefit from the interventions. After trying a variety of different methods for motivating and stimulating the student, a recommendation for dismissal can be made.

Poor attendance and truancy. Students who do not attend school or their therapy sessions regularly are not good candidates for achieving success in therapy. In addition, other students may be denied services if space on the caseload is held for a student who regularly misses.

Student or parents request that services be discontinued. Occasionally, a student or parent requests that services be discontinued. There may be a variety of reasons. When this request is made, it is generally honored.

None of the reasons for completing service can be recommended unless the SLP provides data to support the recommendation. There are many sources of that data including: progress notes, samples of the student's work, teacher's reports, parental feedback, grades, or test results.

Measuring Outcomes

The American Speech-Language-Hearing Association has managed a program to measure treatment outcomes for decades. The program is entitled the National Outcomes Measurement System (NOMS) (ASHA, 1993, 2010). The NOMS has multiple purposes including providing an instrument that enables professionals to create a local and national source of data, confirm and demonstrate the value of our services, provide tools for advocacy and negotiation, enhance opportunities for reimbursement, offer a mechanism for benchmarking clinical progress, and provide guidelines for determining staffing patterns. The NOMS can provide valuable information about speech-language pathology services including the number of treatment sessions the student attended in a given time period, how much progress was achieved, amount and type of services delivered, if the services effectively improved the individual's functional communication status, and the level of satisfaction of the student, teacher, and/or parent. This is valuable information for decision-making and program planning.

ASHA has taken a leadership role by developing such a viable measurement system and facilitating research to determine the usefulness of such a system. In the early 1990s ASHA established the Task Force on Treatment Outcomes and Cost Effectiveness. The task force was charged with creating a national outcomes database for SLPs and audiologists. Health care professionals from many disciplines have embraced this type of efficiency research for years. School-based clinicians just recently began to focus on the importance of gathering data and reporting outcomes.

The overarching goals of outcomes data gathering instruments such as the NOMS are to increase the amount and quality of efficacy research being completed in the profession and to systematize the way that data is collected, reported, and used. The instruments are designed to reflect changes in clients' functional communication skills from admission to discharge, provide information about the number of treatment sessions required, and solicit consumer satisfaction.

In today's business-minded and economical environment, there are increased calls for accountability and documentation of efficiency. Simultaneously, the profession is committed to providing evidence based services. All of these actions will enable clinicians to prove their worth to external constituents. Supporters of the NOMS project continue to promote using this system as an acceptable profession-wide, standardized method for documenting the effectiveness of treatment procedures. Data that are gathered enable clinicians to demonstrate functional changes following intervention. Analysis of the data provides insights into the amount, type and frequency needed to improve speech and language skills. The data gathered will provide SLPs with opportunities for more meaningful discussions and communication with administrators, third-party payers, legislators, other health care providers, families, consumers, and educators. In addition, trends in treatment will be documented.

School-based personnel, like other counterparts in health care settings, are under scrutiny by decision makers who are looking for ways to cut costs, stretch dollars, and reduce expenses. Unless practitioners provide credible data regarding the clients they serve and the procedures they use, service delivery will be greatly impacted. School-based SLPs need methods for documenting progress, measuring significant change, and identifying the service delivery models that are effective.

The NOMS data collection instruments enable SLPs to gather descriptive information about the clients (or students) at the beginning of the treatment period and again at the end. The data gathered by the NOMS for students include: date of birth, school, eligibility for special education and speech-language services, previous treatment, disability codes, and functional communication measures (FCMs). At the end of the treatment period, similar information is obtained including: the amount of services provided, the frequency, the length of services, the service delivery model, changes in the student's functional communication status (changes in behavior), and recommendations for continuation or discharge from services. The NOMS instruments use a seven-point rating scale that has been developed to measure different aspects of a client's functional communication ability at the time of admission and discharge. Several functional communication measures (referred to as FCMs) are listed and describe disorder-specific communicative dysfunction for each student. The seven-point scale ranges from the least functional (Level 1) to the most functional or independent (Level 7). In addition to describing the student's functional skills, the rating also reflects the amount of assistance the student needs to be successful in low and high demand situations (such as learning in the classroom). Children functional at Level 1 need a high degree of support and assistance whereas children at Level 7 do not need assistance to use their communication skills to function successfully in the school setting.

The NOMS data collection process has been ongoing since 1997. In Phase I of the collection process, national data was collected on adults receiving speech-language pathology services in health care settings (Johnson, 1997). Phase II projects were initiated in 1997 to 1998 to collect data on children in kindergarten to grade 12 (Blosser, Subich, Ehren, & Ribbler, 1999). In 2010, ASHA temporarily suspended use of the NOMS for children in kindergarten through grade 12 in order to study findings since its inception and to improve the design and utility for future use. The NOMS Web site remains active and provides results of many studies.

Writing Professional Reports

Prior to enrolling students on the caseload, the SLP should document the nature and extent of the disorder and the appropriateness of speech-language services to treat the disability. Children who do not clearly demonstrate communication impairment should not be included in the caseload. In addition, the impact of the impairment on the student's participation and academic performance must be verified. Goals that are established should make a difference in the student's educational performance. If students will be taken out of the classroom to participate in therapy, the team members should be convinced that it is justified to take students away from their academic subjects. Administrators, parents, and others will want to be assured that you are using therapy time as efficiently as possible.

Progress records for each student in the caseload must be maintained. If progress is very slow or nonexistent, determine what additional steps or alternative strategies can be taken? School districts staff very talented individuals from a large number of disciplines. Students will benefit maximally if SLPs make use of all the knowledge and resources available.

Federal legislation mandates that special educators (including SLPs) provide parents with periodic reports of progress. Undoubtedly many SLPs are very creative in their design of a report card. It is important to use terms that parents can understand to describe the student's speech and language characteristics, goals and objectives of intervention, progress to date, and how that progress is determined. The good news is that periodic records will provide a mechanism for ongoing communication with others on the education team including teachers and parents.

Perhaps the most critical documents the educational team prepares are the Individualized Educational Programs. The purpose and content of the individualized education program documents differ depending on the student's age. The Individualized Education Program (IEP) is for school age students. The Individualized Family Service Plan (IFSP) is for children birth to age three. The Individualized Transition Plan (ITP) is for adolescents transitioning out of school. Regardless of the age, the document must provide information about the students' learning problems and needs (including speech and language impairments); expectations for performance; goals for classroom and all related services (including speech-language therapy); the context and materials for learning; and the role each educator and related services provider is to take. The parents' responsibility is also often described in the IEP, IFSP, and ITP.

Even without demands made by federal mandates for record and report keeping, it makes ethical and professional sense for clinicians to keep an account of a child's progress in therapy. As most clinicians deal with a large number of children, it would be impossible to recall all the facts and details pertinent to each of them.

A sample of the types of forms used to inform parents, document test results, and plan for a student's individualized education and/or transition program can be found in Appendix C. IEPs and other planning forms are discussed in greater detail in other sections of the text.

The speech-language pathologist is responsible to many different people including students, parents, school, administrators, teachers, attorneys, legislators, and fellow speech-language pathologists to name a few. Therefore, records and reports should be written so that they are understandable and contain the type of information others will be able to use to better understand the student and determine whether and what kind of services are required. As stated before, jargon should be eliminated or, at the very least, defined.

The ability to express ideas on paper, as well as verbally, is essential for the speech-language clinician. Some persons seem to be born with this knack, whereas others have to learn it. In any event, the techniques of writing professional reports and letters can be learned. Professional letters and reports must follow a specific framework. In addition, the basic essentials of good writing must be observed.

First, the writing must be clear and concise. Simple terms are much better then complex ones, and simplest and easiest way of saying something is usually the best. Professional vocabulary and terminology must be accurate and appropriate. The beginner who is learning the skill of professional writing should keep in mind the person to whom the report is being written—that is, the reader or listener. This person may be another clinician, the teacher, the family doctor, or the parents. Appropriate word choices should be made in light of the potential reader of the report and the purpose for writing it. Avoid professional jargon when writing to others and do not assume that they know the meanings of technical words.

Remember that reports are written from one human being to another human being. Try not to sound like an institution writing to a human being. Imagine the feelings that parents would experience if they receive a letter from the school clinician stating: "Periodically during the therapeutic intervention the speech-language pathologist will attempt to assess Billy's receptive language abilities by the administration of norm-referenced and criteria-referenced instruments to determine his linguistic status in relation to his peers." Why not state, "While Billy is enrolled in therapy, I will periodically give him probes and tests to find out how well he is progressing in the development of his language skills."

The Progress Report

The progress report covers a span of time, for example, a period of 1 month, 2 months, 6 weeks, 6 months, or a year. These times may vary depending on school policy as the mandate indicates that progress reports must occur as often as regular education students receive report cards. The progress report may be written for the purpose of tracking what was accomplished during therapy sessions. In some schools a case manager is responsible coordinating all of the individuals serving a particular child and reads the progress report to stay on top of how things are going. The progress report should include information such as the specific dates of the therapy, the number of therapy sessions, the name of the clinician, an evaluation of the progress, a listing of the therapy goals and a statement concerning whether or not they are accomplished, intervention approach implemented, the methods of therapy, and the overall results of the treatment to date. In a school the progress report may be written for the teacher's use and should be specific about what was done in therapy and what would be recommended for the teacher to follow up on. Progress reports are usually maintained in the student's school folder (similar to report cards). If the child moves from one school to another the reports may follow to the new school. Progress reports may also be sent to parents. The clinician must be sure the terminology is geared to the parents' understanding. The report card can function as a progress report.

Final Summary Reports

Final reports or ending reports may follow a checklist format or narrative style or a combination of the two. The factual information included in the final summary may include name, date of birth, type of problem, date of the latest service, name of the clinician and supervisor, date when student was first seen, starting date of therapy, and the date and results of reevaluation. Information about the type of therapy, the intervention approach, the setting for the services (classroom or therapy room), and amount of services may also be included. In addition, statements collaborative efforts can also be included. The report should describe the student's progress during the time covered by the report. The rating must be substantiated with specific outcome measures. If using terminology such as "no progress, minimal, moderate, good, or excellent," information must also be provided that defines and explains each category in terms of the amount of improvement the student made on the functional skills that were targeted in therapy. Reports should provide information to explain whether or not the student has achieved the instructional objectives. The contents of the final reports must be as accurate as humanly possible and written so that they will not be misconstrued.

If other services were utilized during this time it would be necessary to include a reference to them and, if available, a summary. Such services would include psychological, social, remedial reading, medical, vocational, educational, and psychiatric. In some cases it might be necessary to attach a copy of the report of those services. The report should indicate whether the service was obtained within the school system or in a community agency.

General Information

Report writing, as the name implies, means reporting the facts without any editorializing. The reader of the report must be able to gain valuable information from the report that enables them to better understand the student and to serve the student in the best way possible based on the information presented.

In writing professional reports the school clinician should keep in mind that opinions, rationalizations, hunches, and unsubstantiated ideas should not be included unless they are labeled as such and add context to the report. They may be included under a section called clinical impressions or a similar category. As long as they are labeled it is permissible to include them.

Risk Management Plan

The school environment is a breeding ground for common pediatric infections. Therefore, schools need to follow procedures to prevent transmission of diseases, protect the health of students and professionals, and ensure individuals' rights to privacy. Some of the common illnesses that are prevalent in schools are flu, measles, chickenpox, colds, skin infections, head lice, pinkeye, and mononucleosis. School clinicians should follow a risk management plan that provides guidelines for infection control procedures.

The ASHA Committee on Quality Assurance (Kulpa et al.,1991) recommended several administrative considerations for clinicians interested in developing a risk management plan for their school. They also suggested supplies necessary for implementing a risk management plan and infection control procedures for decreasing the possibility of transmitting disease through treatment materials, skin contact, and contact with materials and body fluids. Tables 6–3, 6–4, and 6–5 provide an outline of a risk management plan, supplies needed, and procedures to be followed. These procedures are adapted from the Universal Precautions developed by the Center for Disease Control and are applicable to the educational setting.

Table 6–3. Risk Management Administrative Considerations: A Checklist

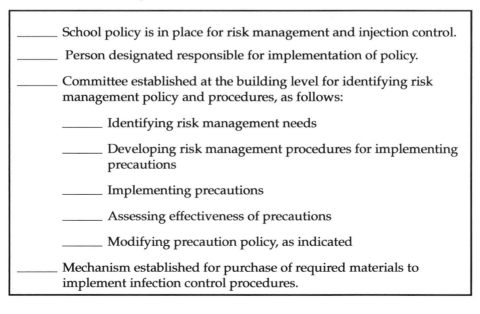

_____ School policy is in place for risk management and injection control.

_____ Person designated responsible for implementation of policy.

_____ Committee established at the building level for identifying risk management policy and procedures, as follows:

- _____ Identifying risk management needs
- _____ Developing risk management procedures for implementing precautions
- _____ Implementing precautions
- _____ Assessing effectiveness of precautions
- _____ Modifying precaution policy, as indicated

_____ Mechanism established for purchase of required materials to implement infection control procedures.

Table 6–4. Infection Control Supply Checklists

The following materials are needed to implement proper infection control procedures.

______ Disposable gloves

______ Alcohol/antiseptic wipes

______ Soap

______ Access to sink/running water

______ Paper towels

______ Disinfection solution (1 part household bleach to 10 parts water)

______ Spray bottle (to mix water and disinfectant solution)

______ Tissue

______ Plastic bags that seal (e.g., Ziploc)

______ Trash bags

______ Household bleach

______ Hand lotion

______ Absorbent powder for bodily secretions

In addition, these infection control materials should be used when implementing procedures that could expose the professional to blood, semen, or other bodily secretions that *contain visible blood* (e.g., oral peripheral examinations, procedures involving tracheostomy tubes, etc.)

______ Mask

______ Goggles

______ Gowns

______ Red trash bags (for disposal of materials that *could be harmful* if handled casually)

Table 6–5. Infection Control Procedures

Decreasing the Possibility of Transmitting Disease Through Treatment Materials

What to Disinfect	*When to Disinfect*	*How to Disinfect*
Evaluation and treatment materials (e.g., toys, games, storage boxes, therapy materials. Work surfaces. Electronic equipment and accessories. Seating surfaces. Materials, supplies, materials, and instruments to examine oral mechanism or ears.	Clean table top and materials after each use. If materials, work surfaces, electronic equipment or seating surfaces contain visible blood, use Universal Precautions.	Use sanitizer, soap and water, or a 1 to 10 solution of household bleach to water, spray, and wipe thoroughly. Use disposable materials (e.g., gloves, etc.) when possible.

Decreasing the Possibility of Transmitting Disease Via Skin Contact

What to Do	*When to Do It*	*How to Do It*
Wash hands (effective if skin is intact). Use gloves (to provide a protective barrier) if your skin or the client's skin is broken.	Before and after seeing each client. After removing gloves. Immediately if in contact with potentially contaminating blood or body fluids. Before touching blood or other body fluids, mucus, or nonintact skin of all clients. When performing an examination of the oral speech mechanism using laryngeal mirrors, middle ear testing, handling or fabricating earmolds and other prostheses. When you have a cut or abrasion. When client has a cut or abrasion.	Use vigorous mechanical action whether or not a skin cleanser is used. Use antiseptic or ordinary soap under running water. Wash for 30 seconds or longer if grossly contaminated. Dry hands thoroughly with a paper or disposable towel to help eliminate germs. Put on hand lotion so hands do not become chapped. Wear gloves.

Table 6–5. *continued*

Decreasing the Possibility of Transmitting Disease by Appropriately Disposing of Materials and Body Fluids

What to Dispose of	*When to Dispose It*	*How to Dispose It*
Dressing and tissues. Urine, feces, sperm, vaginal secretions, menses.	Immediately	Place used dressing and tissues in a plastic bag and tie securely. Discard bags carefully. Wear gloves. Flush urine and feces down the toilet. If it is necessary to use a portable urinal, potty chair, etc., empty it into the toilet and thoroughly clean and sanitize before replacing it or returning it to storage.

DISCUSSION QUESTIONS AND PROJECTS

1. Why must school programs in speech-language be held accountable for students' learning outcomes? To whom are programs accountable?

2. Obtain a copy of a letter written about a student to another educator or health care professional. Critique it based on issues raised in this chapter. Would you make any changes? Find a report that has been written to the speech-language pathologist by another professional. Critique it based on issues raised in this chapter.

3. Start a collection of record and report forms used in the schools. How would you organize the report forms for a school system?

4. Write five outcome-based IEP goals for a student in a school program.

5. Visit ASHA's Web site to learn about the latest reports of findings from the National Outcomes Measures project. Obtain copies of the NOMS. Complete an Entrance form on one of your students. Ask a fellow colleague to do the same. Compare results.

6. Check the clinic at your University or school to see if they have appropriate infection control procedures in place.

7. Discuss procedures you should follow if you learn that a child has a communicable disease. Who should you contact? What precautions should you take? Should services for the child be discontinued?

8. What would you do if a child on your caseload came in for therapy and announced that he has ringworm? What if a sibling of one of your students is reported to have hepatitis?

9. List three essential components that student's SLP records must contain.

7

Establishing the Caseload

Determining the composition of the caseload is one of the SLP's most challenging responsibilities. He or she must make difficult decisions about children who are eligible for services and how to best serve them. Consideration must also be given to implementing the most appropriate procedures for the identification process. The ultimate task of the SLP is to identify and treat those students whose communication problems interfere with educational achievement.

School SLPs are expected to comply with federal and state standards in screening, diagnosis, case selection, and delivery of service. At the same time they are accountable for meeting the local education agency (LEA) requirements as well as the professional code of ethics. In districts where funding is contributed by a number of third-party pay sources (such as Medicaid or insurance), the clinician is also responsible for meeting the requirements established by the payers. Sometimes, these requirements may seem in conflict with one another.

The information in this chapter is presented to help the school SLP carry out the many important processes and formulate the key decisions that become the cornerstones of accountability about the speech-language program and services, including:

- how students are to be identified and referred;
- how they are to be screened and assessed;
- the nature of the disorder or diagnosis;
- the amount of support needed;
- the type of intervention needed;
- whether the expertise of the SLP is required;
- others who should be involved in the delivery of services;
- how much and how frequently the treatment should be delivered; and,
- the most appropriate model and location for services.

The SLP has the major responsibility of determining if a communication impairment exists and its severity. However, the decision about whether a student is eligible for speech-language pathology services or not cannot be made independently. The decision must be made in collaboration with other key team members including the family, educators, school administrators, and others who have critical information to share or who can make significant contributions during the decision making and treatment process.

A Philosophy: The Basis on Which to Build

Knowing who you are and where you fit into the educational scheme provides the basis from which to make many decisions and plans for the speech-language services program. Years ago schools used categorical labels to describe children such as hearing impaired, vision impaired, speech impaired, mentally retarded, orthopedically impaired, developmentally disabled and so on. Class placement, instruction and treatment decisions were made based on these labels. Services were structured around the disabilities rather than individually designed to support the student's success in the learning situation. This psychological-medical orientation failed to provide descriptive information about how the student functioned in learning situations given his or her skills and disability. In other words, categorical labeling did not enable SLPs and teachers to describe a student's communication skills nor understand the impact of the communication impairment on his or her ability to access the curriculum, participate, or perform in class.

To provide appropriate services for children, it makes more sense to describe their communication skills in terms of how they function in high and low demand learning situations, given their impairment. It is important that the classroom teacher as well as the parents understand the connection between the communication impairment and the child's ability to profit from the instruction in the classroom. For example, it is not enough to describe a child as having a brain injury and cognitive-communication disorder and let it go at that. In the school setting, it is necessary to describe how the cognitive-communication disorder affects the child's ability to understand the teacher's classroom instructions; to play with other children on the playground; to monitor his or her own speech and language behaviors; to comprehend reading passages; or to recall information presented in spoken and written forms. The effect of the brain injury on the child's self-image and behavior should also be explained.

Speech, language, and hearing clinicians work in many settings. Clinicians who choose to work in an educational setting have the responsibility of removing or alleviating communication barriers that may hinder the child from accessing the curriculum and benefiting from the instruction offered in the school. She also has the responsibility of evaluating the communication problem and assessing its impact on the learning process. Another responsibility of the school clinician is to serve as a resource person for the classroom teachers and special education teachers who have children with communication disabilities in their classrooms. And, it is of utmost importance to explain all of these concepts for the parents.

Perhaps it is the term "special education" that has led our thinking astray. Special education, in reality, is education that has been individualized for children with special learning challenges. The education of children with disabilities is not something distinct and set apart from education; it is a part of the total school program and responsibility.

Defining the Process and the Terms

Identification refers to locating the preschool and school age students who demonstrate communication impairments or who are at risk for educational or social failure due to inadequate communication skills. Where it is not in conflict with state law and practices and court order, identification would also include those students who are ages 18 to 21. Initial identification efforts in schools are accomplished by referrals and screening programs.

As a starting point, clinicians and educators must establish common operational definitions and terminology for communicating about youngsters with communication problems. The World Health Organization (2011) suggests the following distinctions. Speech-language pathologists work with youngsters with communication patterns that lead to their characterization as *impaired, disabled,* or *handicapped*. Some clinicians don't make distinctions between the three terms. However, The World Health Organization (WHO) provides a definition of the terms that can be useful in determining the extent of services to be provided. According to WHO, *impairment* is an abnormality of structure or function at the organ level. This would include speech, language, hearing, cognitive, and voice impairments. A *disability* is the functional consequence of impairment. People with impairments experience communication problems in the context of daily living situations and activities. A *handicap* is the social consequence of an impairment or disability. Depending of the nature and severity of the impairment, individuals may experience isolation, joblessness, and dependency. Their quality of life is effected (Frattelli, 1999; World Health Organization, 2011).

The term "caseload" refers to the number and type of students that the SLP works with who have Individual Education Programs (IEPs), Individualized Family Service Plans (IFSPs), or Individual Transition Plans (ITPs). Caseload selection refers to the process of determining which students are *eligible* for speech and language intervention services. Not all students referred for services, nor all students who fail screening criteria may necessarily be candidates for the speech-language program or services from the SLP. Those who exhibit communication problems are determined through the following steps:

- *Obtaining appropriate background information*, that is, a case history, including onset, past development, present status, and other relevant information from parents and teachers;
- *Appraising the problem* by observing, interviewing, describing, and testing when appropriate;
- *Diagnosing* which includes making a tentative identification of the problem and determining probable causes.

It should be pointed out that the SLP must use judgment in determining how rigorously these steps are followed. For example, the third-grader that exhibits what appears to be a serious voice problem may be suffering from a cold and sore throat at the time he is observed. That information would preclude interviewing parents or obtaining a case history.

The Prereferral Process

IDEA 2004 established requirements for early intervening services for children in kindergarten through grade 12 who are not currently identified as needing special education or related services but who need additional academic and behavior support to succeed in a general education environment. Many school districts have established a prereferral process called Early Intervening Services as a step that precedes referral for assessment for special education services, including speech-language services. In this process, a school-based interdisciplinary problem-solving team is established to help parents and teachers understand and deal with students who present behavior or learning problems in the classroom. The goal is to identify students who are at risk for failure.

The early intervening process is formalized in some schools and convened on an ad hoc basis in others. The name for the early intervening teams differs from district to district. Common names include Student Support Team, Child Study Team, Instructional Support Team, Student Assistance Team, Prereferral Team, Early Intervening Service Team, or Response-to-Intervention (RtI Team). Regardless of the label, the goal of the team is to provide peer to peer assistance and recommendations regarding how to handle children who exhibit problems in the classroom. Based on the behaviors that the student presents, the team may recommend that the teacher try specific intervention strategies for a specified period of time, collecting data to document the child's response, before referring to a specialist for additional input or evaluation.

Some SLPs participate on the early intervening teams. Others make themselves available to the team on an "as needed" basis. Others may not participate because they are not always available or because the other educators on the team do not clearly understand communication disorders or the SLP's role and potential contributions. Being an active participant on the prereferral team can be very beneficial for increasing teachers' knowledge of speech-language development and problems and recommending strategies that can improve the student's chances of success in the classroom. Prereferral and early intervening services are explored further in Chapter 8.

Identification of Students with Disabilities

Identifying children at risk for communication disability is usually accomplished by utilizing two procedures, either singly or in combination: *referral* and *screening*. The purpose of both procedures is the identification of students with potential communication problems that may impact their educational performance or impairments that are *educationally relevant*.

There is some variability in identification procedures from district to district. In some districts, referral is the primary method of case identification because of its perceived efficiency and effectiveness. Other districts conduct "mass screening" programs where all children of a particular age or grade are screened to determine the potential presence of a communication disorder. Unfortunately, the efficacy research comparing referral to screening for case finding has been somewhat limited. Regardless of whether a student is identified through the referral process or through a screening program, the next step is to determine if further testing by a speech-language pathologist is warranted to determine the presence of a communication disorder.

Referrals for Speech-Language Evaluation

Referrals can be formally solicited at a specified time of the school year as well as invited throughout the school year. The success of any referral system is dependent on forming excellent working relationships with parents and teachers and providing information about communication disorders and referral procedures in a simple and understandable way. So that parents and teachers have a context for making referrals, they must understand the impact of speech and language disorders on the student's school performance, their ability to interact with others, and their ability to communicate wants, needs, and information.

The goal of the teacher or parent referral is for the SLP to become aware of a particular child who is at risk for having a communication disability. The therapist, in the final analysis, is the one who is responsible for determining if such a problem exists. It is, however, up to a team of educators to determine if the student is eligible for services and if an Individualized Education Plan for speech-language services will be developed.

Referrals can be made by anyone who has the child's welfare in mind and suspects a problem. This includes the child's parents, teachers, physician, school nurse, school counselor, principal, peer, or the child. Outside the school, health care specialists, and community service agencies may also advise parents to seek evaluation or treatment for their child. Examples of community service organizations are United Cerebral Palsy, Easter Seals, Autism Speaks, and The Brain Injury Foundation.

SLPs and educators must understand and comply with the school system's policy regarding referrals. The process for referring students for speech-language intervention services should be clearly defined and consistent throughout the school district. Referral forms should be made available to school staff and other individuals. Referrals should be encouraged and invited even though the clinician may sometimes feel that the classroom teacher is referring too many children or referring children who have problems other than those in speech, language, and hearing. The door should always be kept open for referrals throughout the school year because as teachers work with students they may observe communication behaviors that are of concern. Similarly, parents may become concerned when they observe their child struggling. Teachers generally are excellent referral sources because they have a good sense of how children should speak at a particular age or in a particular grade. Because of staff turnover and changes in school practices or service delivery requirements and eligibility criteria, the procedures and opportunities for referral should be presented to the teachers periodically. Written procedures for making referrals should be included in school handbooks and manuals. Forms should be made available on the school Intranet or in the principal's office.

It is especially beneficial if guidelines for making referrals can be presented during a staff meeting or as an in-service presentation. The school clinician will soon learn which teachers in a school are able to identify the children with communication impairments with a high degree of accuracy. Those teachers make great collaborative partners.

Following the initial referral from the classroom teacher or the problem-solving team, the speech-language clinician and fellow team members must make a decision about whether the student is to receive a more complete assessment. According to state and federal laws, parental and/or guardian permission must be obtained before comprehensive testing is undertaken.

Helping Educators Make Appropriate Referrals

Educators and communication disorders professionals must work together to identify children who exhibit inadequate communication skills. The key is to identify those students whose speech and language skills significantly restrict participation in class or interfere with their learning. To help parents and other professionals serve effectively as referral sources, SLPs should take proactive steps to increase their awareness and understanding of the following: how speech and language skills develop; types of communication impairments children present; behaviors and characteristics associated with language, articulation, stuttering, voice, and hearing impairments; terminology used by SLPs to discuss students' functional communication; the many ways that impairments interfere with learning; the SLP's roles and responsibilities; and how speech-language intervention can help.

A systematic referral program can be ensured by providing instructions and guidelines for making referrals during in-service training sessions. Figure 7–1 presents a list of topics that can be discussed during an in-service or preservice presentation to teachers or other groups of people on how to make referrals.

Demonstrating typical disorders can enhance in-service presentations. During the training session, it is helpful to imitate or simulate various kinds of communication problems. A library of audio or video recordings of various types of problems would also be helpful for demonstration. Regional resource centers and universities may have audio or videotapes available for loan to school clinicians for teacher in-service programs. Some publishers sell DVDs that depict various disorders.

Making the Language and Literacy Connection

It is extremely important for educators to understand that communication is the basis for learning and the negative impact

- Normal speech, language, and hearing development.
- Nature and causes of speech, language, and hearing impairments.
- Prevalence and incidence of communication disabilities.
- Terminology used by speech-language pathologists to describe and discuss children with communication impairments.
- Impact of communication disorders on academic performance and social relationships.
- Factors communication disorders professionals consider when evaluating students' communicative performance and determining eligibility for service and discharge from services.
- Referral procedures to be followed.
- The goals of the speech-language intervention program.
- Ways to collaborate with speech-language pathologists.
- What success looks like—the outcomes of speech-language intervention.

Figure 7–1. Topics for in-servicing teachers on how to refer.

speech, language, and hearing impairments can have on academic performance. When explaining communication disorders to teachers, it is especially important to discuss the adverse effect a communication disorder has on the youngster's ability to participate in school activities (oral and written) and learn the general education curriculum.

The overall quality of teacher referrals will improve significantly if teachers become skilled at observing students and relating their communication problems to learning difficulties they may be experiencing. SLPs can help make that connection. In fact, according to ASHA's 2010 Roles and Responsibilities document, the SLP has a responsibility to do so. Provide teachers with instructions for observing the students' skills in the following areas of cognition and communication and explain how the following skills affect classroom performance:

- *Thinking* (organizing and categorizing information; identifying and solving problems; finding, selecting, and using information; and thinking about ideas and events);
- *Listening* (understanding complex sentences and words; understanding main ideas and events; following complex directions; and listening effectively);
- *Speaking* (planning what to say; organizing information in a logical sequence; using grammatically correct sentence structures;

using language to give directions, make reports, tell stories; providing relevant and complete answers);

- *Reading and writing* (comprehension of written language and formulation of written expression); and
- *Survival language* (demonstrating language skills necessary to cope with daily living situations).

Who Can Make Referrals?

Referrals can be initiated in person, by telephone, or in writing. The teacher is able to observe children in a variety of communication-based learning activities. Consequently, the information she has to offer regarding performance is valuable. It is most helpful to provide a simple questionnaire or checklist to assist teachers and others in describing the communication behaviors they have observed, their concerns, and their reasons for referring. Figure 7–2 is an example of the type of checklist teachers might find helpful when observing a child's communication skills. Notice how simple the questions and form are. The initial referral form should be brief so busy teachers can quickly complete it. More extensive information can be obtained through guided teacher observation and specific questions as part of the evaluation process once the child has been identified as exhibiting communication impairment. It is important to note that the teacher's referral activates the IDEA multifactored evaluation process, and parental permission must be obtained to further evaluate an individual student.

Referrals at the Secondary School Level

It is more realistic to use the referral method rather than screening programs in middle schools and high schools. School clinicians, while recognizing the need of improved case finding procedures at this level, point out the difficulties of a screening program because of the complexity of middle and high school class schedules and the greater mobility of high school students, who are changing classes throughout the day. In addition the incidence of communication disorders within the middle school and high school groups tends to be lower.

Screening and referral programs at the high school level are difficult for many of the same reasons. Secondary teachers often do not see students for as great amount of time as elementary teachers see their students. In addition, in many classes, communicative interaction is limited because teachers may teach hundreds of students in the course of a semester and may use a lecture style for teaching. English and language arts teachers may be good referral sources because they are sensitive to communication and they have greater opportunity to hear students communicate during classroom activities. In addition, they are able to observe students' written work. Guidance counselors, coaches, and teachers who sponsor extracurricular activities also converse with students in informal situations with great frequency.

On the high school level, self-referrals or parental referrals are often common sources for identifying individuals with potential communication problems. High school students who have a speech, language, or hearing problem need to know

Teacher's Name ______________________________ Grade or Class __________

As a teacher, you are able to observe students in a variety of communication-based learning activities. Therefore, the information you have to offer regarding speech, language, and hearing performance is quite valuable. This simple checklist is designed to assist you in describing the communication behaviors you have observed for specific children who may be of concern to you.

Instructions: Read the following statements. Indicate the names and ages of any students in your class who demonstrate the speech, language, or hearing characteristics that are described.

	List child's name and age.		
Voice quality is noticeably different from other children (hoarse, breathy, nasal).			
Speech is nonfluent (hesitant, jerky, repetitive, prolonged).			
Child is noticeably frustrated if unable to get message across.			
Pronunciation is difficult to understand.			
Child is unable to ask and/or answer simple questions.			
Child cannot carry on a conversation (relay events, give explanations).			
Child cannot formulate 5- and 7-word sentences; grammar and vocabulary are not age appropriate.			
Generally nonverbal and does not interact with you or peers.			
Has frequent colds or runny nose.			
Attends to speakers face more than expected.			
Frequently responds to statements or questions with "What?" or "Huh?"			
Experiences trouble following directions.			
Primary language spoken by the child or his family is not English.			
Generally appears to be confused during most language-based learning activities (spelling, reading, speaking, writing).			

Figure 7–2. Teacher referral form.

about the services offered if they are to refer themselves. This means that the clinician will have to find ways to let students know the services are available, as well as make it easy for them to refer themselves. Students can be informed of the times and days the speech-language pathologist is in the school building through announcements over the public address system, through the school newspaper, or through signs posted on bulletin boards throughout the building. The message should inform students about the services offered by the speech-language pathologist. It should provide brief explanations of speech, language, and hearing behaviors that may cause concern and which they might want to "check out." It should also describe how to schedule an appointment. In some districts, students may have to inform the guidance counselor of their interest. Middle school and high school students are sensitive about other people knowing they experience difficulties. Therefore, discretion is advised about the testing appointment, location, results, and recommendations. One way to encourage participation is to stress the "self-improvement" aspect of the speech-language program. Students should be guided to realize that good communication skills will improve job opportunities and interactions with their peers.

Screening

ASHA's Preferred Practice Patterns for the Profession of Speech-Language Pathology (2004) explain that speech-language screening identifies infants, toddlers, children, or adolescents likely to have speech-language and communication impairments. Like referrals, screening is a process whereby students in need of further evaluation are identified. Speech-language screening may be conducted by the SLP or by trained paraprofessionals. Screening procedures result in pass/fail decisions and may lead to one of four recommendations: (1) no further steps needed; (2) recommendations to support normal development and prevent speech language impairment; (3) trial use of intervention strategies and monitoring development and improvement over time; or (4) referral for comprehensive speech-language assessment or other assessments or services.

Impairments are likely to interfere with one or more of the following three major components described within the World Health Organization's *International Classification of Functioning, Disability, and Health* (2011) framework:

- Body structures and functions:
  - The intent is to identify and optimize underlying anatomic and physiologic strengths and weaknesses related to communication and swallowing effectiveness. This includes mental functions such as attention as well as components of communication such as articulatory proficiency, fluency, and syntax.
- Activities and participation, including capacity (under ideal circumstances) and performance (in everyday environments):
  - Assess the communication and swallowing-related demands of activities in the individual's life (contextually based assessment);

- ☐ Identify and optimize the individual's ability to perform relevant/desired social, academic, and vocational activities despite possible ongoing communication and related impairments;
- ☐ Identify and optimize ways to facilitate social, academic, and vocational participation associated with the impairment.

- Contextual factors, including personal factors (e.g., age, race, gender, education, lifestyle, and coping skills) and environmental factors (e.g., physical, technologic, social, and attitudinal):
  - ☐ Identify and optimize personal and environmental factors that are barriers to or facilitators of successful communication (including the communication competencies and support behaviors of everyday people in the environment).

- Services may result in a diagnosis of a communication disorder, identification of a communication difference, prognosis for change (in the individual or relevant contexts), intervention and support, evaluation of their effectiveness, and referral for other assessments or services as needed:
  - ☐ Although the outcomes of speech, language, or hearing services may not be guaranteed, a reasonable statement of prognosis is made to referral sources, clients/patients, and families/caregivers.
  - ☐ Outcomes of services are monitored and measured in order to ensure the quality of services provided and to improve the quality of those services.
  - ☐ Appropriate follow-up services are provided to determine functional outcomes and the need for further services after discharge.

Standardized as well as nonstandardized methods are used in the screening process. Given the diversity in our schools, the methods chosen should be sensitive to cultural and linguistic differences. Screening instruments and procedures should be age-appropriate in terms of speech-language and other communication functions and activities. The techniques used should provide insights about the child's oral motor function, communication and social interaction skills, speech production skills, comprehension and production of spoken and written language (as age-appropriate), and cognitive aspects of communication. The SLP and other team members should be able to gain a basic understanding of the student's participation in activities and contextual factors that may affect communication. Children who fail screenings are referred for further evaluation. Parent permission must be obtained before moving forward with the evaluation process.

Mass Screening

Mass screening techniques are employed to screen groups of children to determine those which need additional testing. Mass screening programs are sometimes conducted at the preschool or primary grades. This screening method casts a wide net to see which children stand out as potentially demonstrating speech-language delays, differences, or impairments. Fewer school districts are employing mass screening programs in recent years. The SLP uses the same set of screening procedures with all children who participate in the mass screening program. For example, they may be given a brief articulation screening test and asked to respond to questions and read a passage or tell a story. The clinician then follows up on all the children who do not pass the screening. Further steps are then taken to observe and find out more about the student. The findings lead to a recommendation of whether a more in-depth diagnostic testing is warranted to confirm the presence of a communication disorder, the impact of the disorder on educational performance, and to determine eligibility for intervention services.

Screening is not to be used as an evaluation procedure to determine eligibility for special education or instructional support (related) services such as speech and language services. The intent of screening is to determine if there are instructional strategies that can be used by a member of the educational team (including the teacher and/or the SLP) that would improve the students' classroom performance. SLPs can provide advice and recommendations to teachers of intervention strategies that may help the student.

Although the referral process is the most efficient, there are still times when schools consider "mass screening programs" useful. In those circumstances, school district administrators and the SLP decide when and where the speech-language screening activities will take place and which children will be screened. There are several general factors to be considered before making the decision about the type of screening program to conduct. Determining the answers to the following questions will help use screening time as efficiently as possible:

- What are the goals of the speech-language program?
- Will different populations be served throughout the school year?
- Are speech-language pathology services new to the building, district, or community?
- Will the screening program be conducted by SLPs independently or will there be a team approach involving educators, assistants, or other professionals?
- Are there unique aspects related to the student population (socioeconomic status, mobility, cultural diversity, special education needs) that support the need for screening?
- Have there been significant changes in school personnel or resources?

When the answers to these questions have been obtained, the goals of the screening program can be established. It is important that these goals are not only established, but also provided in writing and made available to the school administration and faculty. When the goals are established, the procedures for carrying out the screening program can be made. The procedures should also be in writing and should be available to administrators, including the director of special education, the director of speech-language services, the elementary and secondary supervisors, the principals of each school, and the teachers in each of the schools to be screened. Parents should be informed of screening programs and procedures. In some circumstances, parental permission may be required. The school district policies should clearly state if parental permission is required or not.

Screening methods should be combined with teacher referrals as well as parental input. The first step in a screening process serves to identify children who potentially may exhibit communication impairments. An observation and follow up discussion would be conducted for those children identified by the screening or by referral as having possible communication problems. The decision to advance to a diagnostic evaluation is made by a team of educators.

Screening programs can be structured in many different ways. One procedure used successfully by many clinicians is to take three to eight children at a time. Prior to starting the screening, the SLP and teacher provide an explanation of what is occurring and what the child is expected to do. While one child is being tested the others observe and generally will know what to do when their turn comes. As each child is finished he or she goes back to the room and gets the next child. This procedure creates little interruption of the teacher's schedule, and the classroom activities go on as usual. A class of 25 children can be screened in approximately 30 to 40 minutes. If instructional aides are available, they may take the children to and from the classroom.

Many school systems employ a team approach, especially in the preschool and kindergarten screening programs. The team members often include the school nurse, psychologist, speech-language pathologist, educational audiologist, occupational therapist, and other specialists who test vision, motor coordination, dentition, general health, and physical well-being. Paraprofessionals or volunteer aides sometimes also assist in this type of screening program. If using assistants in this way, they should be trained and supervised by certified, qualified professionals.

Because the purpose of the screening is detection, not diagnosis, the clinician should strive to resist the temptation to spend more time than is needed with a child who obviously has a problem. The results of the screening task should be recorded immediately after each individual is seen. All absentees should be noted, and arrangements should be made to screen them later.

Getting Ready to Screen

Implementing a screening program requires advance planning and organization. SLPs need to identify the student groups to be screened as well as the tools they will use. Communication with administrators and teachers is essential. Teachers should be informed in advance of the referral and screening program procedures and schedule. This will help them prepare their students and plan for the interruption in their teaching schedule.

Screening Procedures

Screening must be done efficiently and accurately. That is, it must be done with a maximum degree of professional expertise and with a minimum expenditure of time, money, and professional energy. Planning is absolutely essential. In addition to a general plan, there must also be a plan to encompass all the details and follow-up contacts after the screening. Parents should be notified that screening will take place. This can be done by a letter sent home with the children or by announcements in the school newsletter or local newspaper.

Screening of preschoolers is generally completed in the spring or summer preceding their entrance into school. Kindergarten screening is usually done during the first few weeks of school, but it may be done at any time of the year. As mentioned previously, referrals by teachers in the upper elementary grades, middle school, and high school can be obtained with the guidance of the SLP. This process can replace screening at those grade levels.

Screening programs can be carried out by one clinician, by a team of clinicians, or by a team composed of clinicians and trained assistants. If more than one person is involved in a screening program, the procedures should be clearly understood by all to ensure uniform administration and greater reliability.

Screening Instruments

Clinicians use a variety of methods for screening children ranging from observing informal conversations to using formal, standardized screening tests. SLPs may use published or informal screening tools including criterion referenced assessments, checklists, interviews, questionnaires, observations, or clinician-made instruments. There are advantages and disadvantages to each. For example, through observation during informal conversation, one can observe the child's overall intelligibility and the impact of the child's communication skills on communicative interactions. However, this method reduces the quantifiable information, which can be obtained, reduces accountability, and may miss children who are reluctant participants or shy (Westman & Broen, 1989). Formalized methods have the advantage of enabling the clinician to compare the child's performance to others of the same age, implementing the testing consistently across children, and facilitating documentation and accountability.

Instruments for assessing communicative abilities during a screening program differ according to the ages of the children. The instruments should be easily administered and should identify quickly those children who need further testing. In a school screening, whether one clinician or several are involved, the screening devices should be the same, and the standard for judging the results should be consistent from one tester to another. The screening procedures should also take into account differences in ethnic and in socioeconomic backgrounds of the children being tested. The examiners need to keep in mind that they are attempting to detect differences in speech, language, voice quality, fluency, or any other problems in communication that might be potentially limiting to the child's ability to learn in school or function as a useful member of society.

It will be necessary for the school SLP to become familiar with the various speech and language tests. The clinician should find out what the test purports to measure and what it actually measures.

The most appropriate test or tests should be utilized for the particular situation. Check the reliability, norms, and standardization of the test, know the difference between "norm-referenced" tests and "criterion-referenced" tests, and utilize clinical judgment and expertise in synthesizing the information from the tests.

A screening battery carried out by the SLP or as a part of a comprehensive screening program is basically seeking information about a child's oral motor function, communication and social interaction, speech production, voice, fluency, hearing, comprehension and production of spoken and written language, and cognitive aspects of communication. Screening procedures on any age or grade level are subject to some degree of error. Some children will slip by undetected, and others may not be identified correctly. School clinicians and classroom teachers must work together to recognize any of these children.

Teacher Interview Screening

A method that combines screening and teacher referral was reported by Finn and Gardner (1984). Referred to as Teacher Interview Screening, it is comprised of two processes: mandatory teacher inservice programs and the teacher interview. The method utilizes the teacher's knowledge of child development and expertise in observing communication and learning behaviors. This method lays the groundwork for greater efficiency and effectiveness. To facilitate success, teachers in their project were provided with a reference guide that included a communication competence rating scale. Finn and Gardner interviewed teachers and asked them a key question about each student in the class: "Considering the skills outlined on the communication competence rating scale, do you feel this child's communication skills are adequate when compared to his/her classmates?" The teachers and SLP then had three options available to them. They could *pass* the child who had adequate skills, *fail* the child who obviously had inadequate skills, or conduct a *follow-up screening* for those children whose skills were questionable. The follow-up screening in this project consisted of observing the student in the classroom or a more traditional one-on-one screening, depending on the concerns that were expressed.

Finn and Gardner evaluated the effectiveness of the teacher interview, comparing the results to the traditional screening method in terms of cost, reliability and compatibility with intervention philosophies. A two-year study was conducted to determine appropriate cost estimates. The results indicated the total time spent by the staff doing the new screening method was 100 hours and 42 minutes or approximately 13 working days. The traditional mass screening method took 897 hours or approximately 120 working days. Given clinicians' per diem salaries, this amounted to significant savings. Reliability was examined by selecting several of the second grade classrooms. Each child who failed either the traditional screening or Teacher Interview Screening was evaluated and the results were compared. Interpretation of the data showed 84% agreement between the teacher interview and traditional methods of screening. It should be noted that there were no students with disorders (those having a severity score of 4) who were missed by either group. There were no students with a severity of 3 missed by the teacher group, whereas there were 2 children missed in the group screened by the traditional method. With the completion of this project it was concluded that using a well developed teacher interview procedure for screening can be efficient, permit sampling a student's communication skills in his natural environment, and utilize the skills teachers have or can develop to identify students in need of our services. This is the kind of evidence-based study the profession needs to continue to encourage to determine the most effective and cost-efficient methods of conducting our services.

Screening for Phonological Disorders in Primary Grades

Children in kindergarten, first grade, and second grade exhibit many phonological errors. Some of these children will overcome their errors through the process of getting a little older and being exposed to the school environment. However, there are children in this group who will not improve without intervention. Differentiating between these two groups creates a dilemma for the school clinician. Obviously, because of the large numbers, all these children cannot be provided direct services by the SLP. Nor should they be. Through prognostic and predictive testing school clinicians must be able to sort these children into two general groups: those who need direct intervention and those who may modify their speech patterns through indirect methods such as a speech improvement program or instruction provided by the teacher during communication related curricular tasks in the classroom.

Numerous prognostic factors related to phonological errors have been explored including rate of change toward correction, number, type, and/or consistency of errors, phonemic proficiency, and evaluation of the specific sounds or phonological processes exhibited. Clinicians must conduct procedures that will enable them to discriminate between those children who will and those who will not have acquired normal mature articulation by the time they reach the third grade level.

Generally, SLPs take steps to assess the child's degree of stimulability (the ability to repeat sounds, nonsense syllables, words, and a sentence); the ability to demonstrate oral motor movements such as moving the tongue independently of the lower jaw; and the ability to detect errors in the examiner's speech. Some SLPs believe that another effective and reliable predictive variable is the total number of errors in all positions within words produced by the youngster. The persistence of specific types of error patterns may be a predictor. There are several error patterns that are characteristic of children who are unintelligible or phonologically delayed. These include errors involving deletion of phonemes or syllables, change in the manner of phoneme production, substitution of more anterior sounds for more posterior sounds, and change in the phonotactic structure of the word.

Another factor related to the predictability of the correction of functional phonological problems is the inconsistency of errors. It generally has been accepted that the more inconsistent the child's phonological errors, the more possibility there is that he or she will develop through them. The rationale is that the child may be able to produce the sound correctly sometimes but has not learned the appropriate times to produce it. Children exhibiting inconsistent error patterns or phonological processes inappropriate for their age should be further tested with instruments or speech analyses that provide more comprehensive and systematic testing on the way sounds are produced in all possible phonologic contexts. There are several commercial instruments available that can be used to yield helpful information. Care should be taken to learn the premise upon which the judgments will be based (number of errors, type of error patterns, stimulability, and so forth).

There are many resources available in the literature on speech sound acquisition that discuss what can be expected at each age milestone. Many assessment instruments and developmental charts provide estimates of the number and type of correct productions expected for children at various age levels from age 3 to 8.

For older elementary children, the best screening context is spontaneous speech because it is most likely to yield a sample of the child's habitual speech and language. If the child is asked to read words, sentences, or paragraphs, the clinician must be sure that the material is within his or her reading ability.

Screening for Language Disorders

Identifying language disorders in the preschool and school-age child is a complicated, difficult, and often frustrating task. A thorough knowledge of speech and language development is required as well as an appreciation of the fact that both the identification and the assessment of language disorders is a continuous process shared by the persons who are best able to observe the child in many situations. These persons are the parents and the teachers as well as the speech-language pathologist.

In the schools, much of learning is dependent on language abilities: reading, spelling, speech, writing, mathematics, problem-solving, creative thinking, comprehension, and others. An intact language system is important in the learning process. The SLP plays a critical and necessary role in the identification, assessment, and treatment of the student with a language disorder.

Keeping in mind that screening is an identification process, we therefore need to identify the student with the language disorder. The facets of language are reception (decoding) and expression (encoding). The components of language are phonology, morphology, syntax, semantics, and pragmatics. A complete language evaluation should include all of these aspects. On the screening level it is important to ascertain whether or not the language behavior appears to be adequate and commensurate with the age of the student. The Language Arts curriculum can serve as an excellent point of reference for determining if a student's language skills are age appropriate. Teachers have excellent screening and assessment tools that they routinely administer. Students who struggle on those curriculum related tasks may actually exhibit a language disability. An in-depth diagnosis would follow after the child has been identified during the screening process.

One of the most important steps in the identification process is to obtain information from the teacher about how the language impairment may be impacting upon academic performance. Valuable information can be gained by asking teachers to observe their students and respond to a few key questions relating language skills to classroom performance. Figure 7–3 illustrates a simple observation checklist designed to guide teacher's observations and descriptions.

Screening Secondary School Students

Most students with communication problems will have been identified and/or treated by the time they reach middle school or high school. As preparation for the world of work and postsecondary education is of primary importance to secondary teachers, some effort should be made to identify those secondary students who may experience difficulty transitioning from school to postsecondary activities due to communication problems. Teacher referral is one method of identifying students who may be at risk. As a follow-up to receiving a referral, the SLP can conduct an observation screening procedure. There are many opportunities to observe communication while students make oral presentations or participate in class discussions. Screening devices for adolescents often include reading short passages, answering questions posed by the examiner, and recounting events. Voice quality can be noted at the same time. The examiner needs to be aware of the possibility of fluency disorders in adolescents. Verification could be made by interviewing teachers who would be most likely to have heard the student in an informal speaking situation. These teachers might include the physical education teacher, the English teacher, the guidance counselor, and other people active in extracurricular activities.

Students in Special Education Classes

Classrooms in schools throughout the United States are populated with students representing varying levels of learning capability and diverse cultures. Children who present developmental, physical, or mental disabilities such as learning disabilities, developmental delays, cerebral palsy, emotional disturbances and autism may go undetected because the other disabling conditions are more obvious. In some instances, children may have been misdiagnosed as having a particular type of learning disability when in reality their primary problem is a hearing or speech-language impairment.

Children receiving special education services or being considered for placement in special education classes should receive a communication status evaluation as part of the multi-factored assessment process. The evaluations are carried out either at the school site or a nearby assessment center. Many city and county school districts and regional resource centers have centralized diagnostic facilities staffed by professionals with in-depth understanding and expertise. These programs accept referrals from education and health professionals within the district as well as from parents.

STUDENT ____ DATE __________

TEACHER ____ GRADE ________

To the Teacher: Read each of the following statements. Indicate those statements which are representative of the student's speech and language behavior. Refer children who cause you to be concerned for further testing by the Speech-Language Pathologist.

1. _____ In your opinion, the student demonstrates a noticeable communication problem which may be affecting educational performance.

2. _____ The communication problem is most noticeable during:

    _____ Communication tasks (Written ________ Verbal ________)

    _____ Classroom discussion

    _____ Social communication

    _____ Mathematics

    _____ Language Arts

    _____ Spelling

    _____ Oral reading

    _____ Other

3. _____ The student has difficulty understanding subject-related vocabulary.

4. _____ The student has difficulty understanding subject-related concepts.

5. _____ The student has difficulty following written or spoken directions.

6. _____ The student does not understand figurative language.

7. _____ The student has poor reasoning and problem solving ability, showing difficulty with cause/effect relationships.

8. _____ The student's response to questions is inappropriate.

9. _____ The student has difficulty participating in class discussions.

10. _____ The student has difficulty expressing ideas or relating stories and experiences.

11. _____ The student's sentence structure, word choice, or sentence organization interferes with his ability to clearly express the message.

12. _____ The student's speech production (articulation, voice, fluency) makes the conversation difficult for adults to understand.

13. _____ Other students in the class seem to have difficulty understanding the student.

Figure 7–3. Observation to determine language functioning in the classroom.

Limited English Proficiency

Children who live in homes where the primary language is different than English or children who come to school speaking a different language may be referred to as "English Language Learners," "bilingual," "limited English proficiency," or "linguistically different." Teachers often refer these children because they struggle to participate in class due to language barriers and communication breakdowns. They pose unique challenges for educators and SLPs because they may or may not present a communication disability. The SLP must apply the appropriate screening and differential diagnostic screening methods and evaluations. Children's performance may be affected by the selection of test items and materials, performance requirements (e.g., cognitive, motor, and communicative), the verbal style used by the tester, or the testing situation itself.

The SLP's goal is to determine if the child's communication behaviors are due to a disorder or a language difference. The SLP can prepare for this task by becoming familiar with the dialects and languages spoken in the community. Many states and districts have specific eligibility requirements that provide guidance to determine if an English Language Learner qualifies for speech-language services or would be more appropriately served in another way by another type of teacher or specialist with expertise in teaching students English Language Learners. Some characteristics that may point to a disorder versus a language difference are as follows:

- not able to "code switch" and alternate between both languages;
- use the home primary language even in an English speaking setting;
- significant birth or developmental history;
- showing academic difficulty in several subjects;
- processing difficulties;
- social interaction and communication difficulties;
- speech-language production problems in both languages; and,
- requires repetition and modification of instructions.

Alternatives to enrollment in speech-language services with an IEP that educators may consider are speech improvement programs or second language resource support. Options for helping this group of children vary from district to district and state to state. Effective instruction of English Language Learners raises a number of questions that should be discussed with administrators so that appropriate options for educational support or services can be offered. Districts in geographic locations with high foreign populations should also provide teacher training to provide teachers with teaching strategies to help students. The SLP's role is valuable in helping teachers and administrators differentiate disorder from difference in children's language skills.

Children with Hearing Impairments

Hearing impairment may lead to problems for children in the school environment.

Any type and degree of hearing impairment can present a significant barrier to an infant or child's ability to receive information from the environment (Flexer, 1999). Hearing impairment can have harmful effects on social, emotional, cognitive, and academic development. Impairments may limit the student's vocational potential as well. Due to the potential impact of hearing loss on communication development and learning, screening for hearing impairment should be included in the general developmental screening of all children (ASHA, 2004).

The early identification of children with hearing impairments, regardless of the extent of the hearing loss, should be of concern to the educational community. Appropriate intervention can result in improved developmental and learning outcomes. The effects of hearing loss on speech, language, social-emotional, and academic development are well documented (Baker-Hawkins & Easterbrooks, 1994; Bess et.al., 1988; Quigley & Kretschmer, 1982). Flexer (1992) uses a computer analogy to describe the potentially negative effects of any type and degree of hearing loss on academic performance. She states, "data input precedes data processing." In other words, in order to learn, children need to have information or data. In the classroom, the primary way information is entered into the brain is via hearing. If data are entered inaccurately the child will have incomplete or incorrect information to process and their performance will be affected.

Downs et al. (1991) define a hearing loss in children as, "any degree of hearing that reduces the intelligibility of a speech message to a degree inadequate for accurate interpretation or learning." The term "hearing impaired" implies a hearing loss of at least 15 dB HL. A person with a loss of 70 dB or more is considered to be deaf. Millions of school-aged children demonstrate some form and degree of hearing impairment.

There are numerous causes of hearing loss in children including middle ear infections, genetic causes, bacterial infections and viruses, prenatal causes, and noise exposure (Flexer, 1999). The following factors may place infants at risk for hearing loss: family history of childhood hearing impairment; congenital perinatal infection; anatomic malformations involving the face, head, or neck; low birth weight (less than 1500 grams); hyperbilrubinemia (jaundice) at levels exceeding indications for an exchange; transfusion; bacterial meningitis; and severe asphyxia.

Educationally, children with even mild and intermittent losses due to middle ear infection can have difficulties in the classroom. School children with hearing losses may be effected in three ways. They may experience delay in the development of communication skills; they may demonstrate poor academic achievement, and they may become socially isolated and have a poor self-concept due to reduced ability to understand and interact with others.

There are a number of problems a child may encounter in learning language if even a mild hearing loss exists. They may have difficulty abstracting the meanings of words due to inconsistent categorization of speech sounds. The noisy classroom may interfere with reception and their ability to discriminate sounds. They may encounter difficulty with perceiving meanings resulting in confusion in word naming and multiple meanings.

It may be difficult for children with hearing problems to detect grammatical rules or identify relationships between words. Recognition of intonation and stress patterns or the emotional content of conversation will be challenging.

Referrals for Hearing Problems

Teachers and parents are excellent referral sources for hearing problems. As with identifying speech and language disabilities, the quality of the referral will be increased if groundwork is laid in advance. Referral sources should gain an understanding of the importance of hearing for learning, those behaviors which might be representative of hearing problems, referral procedures, and follow-up recommendations. If a hearing loss is detected, the parent should be notified immediately of the results and recommendations. If warranted, the parent will be responsible for seeking medical assistance and informing school personnel of the results of any evaluations. Information about signs and symptoms individuals should consider of significance needs to be provided through in-service meetings or written materials.

The following groups of children are at high risk for potential outer and middle ear disorders: children who experience an episode of acute otitis media prior to 6 months of age; infants who have been bottle fed; children with craniofacial anomalies; ethnic populations with documented increased incidence of outer and middle ear disease; a family history of chronic or recurrent otitis media; children exposed to excessive cigarette smoke; youngsters living in crowded and unclean conditions; and children diagnosed with sensori-neural hearing loss. The history can be obtained by interviewing parents or requesting information in the letter sent to inform them of the screening program and schedule.

Educators and parents can be encouraged to refer children who display the following behaviors:

- *Appearance*—mouth breathing, discharge from the ear canal, malformation of the ear, earwax impaction, damaged or poorly maintained hearing equipment.
- *Behaviors*—constant tilting the head toward the sound source, inability to follow verbal directions, inattention, pulling or rubbing the ears frequently, asking for repetition of words or phrases, misunderstanding conversation of others.
- *Symptoms*—poor language development, buzzing or ringing in the ears, soreness pain in or about the ears.

Screening for Hearing Problems

Because of the importance of hearing to learning, school SLPs or health care professionals need to establish an ongoing identification program that will enable them to screen all children periodically during their school years. In addition, they should work closely with teachers to obtain referrals based on teachers' observations of the student's performance in the classroom. It is also helpful for parents, teachers, speech-language pathologists and others to provide descriptions of the student's listening behavior when making a referral for a hearing evaluation.

Pertinent information about the child's communication characteristics is particularly useful including:

- Child's ability to understand spoken directions and ability to follow directions with spoken words or gestures.
- Child's ability to express needs with gestures, sounds, words, signs and other symbols.
- Ability of listeners to understand what the child is trying to say.
- Child's behavioral response to sounds (startles, blinks, searching for sound, localizing sound, turning head in direction of sounds, etc.)

The members of the ASHA Panel on Audiologic Assessment (1997) recommended guidelines for audiologic screening across the life span. The guidelines consider several aspects related to screening including: (a) the principles of screening; (b) screening test performance; (c) screening program development, management and follow-up; (d) operating definitions; and (e) organizational framework. Screening involves a pass/refer procedure to identify children at risk for significant outer and middle ear disorders that have been undetected or untreated. There are guidelines for audiologic screening of infants and children age birth through 18 years. The guidelines recommend the clinical processes for screening for outer and middle ear disorders among older infants and children and for screening for hearing impairment among newborns and infants (ages birth through 6 months); infants and toddlers (age 7 months through 3 years); preschool children (age 3 through 5 years); and school-age children age 5 through 18 years. It is recommended that infants and children from 7 months through 6 years of age be screened. If it is not possible to screen those children, Bluestone and Klein (1996) recommend that children be screened if they present any of the significant clinical indications. The Panel addressed several aspects of the clinical screening process including: personnel, expected outcome, clinical indications, the clinical process, and pass/refer criteria, follow-up procedures, facilities and equipment, and documentation. They also made a statement about inappropriate procedures. As SLPs should be aware of these recommendations, the key points are highlighted in the following sections.

The student should pass the screening if no positive results exist for test criteria in both ears. He or she should be referred for a medical examination of the ears if ear drainage is observed; if there are previously undetected structural defects; if there are abnormalities in the ear canal; if the tympanometric equivalent ear canal volume is outside the normal range. The pass/refer criteria may need to be modified to optimize performance; but this should only be done by a qualified person.

Screening programs include procedures for detecting impairments of auditory sensitivity as well as peripheral auditory disorders. The goal is to identify individuals with hearing impairments that will potentially interfere with communication and/or individuals with potentially significant ear disorders that have been undetected or untreated. Children who fail the screening should have a complete audiologic evaluation and medical examination.

The screening protocol requires an otoscope or video-otoscope, and a screening or diagnostic tympanometer. You should participate in training to use the equipment. All equipment should be appropriately calibrated and maintained for electrical safety. Appropriate infection control procedures should be followed.

As with the speech-language screening program, mandates requiring that specific age or grade levels be tested vary from state to state. It is a generally accepted practice to screen preschoolers prior to school entrance, children in kindergarten, first, third, fifth, and ninth grades, all new students, transfer students, teacher and parent referrals, and students at risk for hearing loss due to noise exposure or other conditions.

Parents should be informed that the screening is being conducted. There should be an educational component designed to inform parents about the screening and the likelihood that their child might have an ear disorder. The information should be presented in a language they understand. Follow-up procedures should be recommended.

Responsibility for the Hearing Screening and Testing Program

Since the development of an audiologic screening program requires careful planning, implementation, and follow-up, it is recommended that it be designed, implemented and supervised by a qualified educational audiologist. In many school systems educational audiologists are not available, nor do the school systems have access to audiologic services in the community. If an audiologist is not available in the school district or region, SLPs would be wise to seek the advice and direction of a qualified audiologist. In some states school and public health nurses are licensed to conduct screenings in the schools. In many school systems the screenings are carried out by SLPs, nurses, or the cooperative efforts of both, often augmented by volunteers and aides. The personnel who administer the screening program should be adequately trained in the screening and referral procedures to ensure that the results they obtain are accurate and reliable. Ideally, the screening program should at least be supervised by an educational audiologist. Regardless of who implements the actual testing (educational audiologists, speech-language pathologists, or volunteers and aides), it must be implemented according to accepted standards of practice for identification audiometry.

Hearing Testing Environment

School clinicians encounter a number of problems in administering screening programs. One major problem is the lack of an adequate environment that is conducive to achieving reliable test results. It would be extremely unusual to find a space with an ambient noise level meets standards. Testing in an unsuitable room results in a large number of false failures and, eventually, in an inappropriate number of referrals. This can be translated into time wasted by the clinician and both time and money wasted by parents. Middle ear problems are often associated with slight conductive losses, so it is a possibility that many children with middle ear pathologies will not be detected if there is not strict compliance with recommended screening procedures, including using tympanometry procedures.

Advocating for Students with Hearing Impairment

SLPs can provide a valuable service to youngsters with hearing impairment by promoting an understanding of hearing; helping others understand the impact of hearing loss; aiding in screening programs; providing intervention for speech and language disorders; monitoring the functioning of hearing aids and assistive listening devices; and helping teachers employ educational management strategies that improve classroom performance. When audiologic services are not available, the SLP often assumes the responsibility of the hearing-conservation program, including the screening program. Other options include contracting for educational audiology services or sharing service providers with nearby school districts.

There should be a record of identifying information, screening/rescreening results, and recommendations for follow-up. Give complete information about the procedures performed, the results obtained, and the personnel who performed the procedure.

Assessment

According to federal and state laws, all children with disabilities must be assessed before placed in a special education program or before receiving instructional support services such as speech-language intervention. During the assessment process, data and evidence to support the presence of a communication disorder are gathered. Assessment is different from evaluation, which means interpreting or analyzing data. During assessment, information is gathered about the student's communication skills, the demands and expectations of the environment, and the manner and style of communication of the people in the child's environment. It is important to determine how these variables interact with one another. Parents or caregivers must give written permission before their child can be assessed for communication disorders.

Assessment cannot be discriminatory based on race, cultural diversity, or disability. The ASHA Preferred Practice Patterns for Profession of Speech-Language Pathology (2004) specifies the professionals qualified to perform the procedure, the expected outcome(s), clinical indications for performing the procedure, clinical processes, environmental and equipment specifications, safety and health precautions, and documentation aspects. Several recommendations for practice, regardless of setting, are addressed.

Assessment procedures are designed to produce a description of the communication behavior and gather information that will permit conclusions to be drawn about the student's strengths and deficits. It should help define contributing factors and functional implications. The results of the assessment must enable the clinician to determine the student's communication needs and how the communication impairment impacts on the student's educational performance. In addition, it should yield information about the positive and negative factors present in the communication situations that the student encounters.

During the assessment, information is gathered from numerous sources. A case history is completed through interviews and review of available records. The child is observed in the school and class setting so that the communication performance within typical contexts can be determined. Safety and health precautions such as infection control procedures should be followed. After the assessment and evaluation are completed, the clinician should be able to develop a statement of the diagnosis and clinical description of the disorder, make recommendations for type and intensity of intervention, and make appropriate referrals.

Assessments must be administered in the child's preferred communication or linguistic system and consider the child's age, medical status, and sensory status. This was also mandated in the 2004 reauthorization of IDEA. If these steps are not taken, the student may not be accurately assessed and the results will not honestly reflect the child's true achievement and aptitude level. Valid testing methods, standardized and nonstandardized, should be used. The materials, equipment, and environment selected for testing should be appropriate to the student's chronological and developmental age, physical and sensory abilities, education, and cultural/ethnic and linguistic background. For example, testing for a child who does not speak English should be conducted in the child's native language. Native language is defined as the language used by the child, not necessarily by the parents. A child who uses English at school but Spanish at home could be evaluated in English. However, if it is obvious that the child is more competent in Spanish, the testing must be done in Spanish. There are not many SLPs who are bilingual and can conduct assessments in the student's native language. Interpreters can be used to help achieve appropriate testing (Bader, 2011).

Clinicians have successfully used many different methods for assessing students' communication skills. Valuable information can be obtained by interviewing parents and educators. A variety of materials can provide substantial insights into the youngster's capabilities. During any assessment, it is imperative to maintain a perspective that children develop at different rates and that each child is different. Assessment materials and procedures should be individualized and developmentally appropriate. They should yield information about how the student learns and what would be the best way to teach him or her.

Materials commonly reviewed include portfolios of school work samples, language samples, journal entries, audio or video recordings, or class assignments. Student-created materials paint a much broader picture of the skills that are present. Schools maintain educational records that contain significant information. Completion of checklists or developmental scales enables comparison with other children in the same age group. Curriculum-based assessment methods such as reading inventories, proficiency tests, or other performance based reviews permit documentation of the performance within the educational context. SLPs have begun to use dynamic assessment methods that consider how the student performs after they are provided with instructions and assistance. This permits insight into how the student might be able to benefit with intervention. Of course, many norm-referenced and standardized instruments are available for assessing students' communication skills in specific communication domains. Clinician's experience and knowledge of communication development as well as acute observational skills provide a framework for conducting all assessment activities.

The process for learning is equally as important as the content of the curriculum. Cognitive-communication impairments may interfere with the learning process. Any data the SLP can contribute to increase education team members' understanding of this concept will likely result in better program planning for the student.

Documentation of procedures, findings, recommendations, and prognosis should be prepared. If treatment is indicated, recommendations of the frequency, estimated duration, and type of service required should be included.

Multifactored Evaluation

Federal and state laws mandate that each child with disabilities should be assessed in several domains, not just the suspected area of deficit. This is necessary for developing an educationally relevant educational and treatment plan. The evaluation should be multifactored. This means that the evaluation will be conducted by a multidisciplinary team. More than one area of the student's functioning will be evaluated so that no single procedure will be the sole criterion for determining an appropriate educational program placement. This is very important and ensures that students are not misclassified or unnecessarily labeled as being disabled.

The communicative status of all students suspected as having impairments should be at least screened by a speech-language pathologist to rule out the presence of communication impairment. If the screening results suggest a potential communication problem, appropriate comprehensive assessment should be initiated. A key goal is to identify the difficulties the student is having with relationship to the general education curriculum and environment.

Diagnostic-educational teams provide a comprehensive multifactored assessment for children with potentially significant problems, including children with communication problems. The child must be assessed in all developmental domains. The domains include curricular areas that represent early childhood development: adaptive domain, aesthetic domain, cognitive domain, communication domain, sensory-motor domain, and social-educational domain. The areas related to the suspected disability are assessed, and include, if appropriate, assessment of health, vision, hearing, social and emotional status, general intelligence, academic performance and achievement, communicative status, motor abilities, interests, preferences, employability, and adaptive behavior.

Clinicians work in collaboration with other professionals to determine the exact nature of the student's disability and the impact on learning. Professionals from related disciplines will complete many portions of the evaluation. This satisfies the requirement that the evaluation be multidisciplinary. Administration of the assessment protocol should be unbiased and given in such a way that it ensures that the student is not discriminated against regardless of cultural background, race, or disability.

The composition of the team may vary from district to district and is dependent on the characteristics and problems the student exhibits. The following personnel may be represented on multidisciplinary teams: audiologists, guidance counselors, occupational therapists, physical education teachers, physical therapists, physicians, principals, reading specialists, general education classroom teachers, general education curriculum supervisors, school nurses, school psychologists, social workers, special education supervisors and teachers, speech-language pathologists, and vision specialists. Parents, of course, are a required part of the multidisciplinary team. They contribute much to the evaluation process because they possess knowledge about their child's educational, social, and medical history.

Not all children with speech, language, or hearing impairments necessarily require a comprehensive evaluation, but such an evaluation of children with concomitant psychosocial or learning problems can be important in determining recommendations for services or class placement and intervention follow-up. Many types of assessment tools and procedures should be used to gather data during the multifactored evaluation process, including:

- Case history including medical, hearing, and developmental information;
- Assessment of physical and development factors;
- Administration of norm-referenced measures, criterion-referenced measures, standardized tests, and developmentally based tasks;
- Observation of performance in different situations, including the classroom and elsewhere in the school environment;
- Completion of interviews with significant persons including parents and teachers;
- Analysis of class work samples;
- Criterion referenced tests, standardized achievement tests, and other educationally relevant evaluation procedures;
- Review of family history; and,
- Review of school, and medical history.

The data gathered during the multifactored evaluation process are used to determine eligibility for special education or instructional support services, including speech-language intervention. *Thus, it is essential that the SLP and fellow team members know their district's eligibility criteria before assessing.* If standardized tests are administered but the conditions under which they are administered do not meet the standards for that instrument, then a description must be included in the evaluation report indicating the extent to which the administration differed.

Steps in the Multifactored Evaluation Process

Several steps must be followed during the multifactored evaluation process including:

1. Appointing a multidisciplinary team to conduct the assessment.

2. Developing an assessment plan that addresses obtaining a comprehensive description of the problems the student is demonstrating; specifying the information needed; and selecting appropriate evaluation instruments.
3. Conducting the multifactored assessments.
4. Analyzing the results.
5. Preparing a report of findings and reviewing the findings with other team members and the child's parents.
6. Determining eligibility for services.
7. Determining recommendations for placement or services and intervention.
8. Developing a plan for an IEP (Individualized Education Program), IFSP (Individualized Family Service Plan), or ITP (Individualized Transition Plan).

After all team members have completed their evaluation procedures and analyzed their findings, the information gathered by each member should be integrated and synthesized into one report. A sample of the extensive type of information that is generally gathered and analyzed to plan an individualized education program for a student is illustrated in Figure 7–4.

The Speech-Language Pathologist's Responsibility

The speech-language pathologist in the school system has the responsibility of providing diagnostic services for children referred by the multifactored assessment team. This includes all the children identified during speech, language, and hearing screening and those referred by teachers, nurses, parents, and others.

A minimal diagnostic appraisal would include an assessment of the student's articulation abilities and language competencies, fluency, voice quality, and hearing acuity and perception. Figure 7–4 provides a listing of information gathered to make the eligibility determination and develop the IEP. There should also be an examination of the peripheral speech mechanism. It is also important to have additional information, which can be obtained through a case history. Such information would include reason for referral, concerns expressed by parents or guardians, developmental history, family status and social history, medical history, behavioral observations, and educational history. A physical examination may be needed as well as a psychological and educational evaluation.

Parental permission is legally required for the evaluation procedures. Protocols should be developed to ensure confidentiality. The permission must be in writing, and usually a form is utilized for this purpose. In some cases the school system may not be able to provide some of the diagnostic procedures because of lack of specialized personnel or equipment. In this event the school system may arrange to have these procedures carried out by a qualified agency with qualified personnel in the immediate community or nearby. It is the responsibility of the school system to see that the required procedures are carried out. Such referrals are made only after written permission is obtained from parents.

Following is a list of the data sources the team gathers and uses to determine eligibility for services and to develop the IEP.

Identifying and contact information
Background information (health, nutrition, environment)
Academic or preacademic skills
Communication skills
Hearing ability
Motor ability
Behavior
Vision ability
Social/emotional behavioral
Vocational/occupational/transition needs
Medical health
Strengths, interests

Questions the Team Must Answer

- Has the evaluation eliminated lack of instruction in reading or math as a determining factor in reaching a conclusion about the presence of a disability?
- Has the evaluation eliminated English proficiency as a determinant factor in reaching a conclusion about the presence of a disability?
- Has it been determined that this student has or continues to have a disability?
- Describe how the child either meets or fails to meet the definition of the suspected disability for which the assessment was conducted.
- Does information confirm the disability condition has an adverse affect upon educational performance?
- Is special expertise needed to treat this student?
- Is a special instructional or intervention approach required?

Figure 7–4. Suggested components of the evaluation of communication status for disability conditions.

Scanning and Analyzing the Environment and People in the Environment

Clinicians must be prepared to conduct comprehensive assessments of many elements in order to determine a student's communication problems and their im= pact in order to confidently make recommendations for services and intervention. There is a planning concept that businesses and organizations use when determining their strategic business plans for the future. It is referred to as "scanning and analyzing the environment" (Figure 7–5).

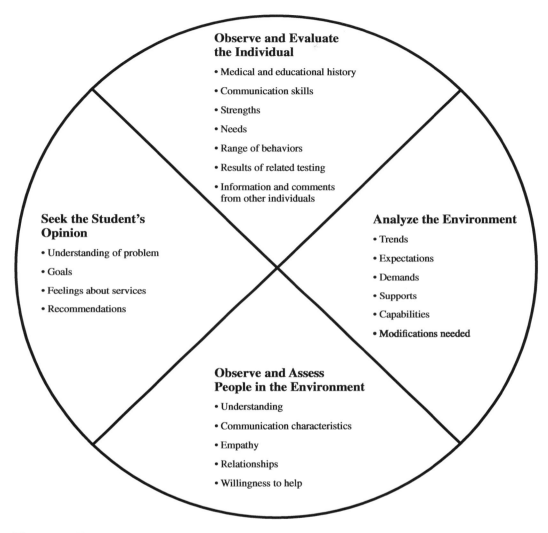

Figure 7–5. Scan and analyze the environment and people in the environment.

Speech-language pathologists can benefit from borrowing this concept. In this process, the SLP obtains a clear picture of the child's communication problems by conducting assessments of the following four aspects:

- *the communication problems the student presents* (medical and educational history; communication skills; strengths; needs; results from evaluation)
- *the environment in which he or she lives, plays, and learns* (expectations; demands; capabilities; aspects that may impede communication; modifications required)
- *the people in that environment who serve as significant communication*

partners (understanding of the student's problem; the partner's communication characteristics; ability to provide assistance)

- *the student's opinion, desires, understanding, and impressions* (understanding of the communication problem; goals; feelings; and recommendations for assistance).

This model is further explored in other sections throughout this book.

When assessing the student's communication skills, it is necessary to gather as much pertinent information as possible through a case history, medical history, and educational history. Information can be obtained by conducting interviews with the parents, the teachers, and if possible, the child. Records and reports can also be useful. Each informant contributes information vital to the construction of a whole picture of the child. For instance, the parents can give background information on the child's development. The teachers may provide needed information on the child's present academic status. The teacher should be interviewed to determine the communication requirements for success within the classroom setting and the student's present communication performance on educational and social tasks. This aspect of the assessment permits the team to determine the student's communication strengths and needs, the range of behaviors exhibited, and the results of tests that have been administered.

Observing the student in the home environment, classroom, and at play as a component of the appraisal process will yield valuable information for formulating the diagnosis and developing an intervention plan. Observations should help the team gain an understanding of the varying demands and expectations present in different situations and the student's capabilities for meeting those demands.

IDEA and best practices for conducting a comprehensive evaluation recommend that the child be observed within the classroom setting. Many districts leave the decision about how to conduct the observation up to the SLP. Other districts have established standardized procedures for conducting the classroom observation. Figure 7–6 illustrates a Classroom Observation Guide that considers the child's performance as well as key aspects in the classroom environment that may influence the student's participation and performance.

Three types of observations are described in a procedure manual prepared for SLPs in the San Diego City Schools (2004–2005). They are *narrative, participant,* and *anecdotal* observations.

- In the *narrative* observation, the SLP passively observes the student and writes notes during the observation. The SLP generally focuses on the context.
- In the *participant* observation, the SLP may engage in the activity being observed. For example they may lead or assist an activity. The SLP makes notes of observations during the activity. However, because he or she is participating, the notes may be briefer than the narrative notes. The SLP may expand on the notes after the observation.

Use this guide when observing a student during a learning activity within the classroom concept. Focus on identifying the demands and expectations of the learning activity and classroom situation. Mark all statements that describe the learning activity, instruction, and classroom environment that you observe. Consider your observations in relation to the student's functional communication skills. Ask yourself—"What modifications in the instructional activity could have led to improved performance?"

Student ______________________________ Date ______________

School ______________________________ Grade/Placement ________

Subject or Learning Activity Observed (Briefly Describe)

Teacher's Instructional Communication

- ○ Provided verbal instructions or explanation
- ○ Provided written instructions or explanation
- ○ Supported instruction with examples, objects
- ○ Explained concepts to increase students' understanding
- ○ Organized flow to instructions
- ○ Used appropriate length and vocabulary level
- ○ Signaled transition from activity to activity
- ○ Confirmed that instructions were understood
- ○ Restated instructions
- ○ Responded to students' questions

Teacher's Location During Instruction

- ○ Front of classroom
- ○ Side of classroom
- ○ Back of classroom
- ○ Meeting with small group of students
- ○ Roaming

Seating Arrangements for Students Participating in the Learning Activity

- ○ Desks in rows or similar arrangement
- ○ Circle
- ○ Large group all students
- ○ Small group/<10 students
- ○ Varies with activity

Figure 7–6. Classroom observation guide. This guide can be used when observing students' performance in the classroom. Focus is on developing a better understanding of the demands and expectations for functional communication skills during classroom learning activities. *continues*

Student Workspace
- ○ Near where the teacher is instructing
- ○ Away from where the teacher is instructing
- ○ Removed from auditory or visual distractions
- ○ Near auditory or visual distractions
- ○ Organized
- ○ Disorganized
- ○ Distracted by other students

Instructional Materials Used During the Learning Activity
- ○ Chalkboard/whiteboard
- ○ Textbook
- ○ Workbook/worksheets
- ○ Objects
- ○ PowerPoint
- ○ Audio recordings
- ○ Other

Student's Options for Response
- ○ Raise hand and speak
- ○ Submit paper product
- ○ Provide explanation
- ○ Engagement in activities
- ○ Presentation
- ○ Follow-up assignment

Pace of Instruction
- ○ Slow
- ○ Average
- ○ Fast

Amount of Time Allocated for the Learning Activity

<15 minutes
15–30 minutes
30–45 minutes
45–60 minutes

- ○ Not enough
- ○ Ample
- ○ Too much

Figure 7–6. *continues*

Method for Assessing Learning ○ Verbal responses/explanations ○ Written responses ○ Quizzes/Tests ○ Demonstration ○ Explain to another person
Classroom Environment ○ Friendly ○ Supportive ○ Relaxed ○ Fast ○ Engaging ○ Formal
Summarize Observations of the Demands and Expectations for Successfully Participating in the Learning Activity. Recommend Modifications and Strategies that Can Lead to Improved Performance.

Figure 7–6. *continued*

- During an *anecdotal* observation, the SLP or another person such as a classroom aide or teacher observes various segments of time in the classroom and writes notes that describe what the child is doing or saying. The notes provide many examples.

The focus of typical classroom observations conducted by SLPs is often on the child and his or her communication performance during classroom activities. Although this is essential, critical information may be overlooked when only the child's performance and behavior is observed. By focusing only on the child, the SLP may miss the opportunity to determine what demands and expectations are placed upon the child and the critical role of the teacher's manner and style of providing instruction. Thus, it is equally important to observe the classroom climate, environment, and those individuals who communicate with the student on a daily basis. This type of environmental observation provides significant information about others' understanding of the student's communication impairment, how that problem impacts on learning, and how their own communication characteristics can help or hinder the child's performance.

This concept is explored further in Chapter 10 which discusses collaborating with fellow professionals. Increasing the child's significant communication partners' awareness of the dynamics of the communication disability and explaining how they might contribute to the child's success by modifying their own behavior will lead to a more effective treatment plan.

The student should also be incorporated into the planning for their own treatment as often as possible and when appropriate. The SLP can contribute to the development of strong self-advocacy skills in the child by providing opportunities for better understanding the disability. If provided with guided questions geared toward the child's developmental age and level of understanding, the student may also be able to contribute to the development of intervention goals and activities. Students can provide information that may be of great value to the clinician. Figure 7–7 illustrates a student interview form developed by Blosser and DePompei (2002). Note how the questions that are asked of students can lead to goals that meet students' needs and interests.

After the background information is obtained, the clinician needs to add to it by describing the problem. Observing the child's performance on appropriate tests that measure the degree of the problem and suggest associated aspects does this. The clinician must be an astute observer and must be able to record information objectively and without bias. In other words, the clinician must be a good "reporter." After all the information has been gathered, the clinician makes a diagnosis of the communication problem (or problems).

A diagnosis, or identification of the problem, is in reality a tentative diagnosis because as a human being grows and changes, the problem changes along with environmental changes and challenges. A diagnosis is much more than putting a label on a person. It is convenient for professional persons to use diagnostic labels when communicating with one another if all parties concerned understand that the label is not the diagnosis. A diagnosis involves weighing all the evidence, discarding some of it as not being pertinent, and keeping the information that merits further investigation.

On the basis of the gathered information, the testing, and the tentative diagnosis, the clinician then determines the prognosis and sets up a long-range plan for the intervention procedures. The long-range plan includes therapy appropriate to the communication problem as well as other strategies and treatment. The school clinician is involved in collaborative team approach with others who are interested in the child's welfare, and these individuals work as a team in establishing an Individualized Education Program (IEP), Individualized Family Service Plan (IFSP), or Individualized Transition Plan (ITP). The school clinician is responsible for the appraisal and diagnosis of the communication problem, but the clinician is a team member in the overall appraisal, diagnosis, and treatment of the child. Final decisions about the student's educational placement rests with the team, including the parents.

Eligibility for Speech-Language Services

The purpose of the assessment and diagnostic procedures is to determine if children are eligible for speech-language services offered by the school district.

Let Us Know How to Help You

You are the best judge of how other people can cause difficulty for you or help you do better. Answer these questions and let's work together to figure out ways to help you talk and listen better.

1. Tell five things that are great about you that you wish other people knew.
2. What problems are you experiencing in class (at home, at work)? Briefly describe the problems you are having (with fellow students, with teachers, with your schoolwork).
3. How do you usually act when you experience problems or frustrations in class (at home, at work)? List some of the ways you behave when you are having problems.
4. What classroom (home or work) situation causes you the most problems?
   - Noise
   - Temperature
   - Pictures and wall decorations
   - Other people in the room
   - Other things
5. List several ways your teachers (family, classroom, coworkers) help you when you experience trouble in class (at home or work).
6. What do you think people should do to help you?
7. List several things your teachers (classmates, coworkers) do to frustrate you or cause you more problems.
8. What do you think people should stop doing when they are around you?
9. At what time of the day do you do your best? Why do you feel this is your best time of day?
   - Early morning
   - Mid-morning
   - Around noon
   - Mid-afternoon
   - Early evening
   - Late evening
10. If you could choose three skills to improve, what would they be?

Figure 7–7. Student interview questions.

The school clinician must be prepared to describe how the student's disability will interfere with his or her ability to benefit from classroom instruction. The final decision regarding eligibility for program services rests with the school team. Four critical questions must be considered by the education team.

1. Based on the diagnosis, does the student present a disability?
2. Does the disability adversely affect the student's educational performance or participation in class and social activities?
3. Are specially designed interventions or instructions and/or related services and supports required to enable the student to access and make progress in the general education curriculum?
4. Is the expertise of a speech-language pathologist required to provide the specially designed intervention or instruction?

IDEA describes a speech or language impairment as, "a communication disorder, such as stuttering, impaired articulation, language impairment, or voice impairment that adversely affects a child's educational performance." States may establish definitions for clinicians and others to follow that differ slightly from the federal definition.

The Individuals with Disabilities Education Act (IDEA) requires that services be based on the individual student's needs that effect participation and progress in the general education curriculum and extracurricular and other nonacademic activities. Decisions regarding the provision of speech-language services or dismissal from services are part of a complex decision making process. Eligibility criteria provide clinicians and other teammates with guidelines for identifying the population to be served. Some districts may refer to eligibility as entrance criteria. The ability to establish and manage a caseload of children with communication impairments begins with understanding the eligibility criteria for receipt of services. All SLPs within a district should follow the district's adopted eligibility guidelines to ensure consistency for decision making across the district. The eligibility criteria that the school team establishes should be standardized within the school district and appropriate to the population served with respect to age, development, culture and/or linguistic diversity, cognitive factors, and health status. Some state departments of education have established eligibility criteria for speech-language intervention programs as well as for other special education programs. ASHA has also provided some guidance on determining eligibility criteria over the past several years. Task forces and committees continue to work on interpretations that are helpful to practitioners. Many articles and documents on determining eligibility are available. Three documents that provide excellent guidance are Roles and Responsibilities of the School-Based SLP (ASHA, 2010), Roles and Responsibilities of Speech-Language Pathologists in Early Intervention: Technical Report (ASHA, 2008) and Admission/Discharge Criteria in Speech-Language Pathology Guidelines (ASHA, 2004).

Eligibility and dismissal criteria can be very valuable when advising teachers and parents about the need for services. In addition, agencies that are charged with reviewing or accrediting programs can also use the eligibility and dismissal criteria for evaluating services or student management. This might include funding sources, governmental agencies, and school district administrators. Clinicians within a district should work together to determine how they will interpret specific aspects of the eligibility and dismissal criteria including terminology and application to certain populations such as adolescents or students with autism.

Determining Eligibility

Eligibility guidelines provide a mechanism to ensure consistency of case identification, prioritization, and selection among clinicians in a district. Guidelines also serve as a framework for evaluation of the demographics of the caseload (incidence, numbers, types of disorders, and severity of students served). A fully certified speech-language pathologist must base eligibility for speech and language services on a comprehensive evaluation. With key input from the SLP, the team then considers the relationship between the student's speech and language disabilities and the adverse effect they may have on the student's ability to access the general school curriculum including academic, social-emotional, or vocational aspects. Thus, the team must consider the need for services as well as the eligibility for services on the basis of federal and state mandates and local policies and procedures (ASHA, 2004).

According to IDEA, a child is eligible to receive services provided by the school when he or she exhibits a speech or language impairment that has an adverse effect on participation and educational performance to the degree that specially designed instruction or related services and supports are needed to help the student make progress in the general education curriculum.

A group of qualified professionals and the parents are charged with working as a team to determine if the child has a disability. They must use information from a wide variety of sources to make their determination. This can include tests, parent input, teacher recommendations, samples of the student's work, observations, and information about the child's health condition, cultural background, and behavior.

Under most eligibility guidelines, children cannot be determined to have a disability if there is a lack of appropriate instruction in reading or math or if the student demonstrates limited English proficiency. This determining factor is extremely important since many SLPs receive high numbers of inappropriate referrals to evaluate and treat students who exhibit reading difficulties or limited English proficiency. For example, teachers may refer students for speech-language services if they present a dialect or demonstrate lack of English proficiency. Although we can be compassionate about the teacher's concern, the student is not likely to be qualified for speech-language services. Instead, the teachers and team should be re-directed to refer the student to an education professional who has expertise in providing educational services and support to English Language Learners and to use a variety of specialized language instruction strategies in their classroom. In order for ELL students to qualify for speech and language services, they must demonstrate the impairment in both languages. Therefore, the student's dominant language must be determined before assessments are conducted.

Adverse Effects

In order to conclude that a disability has an adverse effect on a student's educational performance, the multidisciplinary education team must determine and document that as a result of the disability the student is functioning significantly below age and grade norms for age and grade peers in one or more of the basic skills (language arts, literacy, math, science). SLPs and fellow education team members must document that the impairment adversely impacts educational performance, attracts adverse attention, or significantly interferes with participation, communication, peer interaction, movement, and so forth. Many states have defined adverse effect in their special education policies and procedures.

As an example, the Vermont Special Education Rules (Rule 2362) explain that for all types of adverse effect, significantly below "age or grade norms" means that the student's performance is determined to be among the lowest 15% of students at the child's grade level. On norm referenced tests, adverse effect would be designated by a percentile score at or below the 15th percentile, or a standard score that is at least 1 standard deviation below the mean (typically 85 or below). For adverse effect measures that don't include norm scores (e.g., grades, criterion-referenced tests, work samples, and curriculum-based measures) the multidisciplinary team needs to determine that the student's performance is at a level equivalent to the lowest 15% of grade level peers. It is advisable for team members to cite at least three different measures and document that the adverse effect has been present for at least six months (Vermont Department of Special Education, 2010).

The issue of adverse effect is very controversial and has resulted in many debates among SLPs, educators, parents, and administrators. First and most importantly, each child must be considered individually on a case-by-case basis. Consequently, if two children present an articulation disorder, they are not both automatically considered eligible for speech-language services. The SLP and team have to determine if the education success for each is being impacted by the articulation disorder. The issue is even more complex when you take into consideration the fact that the acquisition of communication skills are required as an integral part of the school's academic curriculum and standards. Therefore communication is considered a basic skill for all students. The logic is that students with speech or language impairments have a disorder that adversely may affect educational performance.

To build a case that a student's disability has had an adverse effect on educational performance, it is advisable for the multidisciplinary team to cite a least 3 different measures and document that the adverse effect has been present for at least 6 months. Figure 7–8 is an adapted version of a checklist that was created by the Vermont Department of Education Student Support Team. It was designed to help teams identify and use a variety of adverse effect measures.

In order to reach a conclusion that a disability has an adverse effect on a student's educational performance, the multidisciplinary education team must determine and document that, as a result of his or her disability, the student is functioning significantly below age and grade norms for age and grade peers in one or more of the basic skills.

Many state and local district's special education policies and procedures provide guidelines for determining adverse effect. As an example, significantly below "age or grade norms" can be interpreted as meaning that the student's performance is determined to be among the lowest 15% of students at his or her grade level. Education team members may use a variety of assessments to determine adverse effect. Following are some examples:

- Norm referenced tests
  - Adverse effect is designated by a percentile score at or below the 15th percentile, or a standard score that is at least 1 standard deviation below the mean (typically 85 or below).
- Measures that do not include norm scores (e.g., grades, criterion-referenced tests, work samples and curriculum based measures)
  - The multidisciplinary team needs to determine that the student's performance is at level equivalent to the lowest 15% of grade level peers.

It is recommended that the team cite at least 3 different measures and document that the adverse effect has been present for at least 6 months.

Following are some questions that can be used by team members to identify and use a variety of adverse effect measures.

YES	NO	Type of Measure
		General Guidelines
		Does documentation of adverse effect make a convincing case that the student's disability has led to basic skill deficits that are preventing access and progress in the general curriculum?
		Is the disability referenced to at least one basic skill area?
		Is the student's performance among the lowest 15% of age and grade level?
		Is the performance documented in reference to grade level norms?
		Has the disability been present for at least 6 months?
		If not present for 6 months, does documentation establish that the disability is not temporary/will escalate without intervention?

Figure 7–8. Documenting adverse effect. Adapted from the Vermont Department of Education (2002). *continues*

YES	NO	Type of Measure
		Test Scores
		Do scores from standards-referenced tests such as state standardized test indicate that the student's performance (e.g., below the standard, little or no evidence) is in the lowest 15% compared to all students at that grade level?
		Are scores on norm-referenced tests (individually administered) or (group administered) at or below the 15th percentile or at least 1 standard deviation below the mean?
		Grades
		Is the student among 15% of students getting lowest grades?
		If student is passing, are grades based on individualized criteria? (15% or less with the greatest needs?)
		When grades from homogeneously grouped classes are used, has adverse effect been compared to average performing students?
		Is the student passing with special education?
		Does documentation shows that removal of supports/services would adversely affect performance?
		The student is passing with special education. Does documentation show a history of adverse effect when services are not provided?
		Does documentation establish the indirect relationship between skill deficits and grades.
		Using Curriculum-Based Measures
		Documentation reference expected performance for average students at that age indicates lowest 15% performance.
		Using Criterion-Referenced Tests
		Does the student lack skills or knowledge typical for grade-level?
		Is the student among the lowest 15% compared to expected grade level peers?
		Does documentation indicate a link between cognitive profile and performance?

Figure 7–8. *continues*

YES	NO	Type of Measure
		Students with Emotional or Behavioral Problems
		Does documentation establish a link between behavior and acquisition of basic skills?
		Is test performance above the 15%ile. Other measures indicate potential behavior problem.
		Refusal or lack of work production is linked by a team member to basic skills.
		Special Circumstances
		Is adverse effect documented in relation to benchmarks for students in restrictive placements and/or placements that have no clear grade/age-level norms.
		Speech/language disabilities: 3 different documentation measures are taken reflecting age and grade-level expectations.

Figure 7–8. *continued*

Classification of Procedures and Communication Disorders

A good place to start any referral, assessment, or eligibility process is to come to an agreement on the definition of terms. Clinicians who work together in a particular school district, region, or state will find it useful to mutually agree upon definitions to be used to describe and discuss children with communication disabilities.

Over the years many ASHA and state licensure committees have reviewed terminology and submitted definitions to their members. Definitions for communication impairments and treatment have been accepted and disseminated for use by federal, state, and local agencies and others concerned with programs for those with communication impairments. The school speech-language pathologist must be able to define and interpret the terminology to parents, teachers, medical personnel, and legislators. Commonly accepted definitions of communication disorders and variations are presented below (ASHA, 1993).

Communicative Disorders

A *communicative disorder* is an impairment in the ability to: (1) receive and/or process a symbol system, (2) represent concepts or symbol systems, and/or (3) transmit and use symbol systems. The impairment is observed in disorders of hearing, language, and/or speech processes. A communicative disorder may range in severity from mild to profound. It may be developmental or acquired, and individuals may demonstrate one or any combination of the three aspects of communication disorders. The communicative disorder may result in a primary handicapping condition or it may be secondary to other handicapping conditions.

Speech Disorders

A *speech disorder* is an impairment of voice, articulation of speech sounds, and/or fluency. These impairments are observed in the transmission and use of the oral symbol system.

1. A *voice disorder* is defined as the absence or abnormal production of vocal quality, pitch, loudness, resonance, and/or duration.
2. An *articulation disorder* is defined as the abnormal production of speech sounds.
3. A *fluency disorder* is defined as the abnormal flow of verbal expression, characterized by impaired rate and rhythm which may be accompanied by struggle behavior.

Language Disorders

A *language disorder* is the impairment or deviant development of comprehension and/or use of a spoken, written, and/or other symbol system. The disorder may involve: (a) the form of language (phonologic, morphologic, and syntactic systems), (b) the content of language (semantic system), and/or (c) the function of language in communication (pragmatic system) in any combination.

Form of Language

1. *Phonology* is the sound system of a language and the linguist rules that govern the sound combinations.
2. *Morphology* is the linguistic rule system that governs the structure of words and the construction of word forms from the basic elements of meaning.
3. *Syntax* is the linguistic rule governing the order and combination of words to form sentences, and the relationships among the elements within a sentence.

Content of Language

Semantics is the psycholinguistic system that patterns the content of an utterance, intent and meanings of words and sentences.

Function of Language

Pragmatics is the sociolinguistic system that patterns the use of language communication which may be expressed motorically, vocally, or verbally.

Hearing Disorders

A *hearing disorder* is altered auditory sensitivity, acuity, function, processing, and/or damage to the integrity of the physiological auditory system. A hearing disorder may impede the development, comprehension, production, or maintenance of language, speech, and/or interpersonal exchange. Hearing disorders are classified according to difficulties in detection, perception, and/or processing of auditory information. Hearing-impaired individuals frequently are described as deaf or hard of hearing.

1. *Deaf* is defined as a hearing disorder that impedes an individual's communicative performance to the extent that the primary sensory avenue for communication may be other than the auditory channel.
2. *Hard of hearing* is defined as a hearing disorder whether fluctuating or permanent, which adversely affects an individual's communication performance. The hard of hearing individual relies upon the auditory channel as the primary sensory avenue for speech and language.

Communicative Variations

1. *Communicative Difference/Dialect* is a variation of a symbol system used by a group of individuals which reflects and is determined by shared regional, social, or cultural/ethnic factors. Variations or alterations in the use of a symbol system may be indicative of primary language interferences. A regional, social, or cultural/ethnic variation of a symbol system should not be considered a disorder of speech or language.
2. *Augmentative Communication* is a system used to supplement the communicative skills of individuals for whom speech is temporarily or permanently inadequate to meet communicative needs. Both prosthetic devices and/or nonprosthetic techniques may be designed for individual use as an augmentative communication system.

Caseload Composition

Caseload composition refers to the specific number of students and the range of communication problems served by a clinician. There is great variability in caseload size and composition from district to district. Therapists often seek guidance regarding the maximum or minimum number of students they can carry on their caseload. They seek that information from ASHA as well as their state associations, licensure boards, administrators, and colleagues. Indicating a specific number of students for a caseload is not necessarily advisable because it does not reflect factors such as the severity of the disorder or the full workload required to carry out the roles and responsibilities.

Although many clinicians desire specific guidance and greater consistency for caseload composition and numbers, the variability is understandable as factors such as demographics, severity, complexity, economics, alternative services and resources that may be available, service philosophy, and state or local mandates differ from place to place. Some state and local education agencies mandate the minimum or maximum number of students that should comprise the caseloads of speech-language pathologists. Thus, the numbers of students served may be different than would be recommended if clinicians were given full control and responsibility for determining caseload composition and size. Due to this situation, SLPs in many school districts may serve very high numbers of students as compared to their peers in other locations. There is little or no agreement at this writing among state and local education agencies concerning what constitutes an ideal or appropriate caseload size.

To determine the SLP's caseload number and type of students to be served, it is important to consider the total *workload* that is necessary to ensure that students receive the full range of services they need. The workload encompasses the time required for conducting evaluations, preparing reports, collaborating with teachers, documenting services, meeting with parents, preparing the classroom environment, training others and more (ASHA, 2002).

Determining Severity

The severity of the impairment is an important factor in determining the need for treatment, the appropriate program placement and/or service delivery model. Therapists must determine the amount, frequency, and intensity of services to provide for children. These aspects of communication should never be considered in isolation. They should be made in relation to the student's age, the demands and expectations of the communication situation, and the impact on learning and performance in the educational setting. These decisions are especially difficult when there are numerous children who present communication disorders.

Severity ranking methods enable the clinician to systematically determine those students who many need the most intense level of services. Unfortunately, there are no nationally accepted procedures or guidelines for rating severity that are common across the profession. Clinicians in different regions in the United States have developed different methods for rating severity. Some methods are very simplistic while others are complex. Many of the severity rating models that have been developed have similar design elements:

- They are based on a continuum of performance model.
- Severity is rated on scale, for example, from "No Problem" to "Mild," "Moderate," or "Severe."
- A combination of objective data is used to determine adverse effect on education performance may include obtaining speech samples, standardized tests, contextual probes, structured observations, classroom work samples, academic results, teacher reports and interviews, child reports and interviews, and parent reports and interviews.
- Descriptive statements are provided about characteristics of the speech-language skill areas to assist the user in deciding the rating number or category to assign. For example, a severity rating scale for

articulation/phonology may consider the aspects of intelligibility, stimulability, phonological processes, error types, and development. The *language* category may consider whether the student presents deficits in language aspects such as semantics, morphology, syntax, or pragmatics. The clinician's determination of severity may be the result of formal or informal assessment measures, impact on educational performance, impact on functional performance, and other factors. A *voice* scale might rate symptoms such as pitch, quality, intensity, or resonance. The tool may ascribe a rating to etiology and physical conditions as well as the effect on communication including the reactions of casual listeners, reactions of significant others, and self-awareness. The *fluency* category would consider aspects such as the interference with communication interaction, the number of stuttered words per minute and percentage of words stuttered, speech rate, duration, awareness, and secondary characteristics. Some considerations should be made for children with disabilities in addition to communication impairments such as mental and developmental disabilities.

The development of eligibility guidelines and severity rating systems should be directed by several guiding principles. In this way, the process of case decision-making will ensure continuity and consistency among all clinicians within the school district. Such a system can help organize the service delivery program according to students' needs. A rationale also can be determined for the allocation of treatment time. There will be accountability for how decisions are made. If a method is appropriately designed, it will incorporate observation of consistent variables by SLPs, teachers, parents, and other professionals without compromising clinical judgment. It will assist the clinician in case decision-making. More importantly, it will drive decisions about who will provide the services; the frequency, intensity, and duration of service; and the delivery model for the least restrictive alternative in a continuum of service delivery options.

Some severity rating scales provide a numerical index to facilitate the rating process. Categories are typically included for: (1) standardized (norm-referenced) test results; (2) nonstandardized assessment results (descriptive); (3) educational relevance and potential impact on educational performance; (4) specific type of disorder; and, (5) prognostic indicators that indicate low potential for success. Following is an explanation of each category.

Standardized Test Results

Students are provided with a complete multifactored, multidisciplinary test battery. A basic numerical factor is obtained from the results of the evaluation. Some protocols assign numeric value to test scores.

Nonstandardized (descriptive) Assessment Results

Clinicians use a variety of methods to collect data about a student's functional communication skills and needs. Common procedures include checklists, interviews, developmental scales, review of student's work, curriculum-based assessment, samples of speech and language performance, and observations in different settings. Again, support for eligibility will increase or decrease based on the findings.

Educational Relevance and Potential Impact on Educational Performance

Upon evaluation of the assessment data and determination of the type of disabilities that are present, the SLP and team should determine how the communication impairment may interfere with the student's learning. Three key educational areas that may be affected are academic, social-emotional, and vocational performance. If the SLP, teachers, and family all agree there is an adverse effect on educational performance, the eligibility for treatment would increase.

Specific Type and Severity of Communication Disorder

Some types of disorders that students exhibit may interfere more with successful educational performance than others. Likewise, the severity of the disorder will cause differing levels of performance and require different amounts of intervention and support. When SLPs complete their evaluation of specific speech and language areas, they are able to discuss the likely impact of the presenting disorder on the student's performance on specific aspects of the curriculum such as reading, writing, oral speaking, mathematics, and so on.

Prognostic Indicators

Some aspects of the student's performance may, in fact, indicate that treatment is not warranted. Prognostic indicators are likely to contribute to a student's success or lack of success. By considering those prognostic factors that do not support treatment, the clinician can provide documentation and rationale for not providing services or for reducing and limiting services to students. Speech-language pathologists also exercise their clinical judgment when determining which children to serve and the service delivery models to provide. Some prognostic indicators that are considered include:

- Chronologic and mental age of the child
- Potential for change due to maturation
- Overall intelligibility and stimulability
- Type of communication problem detected
- Response to intervention methods
- Responsiveness to correction
- Cultural variables
- Gross and fine motor skills
- Auditory memory span
- Orofacial functioning and structure
- Discrimination skills
- Personality and adjustment
- Length of time in therapy
- General health

- Support and cooperation provided by family and teachers
- Academic performance
- Self-motivation.

The diagnostic and eligibility factors determine the type of service that should be provided and lead to recommendations regarding who will provide the services and the frequency, amount and duration of treatment. A student whose communication is within normal limits is not eligible for services. The child with a mild communication delay may be served effectively through indirect or alternative service delivery models such as coaching teachers to use communication strategies. The student with severe disabilities generally needs more direct and frequent services. In all cases, it will be important for the SLP and education staff to plan collaboratively to determine how the student's needs may be best met.

Although a system that is developed for one school system may not be applicable to all school districts, it is important to adhere to a conceptual framework when thinking about how to make caseload selection and service delivery model decisions. Using systematic processes for decision making and standardized practices will enable the clinician to be accountable for the decisions. Ultimately, this type of information is necessary in order to document the importance and effectiveness of the speech-language intervention program. Data generated will help the clinician support discussion of changes in program design and implementation of new service delivery models. One excellent example of a rating scale designed by a team of SLPs is illustrated in the Communication Rating Scales (North Inland SELPA, 2007; Selk, Bartz, Birrenkott, & Olmos, 2008). Tables 7–1 to 7–5 present examples of articulation, language, voice, and fluency scales.

Table 7–1. Communication Severity Scale: Articulation/Phonology. Reprinted with permission from North Inland SELPA.

COMMUNICATION SEVERITY SCALE

ARTICULATION/PHONOLOGY

Date ____________

Student ____________

Birthdate ____________ Age ________

	No Apparent Problem/Discrepancy	Mild	Moderate	Severe
Sound Production[1, 2]	0 No phoneme and/or phonological process[1] error(s), or student's speech is characterized by error(s) that are consistent with normal development.[2]	1 Speech is characterized by phoneme error(s) 1 year below developmental age/chronological age. 1 phonological process error 1 year below normative data.	3 Speech is characterized by phoneme error(s) 1-2 years below developmental age/chronological age. 2 phonological process errors 1 year or more below normative data.	5 Speech is characterized by phoneme error(s) more than 2 years below developmental age/chronological age. More than 2 phonological process errors 1 year or more below normative data.
Stimulability[3]	0 Phoneme and/or phonological process error(s) are stimulable for correct production in several contexts. Targeted sound(s)/phonological processes are adequate for speech production at the sentence level.	1 Phoneme and/or phonological process error(s) are stimulable in at least one context. Targeted sound(s)/phonological processes are adequate for speech production at the word level.	3 Phoneme and/or phonological process error(s) approximate correct production. Targeted sound(s)/phonological processes are adequate for production in isolation or at the syllable level.	5 Most phoneme and/or phonological process errors are not stimulable for correct production.
Intelligibility/Effect on Communication[2]	0 Inconsistent phoneme and/or phonological process error(s) do not affect intelligibility. The student's speech error(s) do not interfere with social/emotional, educational, and/or vocational functioning.	1 Connected speech is more than 80% intelligible; error(s) may be noticeable to listeners. The student's speech errors have minimal impact on social/emotional, educational, and/or vocational functioning.	3 Connected speech is between 50-80% intelligible when context is unknown. The student's speech error(s) interfere with social/emotional, educational, and/or vocational functioning.	5 Connected speech is less than 50% intelligible, although isolated words may be intelligible. Gestures/cues are usually needed. May severely detract from content. The student's speech error(s) seriously limit social/emotional, educational, and/or vocational functioning.

[1] Phoneme and/or phonological process disorders must be present in 2 or more positions of a word to be considered as errors.
[2] Do not include regional or dialectal differences without applying other environmental/cultural considerations.
[3] Check Stimulability only for sounds at or below chronological or developmental age.

Table 7–2. English Learner Analysis. Reprinted with permission from North Inland SELPA.

ENGLISH LEARNER ANALYSIS

	Normal 0	**Emerging 1**	**At Risk 2**	**Significant 3**
# of Years in USA	____Newcomer	____1-2 years	____2-3 years	____More than 3 years
Educational History	____Change in language instruction within 2 years ____Responding to basic instruction ____Appropriate response to instructional strategies ____ELD (English Language Delivery) services for less than 1 year	____Consistent language of instruction for at least 2 years ____Responding to 2 or more subject areas ____Slow Response to instructional strategies ____ELD services for 1-2 years	____Consistent language of instruction for more than 2 years ____Responding to less than 2 subjects ____Limited response to instructional strategies ____ELD services for 2-3 years	____Consistent language of instruction for more than 3 years ____Not responding to 3 or more subjects ____Not responding to instructional strategies ____ELD services for more than 3 years
Language Development	____L1 proficient within expectancy according to developmental/ chronological age ____L2 proficient within expectancy guidelines *(i.e., L2 Acquisition Stage I-II) ____Overall bilingual communicative skills are within expectancy with teachers and same language peers ____Appropriate use of classroom Discourse Skills	____L1 slow and/or inconsistent rate of progress ____L2 acquisition slow and/or inconsistent rate of progress *(i.e., L2 Acquisition Stage I-IV) ____Overall communication demonstrates mild difficulty in receptive skills in L2; slow or arrested development in L1, or both languages (reported) ____Emerging use of classroom Discourse Skills	____L1 slow and limited progress according to observable/reported peer/family interaction ____L2 acquisition limited progress *(i.e., L2 Acquisition Stage I-III) ____Overall communication demonstrates moderate difficulty in receptive skills and expressive skills; plateau in both languages for more than one year (observable) ____Minimal use of classroom Discourse Skills	____L1 no growth/regression according to measures, peer/family interaction ____L2 acquisition arrested / regression *(i.e., L2 Acquisition Stage I-II) ____Overall communication demonstrates significant difficulty in either or both receptive and expressive skills (reported and observable) in L1 and L2 ____Ineffective use of classroom Discourse Skills
Levels of evidence (academic/ language measures & analysis)	____1 year or less below A.G.E. ** (Adjusted Grade Expectancy) ____Presents with weakness, yet steady progress Progression in Academic and Language measures: ____ ____ ____	____1-1½ years below A.G.E. ** ____Presents with 2 or more areas of strengths Progression in Academic and Language measures: ____ ____ ____	____2 years below A.G.E. ** ____More weaknesses than strengths Progression in Academic and Language measures: ____ ____ ____	____More than 2 years below A.G.E. ** ____Weaknesses significantly effect strengths Progression in Academic and Language measures: ____ ____ ____

If majority of observations fall within 2 and 3, evaluation may be warranted.

* **TESOL** (see the following chart)

** **A.G.E. – highest grade level of instruction in L1**

Table 7–3. Communication Severity Scale: Voice. Reprinted with permission from North Inland SELPA.

COMMUNICATION SEVERITY SCALE

VOICE

Date ______________

Student ______________

Birthdate ______________ Age ________

	No Apparent Problem/Discrepancy	Mild	Moderate	Severe
Characteristics	0 Slight pitch, quality, intensity, and/or resonance variations may be present.	1 Voice quality may be harsh or raspy; occasional pitch breaks may occur. Intensity differences may be intermittent. Pitch may be inappropriate for age/sex. Resonance may be slightly hyper/hyponasal. Voice difference calls attention to itself.	3 Frequent pitch breaks interfere with vocal continuum. Hyper/hyponasality interferes with intelligibility. There is an intermittent, noticeable difference in the intensity or quality.	5 Persistent, noticeable differences in pitch, intensity, quality, and/or resonance are evident in a variety of settings. Vocal production is extremely limited or non-existent.
Etiology-Current Physical Conditions	0 Physical factors influencing quality, resonance, or pitch, if present at all, appear to be temporary and may include: allergies, colds, abnormal tonsils and adenoids, short-term abuse, or misuse.	1 Laryngeal or structural pathology may be suspected. Physical factors may include nodules, polyps, ulcers, edema, palatal insufficiency, etc. Medical evaluation usually indicated. Medical evaluation always required if increased tension is the appropriate intervention.	3 Probable presence of laryngeal or structural pathology. Physical factors may include nodules, polyps, ulcers, edema, partial paralysis of vocal folds, palatal insufficiency, enlarged/insufficient tonsils and/or adenoids, neuromotor involvement, hearing impairment, etc. Medical evaluation required.	5 Physical factors include laryngeal pathology, hearing impairment, neuromotor involvement of laryngeal muscles, cleft palate, etc. Possible psychosomatic factors. Medical evaluation required.
Effect on Communication	0 The student's voice does not interfere with social/emotional, educational, and/or vocational functioning.	1 Distracting to some listeners. The student's voice difference/disorder has minimal impact on social/emotional, educational, and/or vocational functioning.	3 Distracting to most listeners. The student's voice disorder interferes with social/emotional, educational, and/or vocational functioning.	5 The student's voice disorder seriously limits social/emotional, educational, and/or vocational functioning.

Table 7–4. Communication Severity Scale: Fluency. Reprinted with permission from North Inland SELPA.

COMMUNICATION SEVERITY SCALE

FLUENCY

Date ____________

Student ____________

Birthdate ____________ Age ________

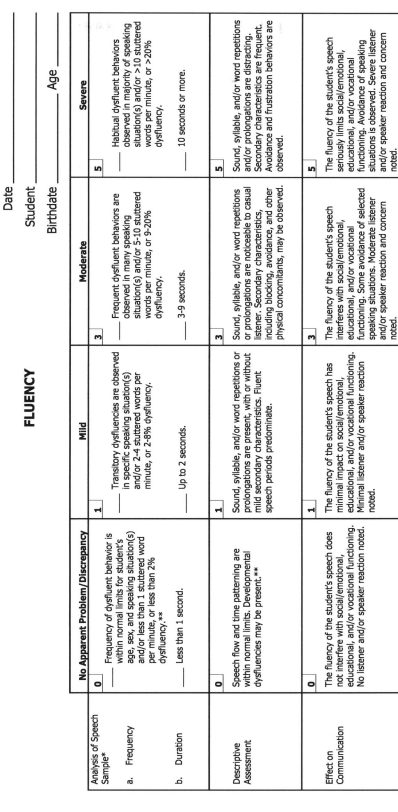

	No Apparent Problem/Discrepancy	Mild	Moderate	Severe
Analysis of Speech Sample* a. Frequency b. Duration	0 ____ Frequency of dysfluent behavior is within normal limits for student's age, sex, and speaking situation(s) and/or less than 1 stuttered word per minute, or less than 2% dysfluency.** ____ Less than 1 second.	1 ____ Transitory dysfluencies are observed in specific speaking situation(s) and/or 2-4 stuttered words per minute, or 2-8% dysfluency. ____ Up to 2 seconds.	3 ____ Frequent dysfluent behaviors are observed in many speaking situation(s) and/or 5-10 stuttered words per minute, or 9-20% dysfluency. ____ 3-9 seconds.	5 ____ Habitual dysfluent behaviors observed in majority of speaking situation(s) and/or >10 stuttered words per minute, or >20% dysfluency. ____ 10 seconds or more.
Descriptive Assessment	0 Speech flow and time patterning are within normal limits. Developmental dysfluencies may be present.**	1 Sound, syllable, and/or word repetitions or prolongations are present, with or without mild secondary characteristics. Fluent speech periods predominate.	3 Sound, syllable, and/or word repetitions or prolongations are noticeable to casual listener. Secondary characteristics, including blocking, avoidance, and other physical concomitants, may be observed.	5 Sound, syllable, and/or word repetitions and/or prolongations are distracting. Secondary characteristics are frequent. Avoidance and frustration behaviors are observed.
Effect on Communication	0 The fluency of the student's speech does not interfere with social/emotional, educational, and/or vocational functioning. No listener and/or speaker reaction noted.	1 The fluency of the student's speech has minimal impact on social/emotional, educational, and/or vocational functioning. Minimal listener and/or speaker reaction noted.	3 The fluency of the student's speech interferes with social/emotional, educational, and/or vocational functioning. Some avoidance of selected speaking situations. Moderate listener and/or speaker reaction and concern noted.	5 The fluency of the student's speech seriously limits social/emotional, educational, and/or vocational functioning. Avoidance of speaking situations is observed. Severe listener and/or speaker reaction and concern noted.

* Recommended Procedure: Tape record speech sample of 150 words minimum for calculations. Average three longest blocks to determine duration.
** See Continuum of Dysfluent Behaviors.

IMPORTANT NOTE: Special consideration needs to be made for preschool or beginning stutterers. They should be monitored frequently and carefully if not enrolled for direct or indirect treatment.

Table 7–5. Communication Severity Scale: Language. Reprinted with permission from North Inland SELPA.

COMMUNICATION SEVERITY SCALE

LANGUAGE

Date ____________________

Student ____________________

Birthdate ____________ Age ________

* Standard scores are based on a mean of 100 and a standard deviation of 15. The standard score may be a receptive, expressive, or total language quotient. For students who are English Learners, the evaluation needs to be conducted in their dominant language ____________________.

	No Apparent Problem/Discrepancy	Mild	Moderate	Severe
FORMAL ASSESSMENT Comprehensive, Standardized Measure(s) and Scores	0 Standard score* of 78 or above. Less than 1.5 SD below test mean for chronological age or developmental level.	1 1.5-2 SD below test mean/cognitive level in one or more ___ Semantics ___ Morphology ___ Syntax ___ Pragmatics	3 2-2.5 SD below test mean/cognitive level ___ Semantics ___ Morphology ___ Syntax ___ Pragmatics	5 > 2.5 SD below test mean/cognitive level ___ Semantics ___ Morphology ___ Syntax ___ Pragmatics
INFORMAL ASSESSMENT Check descriptive tool(s) used: ___ Communication Sample ___ Checklist(s) ___ Observations ___ Family/ Educational History ___ Other	0 Language skills are within expected range for chronological age and/or developmental level.	1 *At least one of the following areas is deficient.* Check area(s) of weakness: ___ Sentence length/complexity ___ Word order/syntax ___ Vocabulary/semantics ___ Word finding ___ Word form/morphology ___ Use of language/pragmatics	3 *At least two of the following areas are deficient.* Check areas of weakness: ___ Sentence length/complexity ___ Word order/syntax ___ Vocabulary/semantics ___ Word finding ___ Word form/morphology ___ Use of language/pragmatics	5 *At least three of the following areas are deficient.* Check areas of weakness: ___ Sentence length/complexity ___ Word order/syntax ___ Vocabulary/semantics ___ Word finding ___ Word form/morphology ___ Use of language/pragmatics
FUNCTIONAL/ EDUCATIONAL LANGUAGE SKILLS	0 Functional language skills within expected range for chronological age and/or developmental level.	1 The student's language deficits have minimal impact on social/emotional, educational, and/or vocational functioning.	3 The student's language deficits impact social/emotional, educational, and/or vocational functioning. The student may require more cues, models, explanations, and checks on progress or assistance than typical student.	5 The student's language deficits severely impact social/emotional, educational, and/or vocational functioning. The student does not perform effectively most of the time despite the provision of general education modifications and supports.

Describing Functional Communication

Identifying the nature of a student's communication impairment is important. However, describing how the student functions provides key information that can be used for planning appropriate services. The National Outcomes Measurement System (NOMS) is an instrument that was developed by ASHA decades ago to provide a framework and process for clinicians to obtain and report data about treatment outcomes. The NOMS represents a national effort to develop a common language for describing and rating students' functional communication skills. There are adult as well as pediatric versions. In 2010 use of the NOMS that had been designed for use in school-based programs was suspended so that a team of leaders in pediatric and school service delivery could review how clinicians had used the tool and create new methods for proving the value and benefits of speech-language services. Even though the NOMS was pulled for review and improvement, there are many positive aspects about the NOMS process that bears discussion. Most importantly, the NOMS design offers a systematic method for measuring specific aspects of a student's functional communication. The NOMS Functional Communication Measures (FCMs) provides a mechanism for school based clinicians to report descriptive data about their caseloads and service delivery models. It could also be used to measure the effectiveness of treatment over time.

The NOMS includes a 7-point rating scale ranging from least functional (1) to most functional or independent (7). Functional communication is defined as the ability to convey or receive a message regardless of the mode of communication. Guidelines are provided for measuring each aspect of functional communication skills: composition, fluency, emergent literacy, intelligibility, pragmatics, reading comprehension, speech sound production, spoken language comprehension, spoken language production, voice, word recognition, and writing accuracy. The NOMS definitions provides a way for determining the functional status measures considering the support required to assist the student in becoming a functional and independent communicator. The NOMS also considers the verbal, comprehension, pragmatic, or vocal demands placed on the student in variety of situations including educational, social, and extracurricular activities. The explanations for each of the seven levels for each of the functional communication measures enable the user to rate the student's functional communication from very dependent to consistently independent. As an illustration, following are some examples of the type of terms that are used to describe the student's functional communication at Levels 1, 4, and 7.

> *Level 1:* Rarely grade or age appropriate; not functional for communication; not understandable to familiar listeners; unaware of incorrect productions; avoids spoken interactions.
>
> *Level 4:* Usually age appropriate in low demand educational activities; occasionally age appropriate; usually successful when maximum support to

reduce the verbal demand is provided; ability to participate is occasionally limited; rarely self-monitors.

Level 7: Consistently grade level; consistently appropriate; consistently successful; speech does not call attention to itself; self-monitoring is used as needed; consistently understood by listeners; not dependent on others.

The intent of the NOMS and Functional Communication Measures is to provide SLPs with a tool that will enable them to measure change in functional communication abilities over time from entrance to dismissal from speech-language services. In other words, the NOMS is a valuable tool for measuring outcomes. As the NOMS project continues and the results are verified through additional research, there will be opportunities for determining how these instruments can be used to describe students' communication behaviors and make clinical decisions.

Clinical Judgment

Regardless of the rating procedure or scale used, we cannot dismiss the importance of clinical judgment. In conjunction with assessment methods, the speech-language clinician needs to consider the following factors:

- The consistency of the inappropriate communication patterns;
- The student's ability to interact verbally with others;
- The effect of the communication problem on school performance;
- The possible impact of the communication problem on the listener;
- The ability of the student to communicate well enough to satisfy his or her needs;
- The status of speech and language stimulation in the home;
- The student's response to stimulation of the deficit in speech and language structures;
- The student's chronologic age in comparison with the expected age for developing the communication skills that are in deficit or missing.

Matching the Right Student with the Right Services and Intervention

After the assessment data has been gathered, the clinician evaluates the data and comes to a conclusion about the nature and severity of the communication disorder. It is, at this point, that the SLP and fellow team members (including educators and family) face three difficult tasks. First, the team must determine if the student meets the *eligibility criteria* for treatment and services. Second, the child's *functional communication level* should be established. Third, the *intervention and service delivery model* most appropriate to meet the student's needs must be determined. The type of services to be provided as well as the service providers and the frequency and intensity of treatment are critical aspects of establishing the SLP's caseload, schedule, and workload.

Educational colleagues and school administrators responsible for determining policy for special education programs in the district should be aware of the decision-making criteria that SLPs follow to determine eligibility, severity, and priority case selection. The case identification and selection system and procedures should be in written form and made available to administrators and educators within the district in order to improve accountability and understanding of the functioning of the program. If the case selection system is understood, then the cooperation of other school personnel can be readily enlisted. The principal is a key figure in the success of SLP and other related services programs. Teachers who are familiar with case selection procedures tend to work collaboratively with clinicians and assist children in their classroom. Having a documented eligibility and case identification system is also useful for helping parents understand the rationale for recommendations regarding their child's program. This knowledge also helps others understand why some children are not eligible for services should questions arise.

Service Completion: Discharging Students from Therapy

In the process of selecting students for therapy, diagnosing, providing therapeutic intervention, and maintaining students in therapy, sometimes too little attention is paid dismissal or discharge from services. It is important to continuously reevaluate whether or not as student should continue to receive speech-language services, discontinue services, or be provided with another type of services that may be more appropriate given the student's performance.

Initial discussions about dismissal from services should begin when the student is first determined eligible for services and the IEP is formulated. Make goals of the speech-language intervention services clear to parents and teachers at that time. Help them realize that success means dismissal from therapy. The question of when a child should be exited from treatment may be predicated on when the pupil reaches maximum anticipated performance or when the student's communication problem has been completely improved. Here are a few important points to highlight in your conversation with parents and teachers:

- The student should be dismissed when his or her impairment no longer creates an adverse effect on education.
- The focus of services may be to reduce the effect of the impairment.
- Dismissal may occur before a student demonstrates complete mastery of all targeted skills. In other words, intervention should not be expected to continue until performance is perfect or 100% accurate.
- As the student improves, the context and/or location of the services may shift from the therapy room to other contexts such as the classroom or resource room and more people will be engaged to give the student experience at using

improved communication skills with others.

After the student has been placed in a therapy program the short- and long-term performance objectives are identified and written in the intervention plan. The objectives are based on characteristics identified through testing, observation, comments from parents and teachers, and discussion with the student.

The desired outcomes of treatment are a statement of what the student should be able to do at the termination of the treatment program. The short-term objectives are the steps through which the student must progress successfully to reach the long-term objectives. This, in effect, means that long-term (or terminal) objectives constitute the exit criteria, or the point at which the student is dismissed from therapy. This is part of the intervention plan (IEP, IFSP, or ITP).

Obviously, the nature of the disorder will have a direct bearing on the expected outcome of treatment. For example, a student with cerebral palsy and apraxia may not be expected to attain "normal" speech patterns, depending on the extent of the involvement. This dismissal point for this student may be "adequate" speech or understandable communication using an augmentative device. A student with a phonological problem potentially may be able to attain a more complete mastery of the distorted sounds, and the dismissal point for this student would be when the student could use the sounds correctly.

Dismissal from services is covered in IDEA (2004) regulations. Unless the student graduates from secondary school or has reached the age of 22, reassessment of a student is required. SLPs must develop criteria for service completion that is unique for each student and terminate therapy when these criteria are met. This means that dismissal from therapy may occur at any time during the school year. This is a change in practice for some clinicians who are used to carrying students on their caseloads throughout an entire academic year. Students who have not reached optimum improvement at the end of the school term are often continued into the following term. Students who transfer to another school are referred to the SLP in that school system. Parents should be urged to inform the new school that their child has been in therapy and they wish it to continue. In this situation, the referring clinician secures the proper release forms to transfer the student's therapy records to the new school.

When a dismissal is made, the child should be scheduled for periodic rechecks to find out if the skills developed in therapy are being maintained. The classroom teacher and parents can be called on and coached to observe the student's communication and report on progress as well. When engaging others in this way, it is helpful to be very specific about what communication patterns sound like.

Four steps that practitioners follow when determining if services should be continued are as follows:

- Hold a reevaluation planning meeting to review existing current data regarding the student's progress and performance.
- Determine what additional data may be needed to make the decision (standardized and nonstandardized assessments, curriculum-based assessments, student work portfolios).

- Conduct additional assessment procedures recommended by the IEP Team.
- Include the family in the planning and discussions.

When the student has reached the optimum levels of performance, it is time for dismissal. The criteria for dismissal are unique to each child and must be carefully established, evaluated, and reevaluated during the course of treatment. If necessary, they must be adjusted or modified in the light of more knowledge about the student. In addition to providing rating scales for determining selection for the caseload (eligibility criteria), it is also important to provide clear guidelines for determining readiness for program completion (dismissal criteria). Some examples of dismissal criteria are listed below:

- Speech and language goals and objectives have been met.
- Speech and language skills are developmentally appropriate or are no longer academically, socially, personally, or emotionally affecting the student. Documentation must be present by one or more of the following: student, teachers, parents, speech and language clinician.
- The student has made minimal or no measurable progress after one academic school year of consecutive management strategies. During that time, program modifications and varied approaches have been attempted and a second opinion has been obtained.
- Maximum compensatory skills have been achieved or progress has reached a plateau due to cognitive ability level, structural deviations (e.g., severe malocclusion, repaired cleft lip or palate, physical condition of the vocal mechanism, or other physical deviations or conditions); or neuromotor functioning (e.g., apraxia or dysarthria).
- Limited carryover has been documented due to the student's lack of physical, mental or emotional ability to self-monitor or generalize the behavior in one or more environments.
- Due the nature of the student's impairment, he or she could be served better elsewhere.
- Lack of progress or inability to retain learned skills due to poor attendance and participation, although program IEP goals and objectives have not been met. Poor attendance and participation records should not stand alone, rather it is the lack of progress or retention which is of primary concern when utilizing this criteria.
- The student has graduated from high school or has reached the age of 22 years.
- Individuals who are significant in the child's life no longer see a need for services.
- Associated and/or disabling conditions prevent the student from benefiting from services.
- The student uses assistive technology aids appropriately, effectively, and independently.

Who Determines Eligibility or Dismissal?

A placement team composed of those individuals with the greatest knowledge of the child must always make the decision regarding eligibility for services and appropriate placement of the child with disabilities. This includes the child's parents. The parent need not be the natural parent of the child as long as he or she meets the legal qualifications of the parent surrogate. The federal law also specifies that the team should include a representative of the local educational agency, the teacher, and if appropriate, the child. Although the law does not state that other individuals are required to be present, good educational practice would suggest that other team members also attend. This list would include those persons who by virtue of their professional backgrounds and the child's unique needs would reasonably be expected to be involved. It might include the principal, psychologist, reading teacher, occupational therapist, physical therapist, vision consultant, and speech-language pathologist and audiologist. The results of the multifactored evaluation and the possible placement options should be available when the placement team meets.

Coordinator of the Placement Team

The representative of the local educational agency usually is the case manager and coordinator, and as such arranges for the meeting, presides over the meeting, determines that all necessary persons are present, and acts as spokesperson for the school system. The chairperson presents the necessary information and data or calls on the person responsible for presenting it. The chairperson also has the responsibility of informing the parents of their rights. Setting the tone of the meeting and seeing that all the basic ingredients of the Individualized Education Program are present, and that the procedures are carried out according to state and local guidelines, are also within the responsibilities of the chairperson.

The Teacher as a Team Member

The teacher is the person most responsible for implementing the child's educational program. The teacher in the case of the child with communication handicaps may be the speech-language and hearing clinician or the classroom teacher. The teacher's responsibilities as a team member at the meeting include explaining to the parents the learning objectives, curriculum and various techniques that are used to meet the annual goals. The teacher will also explain to parents why one particular strategy was used instead of another. In addition, the teacher will answer questions parents might have about events that occur within the classroom. In effect, the teacher is the main emissary between the school and the parents.

Speech-Language Pathologist's Role on the Team

The role of the speech-language clinician on the placement team may vary according to state regulations and the guidelines and practices of the local education agency. If the child in question has a communication problem, the person providing the language and speech services in the school needs to participate in the placement process. Although the full placement team has the responsibility of developing an educational program for each pupil, the school clinician should be prepared to provide input into the process of establishing goals, objectives, prognosis, and intervention strategies. The school clinician will also be responsible for reporting to the placement team the results of any diagnostic and assessment testing and may recommend further testing.

Family as Team Members

Family members can provide insights about the home situation, the impact of the disability on interactions and home activities, and factors that may be contributing to the child's problems. Making family team and members gives both family and speech-language pathologists, as well as other members of the team, an opportunity to observe each other's interaction with the student, The family may be team members in the actual diagnosis, treatment, and carrying out of the IEP, IFSP, or ITP. Furthermore, the more the caregivers are included in these processes, the smoother and the more consistent is the delivery of instruction to the child. Both family and SLPs gain from the insights of the other, and both will be able to use each other as a source for added ideas. Also, family and SLPs will be able to keep each other informed about the progress of the child.

Reports to caregivers, both oral and written, should be in clear, understandable language and not in professional terminology, sometimes referred to as jargon. Clear explanations of the diagnosis and treatment strategies should be made to caregivers. The SLP should make it plain to caregivers that diagnosis is an ongoing process and that, as the child changes and progresses, the assessment of his or her condition will change.

Speech-language pathologists should avoid labels as much as possible when talking with family. If labels have to be used, it should be made clear to family that the terms are merely words for explaining the communication disorder.

The Placement Team's Purpose

The ultimate result of the placement meeting is to develop an IEP, IFSP, or ITP for the child and to achieve agreement to that plan by the parents and professionals. The plan must be a written document, prepared and distributed according to the policies of the state and local education agencies. Policies also regulate who shall have access to the report and how copies shall be made available. A copy of the report is made available to the parents. All placement team members sign the report.

In most cases the speech-language pathologist is a member of the team if the child displays communication difficulties. If the clinician is not on the team (an unlikely, but not impossible, situation), a copy of the document should be made available.

Ethics and Responsibilities

Selection of testing procedures and, ultimately, of those students who will or will not receive services in our programs should be guided by professional ethics and standards of practice. For example, if during the testing session with a child another area of testing is identified, it is the SLP's responsibility to refer that child for services by the appropriate professional. This may mean a medical referral for a physical condition observed, the school psychologist for a learning disability detected, or the guidance counselor for a suspected emotional or social problem. This necessitates looking at the "whole child" not just the speech and language behaviors displayed. Children are complex creatures. We cannot diagnose or treat them in isolation. We must report the total picture that we observe when we create our description of the child's behaviors and needs (Peterson & Marquardt, 1990).

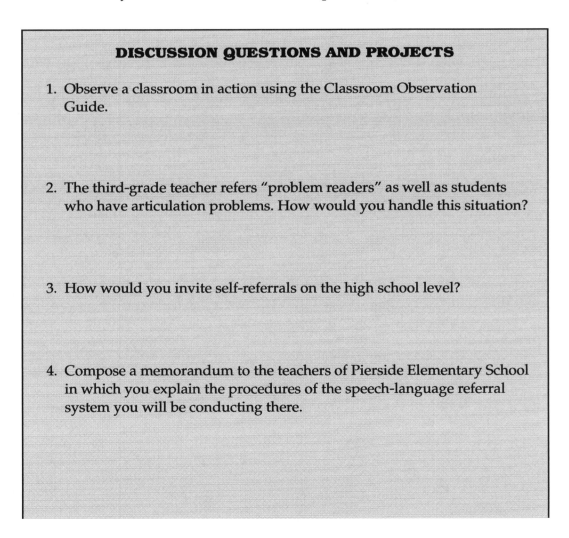

DISCUSSION QUESTIONS AND PROJECTS

1. Observe a classroom in action using the Classroom Observation Guide.

2. The third-grade teacher refers "problem readers" as well as students who have articulation problems. How would you handle this situation?

3. How would you invite self-referrals on the high school level?

4. Compose a memorandum to the teachers of Pierside Elementary School in which you explain the procedures of the speech-language referral system you will be conducting there.

5. Interview a school-based SLP to find out what procedures are used to identify, select, and prioritize students for the speech-language caseload.

6. Survey several SLPs in the schools to find out how they identify students who may have a hearing loss.

7. Find out how preschool children with communication disorders are identified in your area.

8. Using the Communication Severity Scale, determine the level of severity of two of the students on your caseload.

9. Develop a library of examples of speech and language disorders.

10. Develop a list of materials that can be incorporated into a presentation to parents and/or teachers.

8

Considerations for Service Delivery and Scheduling

The roles and responsibilities of the speech-language pathologist working in the educational setting have changed greatly in the past few decades. IDEA mandates that, as a related service, speech-language therapy must support the student's IEP by addressing the necessary skills in the least restrictive environment. Intervention and services should be designed to help the student achieve as much as possible from his or her education or special education program. The SLP's roles will continue to change as our understanding of the needs of children with communication disabilities expands, as the impact of communication impairments on learning becomes more clearly defined, and as service delivery methods improve. SLPs can no longer implement their programs in isolation from the rest of the educational system. Speech-language pathology services are an integral part of the total educational program for children with disabilities. Clinicians have increased responsibilities for demonstrating how communication disabilities impact the learning process across the curriculum, especially in the area of literacy. There is a demand to design programs that will increase children's potential for success within the educational setting.

Federal legislation greatly impacts the role of the speech-language pathologist in education. The laws specify requirements for identifying children with impairments, providing appropriate services based on individual needs, incorporating parents into the planning process, collaborating with fellow educators, and making available a broad range of service options. Legislation fosters change in the way speech-language services are provided. Schools are required to align all programming, including speech-language assessment and intervention services with the curriculum and state education standards. Schools are continually challenged to adhere to state standards and comply with federal legislation. As discussed in Chapter 3, the push for high quality education standards resulted in the creation of The Common Core State Standards for English Language Arts and Literacy in History/Social Studies, Science and

Technical Subjects (2010). As members of the education community, school-based SLPs can contribute much to ensuring that students access the curriculum and achieve success.

Service delivery refers to how services will be provided for children. Service delivery options must be determined in collaboration with other members of the student's IEP team. The decision of how services are delivered can only be made after the team has jointly addressed what the student's impairments are, the resulting impact on school performance, whether the expertise of an SLP is required, and what specialized interventions will be necessary to support the student and meet his or her needs. In this chapter, a range of service delivery options for children with communication disabilities are explored. Emphasis is placed on determining ways to match students with the right interventions and service delivery. Children may present communication "differences," "deficits," or "disorders." Explanation is provided of a wide range of options for delivering services to meet the needs of this range of communication skills. For example, children with speech and language *difference* are likely to benefit from teachers using specialized strategies for working with English Language Learners during classroom instruction. Children with mild *deficits* often show change when they participate with other children in a speech-language improvement program. Children with communication *disorders* that affect their educational progress or attract adverse attention benefit from more frequent and intense services. In those situations, an IEP is developed and an individualized plan of intervention is initiated.

The many different contexts for service delivery are briefly described. The definitions of communication disorders and an understanding of the range or continuum of service delivery alternatives may be considered the building blocks of good program development and management. The complex issue of determining what to do with children placed on the caseload and how to individualize intervention and services are explored. In addition, scheduling alternatives and other important variables when scheduling various age or disability groups are presented.

Speech-language pathologists and special educators have vigorously debated the effectiveness or efficiency of many of the service options. There is not always agreement among professionals on a right or wrong approach. However, there is consensus that the approach selected must be designed to meet each individual student's needs. Fortunately, the discussions continue and often generate more evidence. Eventually, some common ground may be reached.

Classification of Procedures and Communication Disorders

It is beneficial to use terminology that is standardized and consistent when discussing or describing communication impairments and procedures to others. The World Health Organization's *International Classification of Functioning, Disability, and Health: Children and Youth Version* (ICF-CY) is the system of assigning codes to diagnoses and procedures used in health settings for billing and record keeping (National Center for Health Statistics, 2010; World Health Organization, 2010). The codes specify the Body Structure, Body Function, and Activities and Participation that are addressed by individual intervention approaches (McCauley & Fey, 2006; Williams, McLeod, & McCauley, 2010). The terms can be used by SLPs within speech-language programs in school settings as well, especially by those clinicians who work in school districts that bill Medicaid for services. The ICF-CY nomenclature and classification system can be used to uniformly describe the communication disorders they treat and the procedures used for assessment and therapy. The system is especially valuable for clinicians interested in analyzing their service programs, generating research data about their caseloads, or developing a computerized information management system. The Classification System can be accessed on the ASHA, the Center for Disease Control and Prevention or the World Health Organization Web sites.

ASHA has also developed a resource describing practice approaches that are essential to good service delivery. Referred to as the Preferred Practice Patterns for the Profession of Speech-Language Pathology, these statements define universally applicable activities that are directed toward providing service to clients/patients (The American Speech-Language-Hearing Association, 2004). This includes the requisites of practice, the processes to be carried out, and expected outcomes. The idea behind the Preferred Practice Patterns is to provide an informational base to promote the delivery of quality care. They are flexible and yet definitive enough to enable decision-making for appropriate clinical outcomes. They reflect the generally accepted professional response to a particular set of client characteristics or circumstances. School-based clinicians can use the Preferred Practice Patterns as a tool for discussing common practices that can be utilized throughout the school district or for discussing service delivery needs. In addition, they can be given to administrators to promote better understanding of the profession. The Preferred Practice Patterns are reviewed and updated periodically. The Communication and Language Intervention Series (Williams, McLeod, & McCauley, 2010; McCauley & Fey, 2006) also provides a comprehensive resource that describes intervention methods and key service delivery recommendations for speech and language disorders.

Inclusion

SLPs seek ways to incorporate inclusive models of service delivery that merge speech and language services with educational programming. Inclusive practices are based on the unique and specific needs of the individual and are provided in a setting that is least restrictive (ASHA, 1996). The term inclusive practices means that the services are designed to meet the unique needs of the student and his family. There are many factors that are considered when designing the intervention and services. They include but are not limited to, age, communication competence, type of disability, language and cultural background, academic performance, social skills, education concerns, and attitudes. Inclusionary practices have been mandated by IDEA since 1997.

Clinicians strive to develop services and acceptable service delivery environments for all children with special needs, especially those who demonstrate severe disabilities such as autism spectrum disorders. Personnel working in educational settings must demonstrate that their services will support the student so that he or she can participate to the maximum extent possible in social and learning contexts (Hales & Carlson, 1992). These directions would indicate that the general education classroom should always be considered the first step in the options for service delivery for students with communication disabilities.

Clinical effectiveness is defined in terms of helping students reach measurable, functional outcomes so they can participate in school, community, family, work, and play activities. Service delivery has been expanded to encompass all settings. These issues are causing practitioners to seek different options for serving their caseloads.

One major challenge that poses a barrier to accomplishing goals for inclusion continues to be the relationship between the classroom teacher and the speech-language pathologist. Teachers may lack the understanding and preparation they need to provide assistance to students who are in their classes. In addition, SLPs are not always aware of the curriculum or other aspects of educational programming that make a difference to student learning. Evidence about the amount and type of intervention that is needed to change a student's communication behavior is not yet conclusive. Unfortunately, there are not common guidelines for decision-making. The least restrictive environment is mandated by law. But it appears that clinicians and educators continue to struggle with how to interpret this mandate for students with communication impairments and other disabilities. There are some who believe that the law is being overinterpreted by educators. The legislation really mandates that children are supposed to be served by the best intervention model *for them*. For some children, this will be through an inclusive approach within in the classroom setting. For others, it will mean pullout programming or some other model. In many cases, it makes sense to either combine models or move from a pullout model to an inclusion model. SLPs are charged with using their expertise and clinical judgment to determine the most appropriate model for each child. Offering a continuum of services is really the intent of the law.

Typical Service Delivery Options

Before a comprehensive speech and language intervention program is organized by the school clinician, some basis must be established for its implementation. The ASHA Preferred Practice Patterns (2004) state that a "variety of service delivery models and supports may be utilized including direct service; indirect service through consultation and collaboration; service by support personnel with appropriate supervision; service by transdisciplinary or interdisciplinary teams; and service mediated by technology such as telepractice" (p. 5). No one service delivery model should be used for treatment. Rather, the model selected should be based on the needs of the person served.

Numerous models for delivering speech-language pathology services are being practiced in schools across the country. Service delivery models are designed based on the requirements of the federal and state laws, the needs of the school district, the unique demographics of the community, specific needs of the populations to be served, and the insights of professionals. There are variations in service delivery models from school district to school district. Differences may be due to the populations served, intervention goals, funding capabilities, administrative support (or nonsupport), and professional expertise and energy. Service delivery recommendations may range from no service, to monitoring behavior, to engaging educators and parents in implementing strategies, to structured therapy in the classroom or therapy room, to special education placement. Or, the above models may be combined to meet the student's needs.

Two of the greatest complications in determining the model of service delivery are the daily school schedule and the logistics of getting services to the students. In order to participate in speech-language intervention, services must fit into the school day. They may be integrated into classroom learning activities or woven into the students' academic and extracurricular schedule. Unfortunately, many students may miss valuable academic lessons and class time in order to participate in therapy sessions. This poses a great dilemma for SLPs and educators. Many models have historical roots; with patterns of service delivery being passed from clinician to clinician through the ages. The literature on school-based service delivery provides some insights about some common models that are in place. More research is needed to define and create service delivery models that are proven to be efficient and effective.

The laws regulating special education are very clear on several major points. First, services must be delivered in the least restrictive environment (LRE). Second, regardless of the model implemented, the school district should make available a continuum of service delivery options for providing services. Third, the service delivery model selected should be appropriate for the student's unique characteristics and needs. And, last, all services must be educationally or functionally relevant and help children make progress and achieve their educational goals.

IDEA requires that children with disabilities be educated, to the maximum extent appropriate, with children who are nondisabled. Least restrictive environment (LRE) is the term that is used. Special classes, separate schooling, or removal of children with disabilities from the regular education environment occurs only if the nature and severity of the disability is such that education in regular classes with the use of supplemental aids and services cannot be achieved satisfactorily. The LRE for students with communication impairments and other disabilities is stated in the Individualized Education Plan. Therefore, when the IEP is created, care must be taken by the SLP and other educators to determine the most appropriate learning environment, the rationale for the recommendation, and how the environment should change over time depending on the student's acquisition of skills and performance.

This leads us to conclude that multiple, alternative forms and modes of service delivery should be implemented based on the student's needs and preferences. Our service delivery models or paradigms should reflect the flexibility we need to best serve our students. As communication does not occur in a vacuum, we must pay particular attention to managing the physical and interpersonal environments in which students learn, live, play, and work (National Joint Committee for the Communication Needs of Persons With Severe Disabilities, 1992). By incorporating meaningful communication partners, including teachers and parents, services can be more effective (Blosser & DePompei, 2002; Cirren & Penner, 1995; Flynn, 2010).

Over the past several years, there have been many discussions of models for delivering speech-language services (ASHA, 1991, 1999, 2010; Blosser & Kratcoski, 1997; Crais, 1991; Creaghead, Esotmin, Freilinger & Peters-Johnson, 1992; Dodge & Mallard, 1992; Flynn, 2010; Holzhauser-Peters & Husemann, 1988; Montgomery, 2009; Montgomery & Blosser, 2010, Moore & Montgomery, 2001; Nelson, 2009; Simon, 1987; Vicker, 2010). An evidence-based systematic review of the effects of different service delivery models on communication outcomes for school-age children was completed by an ASHA appointed team of experts in school service delivery (Cirrin et al., 2010). The team reviewed peer-reviewed articles from the last 30 years that addressed the effect of various service delivery models and intervention outcomes. They conducted their review following explicit procedures and criteria defined in the Evidence-Based Systematic Review (EBSR) process. The results of the review indicated that the current evidence base does not support any particular service delivery model as preferable for meeting the communication needs of elementary school-age children. They indicated that the services for each student must be based on the specific needs of each student and that SLPs and their education colleagues must rely more on reason than research to make decisions about service delivery for individual students. The researchers concluded that further research is needed to determine effective service delivery options for school-age children.

The service delivery model and setting for the service should be based on the individual needs of the student. Using the IDEA least restrictive environment and the continuum of services recommendations as our guideposts, it seems logical to first consider providing services to students within their classroom setting and then move to other environments that would be considered more restrictive such as the therapy room or specialized programs within or outside the school district. Many school service delivery experts suggest that some students may require direct, individualized instruction that can be best accommodated in the speech-language therapy room. Then, after the targeted speech-language behaviors are established, the student can be moved along the continuum of service delivery back to less restrictive settings such as the classroom.

A Menu of Service Delivery Options

Service delivery options are often presented as though they are discreet programs with unique characteristics. In fact, they are often artificially presented in a hierarchical structure based on factors such as frequency of services, location of services, and amount of direct contact between the speech-language pathologist and student. Discussions of the range of service delivery options for speech-language therapy service delivery are generally assigned labels such as direct therapy; pullout services; integrated services, home-based intervention; residential services; parent training programs; diagnostic intervention; center-based; classroom-based; 3:1 service delivery; consultation/collaboration model; resource rooms; self-contained classrooms; community-based; in-service education programs, and many more.

Key Service Delivery Variables

Trying to sort through and understand service delivery using terms such as these can be difficult. The task can be simplified by understanding the key service delivery variables that can be manipulated to meet a particular student's needed. Here are some of the most important variables that an SLP must consider when recommending services:

- The type and severity of the student's communication disability, including amount of assistance needed and impact on performance;
- The frequency, intensity, amount, and duration of the services;
- The roles performed by the clinician (direct or indirect; generalist or specialist);
- The roles others play and ways they can support speech-language development and improvement;
- The location of the service (therapy room, classroom, resource room, other school contexts, the community);
- The purpose of the service (screening, assessment, intervention, generalization);
- The presence of peers and the number of peers who participate (individual, small or large group, peers within the classroom); and,
- The scheduling format (block, 3:1 model, intensive).

Unfortunately, there is limited consensus concerning the definitions of many of the service delivery models used by SLPs in the schools. It is even more unfortunate that there are not many commonly shared definitions of service delivery models among professionals and educators. This presents a problem for educators, parents, administrators, and third-party payers. There is often confusion and misperception about the type of service to be provided, the reason that a particular model is selected, and the appropriateness for the student. Unfortunately, many parents and teachers are led to believe that one option is better than another and that more time with the SLP directly providing the majority of the services is preferable to incorporating other people (such as teachers) or providing services in different environments (including the classroom). This "more is better" concept has restricted the acceptance of expanded or alternative service delivery models. It has also limited the involvement of others who are significant in the student's life and who can contribute to improving the student's communication skills.

In lieu of definitions that are uniformly accepted by all professionals, the following are several representative descriptions of service delivery models that have appeared in the literature (ASHA, 1993, 1996; Cirrin et al., 2010; Flynn, 2010; Homer, 1997; Montgomery & Blosser, 2010; Soliday, 2010). These are provided only as a frame of reference for the discussion of the concept of options for service delivery. The order of presentation of the options is not meant to suggest that one model is better than another or that there is a prescribed hierarchy or transition from one model to the next. Rather, it is hoped that the list and these explanations will serve as an illustration of the many options from which SLPs can select the best service model for students based on their individual characteristics and needs.

Monitoring Speech-Language Behavior

Not all students must be seen directly or on a routine (daily, weekly, monthly) basis. For example, children who demonstrate developmental delays but do not warrant direct intervention can be monitored for a period of time until the clinician and education team determines that intervention would be beneficial. In some situations the student's needs may be met by a teacher but the SLP is needed to occasionally monitor progress or recommend modifications. When monitoring students, the SLP observes the student's communication behaviors over a specified period of time. She may be monitoring to see if children with immature speech and language patterns show change over time (thus decreasing the need for therapy). She may be watching to see if the student's behaviors change when stimulated or motivated by a certain situation or person. In addition, children who have been enrolled in therapy and are dismissed may be monitored for a specified time period to determine if generalization has occurred and new patterns are stabilized.

Traditional Model of Service Delivery

As a context for this discussion about service delivery models, it is important to understand that the most frequently used model of service delivery is the "pullout model." As a basis for comparison with other models, the pullout model is frequently referred to as the "traditional" model of service provision. In this model, the SLP sees children individually or in small groups in a special location separate from the educational activities, often referred to as the Speech-Language Therapy Room. Pullout refers to removing students from the classroom for a specified amount of time and conducting individualized or small group intervention or instruction on specific tasks in a site other than the classroom. Pullout is the approach that most educators and administrators expect to be used when a student requires speech-language services. In fact, it is the "default" model. Because the pullout model is used so frequently, many parents have come to expect it as well.

Although this model is the most typical model of service delivery, it is certainly not the only model. Breaking this tradition and expanding service delivery to include numerous other options, providers, and locations has been a challenge for many practitioners. The challenge is complicated by the fact that evidence proving that any of the numerous service delivery methods are equally or more effective than another is lacking (Cirrin et al., 2010). Although logistically the pullout model may present a convenience for organizing the speech-language pathologist's schedule, there is little evidence to indicate that this model of service delivery is comparatively more effective or efficient than other models for accomplishing goals and changing students' communication behaviors. In other words, implementation of the pullout model does not necessarily ensure that the student will acquire new speech and language skills or generalize skills being addressed in therapy sessions to other situations. The pullout model, in fact, is actually one of the most restrictive service delivery models rather than the least restrictive model as mandated by IDEA. Therefore, it should not be the first choice.

The pullout mode of delivery has historically been referred to as the primary model used by the speech-language pathologist to deliver service in a school setting. Surveys of school-based SLPs indicate that nearly 85% of school clinicians report using this model. When the pullout model is implemented, speech and language services are provided as a supplementary service to regular or special education programs. The student leaves the classroom to receive direct intervention from the speech-language pathologist. Pullout intervention may be aimed at an individual student or a group of students. Criteria for grouping students into a particular session may include age, grade level, type and degree of communication disorder, and functional level. Traditionally sessions are scheduled for an average of once or twice per week for an individual student or group of students. Group size may average from two to four students but may include as many as ten students. The number of sessions per week, length of time per session, and number of students per session are influenced by the nature and degree of the students' problems and the speech-language pathologist's caseload demands. Again, there is limited evidence to guide decisions about the frequency, number, length of sessions, intensity, or scheduling of services (Warren, Fey, & Yoder, 2007). The average pullout session is 30 minutes twice per week. This totals only about 32 to 36 hours of therapy per year. Creative use of learning centers, technology, and speech-language pathology assistants are sometimes used by clinicians to maximize the benefits of pullout intervention. Unfortunately, the pullout method does not automatically promote much interaction and collaboration between the SLP and teacher.

The pullout model has become the norm in many school districts. Clinicians may be stuck in a routine that does not enable them to evaluate each child to determine the most appropriate service delivery model from a creative, flexible, unique point of view. It is this scheduling pattern that has restricted many clinicians from implementing a more individualized, variable service delivery approach. Clinicians must ask themselves: *How can it be that the majority of students served need to receive direct services twice per week (Monday or Wednesday; Tuesday or Thursday) for one half-hour? This scheduling pattern defies the notion that the intervention model selected should match the student's needs. Doesn't it make more sense to consider alternative approaches that are suited to each child's individual needs?*

Although the typical pullout therapy session is scheduled twice per week for 30 minutes each session, there is no reason that the time frame can't be modified to increase or decrease intensity and frequency. In fact, many clinicians have begun to modify the amount of time scheduled for services. For example, some clinicians see children every day for 5 to 10-minute sessions. Two programs that represent this model are Speedy Speech (2011) and 5 Minute Kids (http://www.5minutekids.com, 2011). Instead of lasting the full school year, the sessions are scheduled for blocks of time such as 8 or 10 weeks. At the end of the time period, the child's performance is evaluated and a decision is made to continue or discontinue the services at that same level of intensity and frequency.

Collaboration

The term collaboration means that the SLP works closely with other educators and family members to facilitate better understanding of a student's communication impairment, to determine how learning is affected, and to jointly implement strategies for helping the student improve communication and learning (ASHA, 1996). Collaboration implies a partnership and willingness to work together. The collaborative partners jointly determine goals and objectives for intervention, including the service delivery and environment where services are provided. Collaborative services may include instruction of the student's communication partners and may focus on how to facilitate functioning, modify barriers to successful communication, or increase participation.

Descriptions of service delivery models frequently list collaboration as though it is a unique and separate model. However, a different view of the collaboration is recommended. It is suggested that collaboration is *essential*. Speech-language services should *always* include collaboration with significant individuals in the student's life. Without collaboration, we are truly providing services in a vacuum. With collaboration, we have a better chance of having the skills we are targeting support educational success and transfer into classroom, home, and other communicative situations. The power of speech-language intervention services multiplies when the frequency of intervention occurs throughout the school day and home activities.

Here is an example of how collaboration can work: The speech-language pathologist observes a class and identifies critical information about communication within that classroom that can contribute to creating an intervention plan for the student. The SLP describes the communication demands during instructional assignments, the various levels of speech and language competence among peers, and the student's overall communication during the learning activity. Following analysis of the information, the speech-language pathologist meets with the teacher to share observations and recommendations to enhance the students' language skills and incorporate language development into the curricula. The speech-language pathologist demonstrates and recommends specific teaching strategies and techniques and may provide supplementary materials to the teacher.

When an IEP is developed for a student, goals and objectives are indicated linking the student's language performance with the educational curriculum. The speech-language pathologist may suggest specific strategies to the teacher so he or she can help the student reach the goals and objectives specified in the IEP. Following are some examples of successful collaboration. The SLP explains or demonstrates specific techniques that the teacher, tutor, peer, or parent can use to assist the student in carrying appropriate language skills into everyday life. The SLP provides informal analysis and suggestions for modification of the classroom environment, the teacher's communication style and delivery, or student-learning strategies. Language materials that may include pictures, word lists, and so forth, for others to use with preschool, kindergarten, or high-risk students are provided on a routine basis. The SLP may demonstrate language and speech enrichment sessions in the classroom as needed.

The collaborative model is sometimes referred to in the literature on service delivery as an "indirect service delivery model." Again, this notion doesn't make sense because collaboration should always take place and should be documented in the IEP in combination other service delivery models. This simple action will enable the SLP to create the framework and justification for working with significant people in the student's life and for implementing a variety of service delivery options along a continuum over the period of time that the student receives services. A range of services can be offered depending on the student's changing needs and skills.

Integrating Therapy into the Classroom

In this model, treatment is provided in the classroom, which is considered the least restrictive environment. Many of the interventions that are offered in the therapy room can also be delivered within the classroom setting. Even better, when classroom teachers learn how to modify the instructional environment or their instructional communication to support the student effectively throughout the day, the amount and quality of services can is multiplied. Many terms are used to describe services that are integrated into the classroom. For example, some SLPs refer to this model as classroom-based, push-in, curriculum-based, transdisciplinary, integrated, or inclusive programming.

The variety of labels used for providing services in the classroom environment exemplifies the inconsistency SLPs exhibit when describing service delivery options to parents, teachers, and others. Of all of the terms and definitions for service delivery, integrating services into the classroom seems to simultaneously create interest and concern for SLPs. They are interested because the classroom is the natural environment for students. They are concerned because they are not always sure of what to do or how to provide services within the classroom setting once they get there. In addition, teachers may lack understanding of what the SLP is trying to accomplish by offering services within the classroom.

It often appears that each therapist and each school district defines classroom-based service delivery differently and place different expectations of the SLP for goals, scheduling, types of children served, and types of activities conducted. For example, one clinician may interpret classroom-based model to mean that the SLP incorporates classroom-based materials in therapy. A second clinician may define classroom-based as working collaboratively with the teacher. In a third interpretation, the clinician may be working with a small group of children within the classroom structure. A fourth SLP might present a language or listening-based lesson to an entire class to demonstrate how to elicit appropriate speech and language from a particular student during a classroom lesson. A fifth interpretation describes classroom-based as team teaching or co-teaching.

This much confusion about service delivery is especially troublesome when a team of educators is trying to develop an IEP for a student with a communication disorder. Imagine how confused the parents must be when they try to understand what services will be provided to help their child! In fact, the term is so confusing that sometimes parents resist the recommendation that a classroom-based service delivery model be provided for their child.

A more positive approach to explaining an integrated classroom-based service delivery model is for the SLP and teacher to collaborate to jointly exchange information, establish goals, modify instructional strategies, and evaluate progress. The following reasons for incorporating services into the classroom can contribute to developing a convincing discussion during the development of the IEP and for planning sessions.

- Classroom-based services facilitate the provision of speech-language services in the "least restrictive environment" within the school setting.
- Teachers and SLPs can gain a better understanding of how the student's disability impacts on his learning performance and success.
- Treatment will be more relevant to the student's needs and take into consideration what the student needs in order to succeed in the general education curriculum.
- Teachers and therapists can work closely to determine goals, curricular challenges, modification strategies, progress, and problems.
- The classroom is a more "natural" learning environment for the student. Students learn the speech and language skills they need when they need them.
- Therapists can model treatment and intervention strategies and techniques for the teacher, demonstrating how to employ the technique during instruction within the classroom situation, thus extending the number of people and opportunities for helping the student.
- Teachers can observe what the therapist does to elicit, modify, and reinforce speech and language skills.

- Classroom materials can be used during the treatment or classroom session (such as class assignments, workbooks, textbooks, etc.) so that the student can learn to practice his new skills in the context in which he learns.
- Assessment and intervention can be incorporated into a variety of learning routines.
- Assessment and intervention strategies can be selected and planned with the student's specific disability and learning needs in mind. SLPs can determine if those strategies are appropriate and if they work.
- Targeted skills can be reinforced.
- The classroom fosters social relationships and, therefore, the practice of social communication.
- Conducting services in the classroom enables students to continue to participate in classroom activities so they don't miss out on valuable instruction time.
- There are increased opportunities for practice.
- Problems can be addressed as they arise.
- Teachers can observe what therapists do to help students. They can then repeat the techniques during their own instruction.

Many clinicians ask what they are supposed to do once they are in the classroom. If the SLP isn't sure, it can be concluded that the teacher doesn't know what is supposed to happen either. SLPs may be unsure of their role and how to provide speech-language oriented services within the classroom environment. Friend (2010) suggests several ways that teachers and SLPs can partner in the classroom:

- One teach, one observe
- One teach, one drift and assist students
- Station teaching with each teaching at a separate center
- Parallel teaching with each instructing half of the class using the same material
- Remedial teaching where one presents material while the other re-teaches previously taught material.
- Supplemental teaching which is when one presents a lesson in a standard format while the other adapts the lesson.
- Team teaching with both sharing the teaching time.

By simply planning to use the time in the classroom together wisely and remembering the distinct roles and responsibilities of each professional, the SLP and their teacher partner will come to know a little more about each other's perspective, challenges, teaching goals, and instructional strategies.

Working with students is only part of the treatment dynamic. Working with classroom teachers is extremely important. Teachers and SLPs can join forces and share the responsibility. The classroom teacher possesses expertise in curriculum, classroom management, and large group instruction. The SLP knows about communication development, communication disabilities, and individualized intervention strategies. Together, these skill sets are powerful. Through collaboration, teachers and SLPs can learn to complement each other to achieve their respective goals for the student.

Consultation

SLPs may provide consultation services to support student success and generalization of skills into the learning situation. When consulting, the SLP acts as a resource to educators and fellow IEP team members. Consultation engages others in school as appropriate. Consultation is generally problem-oriented. Consultation may take place in or out of the classroom. Some examples of expert consultation include observing students upon request, programming alternative communication devices, engineering the classroom environment so that it is right for the student's needs, teaching intervention strategies, and referring to other professionals. In some districts, SLPs initiate a consultant model when students are dismissed from therapy so they can monitor the student. They periodically check on a student. The frequency of consultation can vary from one time per week to four times per year depending on the support needed by the educational team or student. Consultation services should not be random. Rather they should be planned and purposeful. Consultation generally is combined with other services and should be documented on the IEP. When consulting, the SLP may provide recommendations to the student, educators, and/or parents.

Community-Based Intervention

Programs for children with low-incidence disabilities emphasize community-based instruction. In this model, the speech-language pathologist collaborates with the special education teacher and other staff members to assist the student in utilizing functional speech and language in community settings. As part of their school program, severely involved students learn how to function in typical situations within their own home or communities. The speech-language pathologist provides direct or indirect services to students on-site in community settings such as restaurants, stores, libraries, banks, post offices, and so forth. The speech-language pathologist helps students communicate, monitors their progress, and assists in planning instruction and reinforcement. As a collaborator in a community-based intervention program, the speech-language pathologist assists the teacher, occupational therapist, physical therapist, or other staff members in developing plans and strategies to encourage the growth of the students' functional communication areas.

Because the school is a community site, emphasis can be placed on development of the student's functional communication skills and carryover of those skills into everyday home, community, and work life. For younger children, the playground, lunchroom, and gym are all considered part of their community. The speech-language pathologist can enlist the support of many resources in the school to aid in development of a student's communication skills. In community-based sites, the speech-language pathologist analyzes the experience and site to identify relevant vocabulary to be learned. He or she develops language concepts relevant to assigned tasks, and guides staff in using instructional language most likely to clearly convey instructional messages to students. SLPs should also be involved in transition programs that prepare high school students for graduation and work experiences. For example, the SLP can contribute by helping a student complete job and college applications or prepare for interviews.

Speech-Language Pathology Assistants (SLPAs)

Speech-language pathologists in several states have begun to utilize SLPAs in order to expand the amount of therapy they can provide to students or to reinforce skills. In order to increase the possibility that the SLPA will have a positive influence on the students, it is imperative to prepare them for their role and responsibility by providing training, resources, structured manuals, and materials. As with classroom teachers, instructing SLPAs to use specific strategies can be a valuable investment of time. The SLPA's scope of practice is very clear. For example, they cannot diagnose a student or determine the treatment plan. If they stay within the scope, they can contribute much to the SLP program. ASHA has developed guidelines for the scope of practice and supervision of SLPAs. However, states regulate the role and supervision of SLPAs in schools and other settings through specific licensing policies and procedures.

Matching Service Delivery Options to Individual Student's Needs

If service delivery approaches are to be effective, the various options will not be mutually exclusive and the clinician will be able to use them individually or in combination to best serve the needs of a particular student. The service delivery option selected should be the most appropriate to meet the child's needs and should be the least restrictive in terms of promoting inclusion and enabling the child to participate in the activities of the school as much as possible.

Consideration should be given to the student's level of functioning and should serve children and youth with communication disabilities ranging from severe disorders to developmental problems. The model needs to be applicable to children of all ages in regular education as well as special education programs. It should also make provisions for providing preventive services to the overall school population.

The service delivery options and the SLP's caseload should be based on several variables relating to the student and personnel available. This includes the type and severity of the student's communication impairment; the effect of the communication disorder on academic performance; the relationship of the communication disorder to other learning conditions; the stage of development of the communication disorder; the student's history in the speech-language intervention program; the amount and type of services needed to implement intervention strategies; and scheduling opportunities. (ASHA, 1984; Eger et al., 1990). The frequency, intensity and duration of services required to provide individual assistance to a student should be based on that student's particular needs. Because students' needs are constantly changing, these factors must be continually re-evaluated and the program adjusted periodically. Consideration should be given to the number of children who can be adequately served using particular service delivery options or combination of options. However, the service delivery model selection should not be driven by the lack of time to accommodate a specific model. Federal, state, and local requirements for serving students with communication disorders must also be considered.

Decisions regarding a group versus individualized or combined group/individualized program should be based on student need rather than factors such as administrative direction and time or budget constraints. That is why service delivery models where each student receives the same type of intervention for the same amount of time (twice per week for 30 minutes each session) are not appropriate. The service delivery models selected should allow adequate frequency and intensity of help to achieve optimum progress. As with group size, decisions regarding the length and frequency of intervention should be based on the student's needs and clinical factors rather than budgetary and administrative issues. The option selected should provide students with the best chance for functioning successfully within the school setting and in their future lives.

Determining the Amount, Frequency, and Duration of Services (Dosage)

School teams struggle with how to determine and state the amount of services each child needs in order to improve his or her communication skills. In addition, they must also recommend the frequency for providing the services and the time frame or duration. Together, these elements are sometimes referred to within the communication disorders literature as the "treatment intensity" or "dosage" (Williams, McLeod, & McCauley, 2010). One of the SLP's responsibilities is to recommend the dosage of services for the IEP. The most important responsibility for SLPs is to be clear about the rationale for recommending a particular amount of time, frequency, or duration for services. As mentioned previously, evidence to guide decisions about the dosage is lacking.

Unfortunately intervention research has not conclusively indicated the intensity or dosage for remediating different types and severity of impairment. The intensity or dosage is very individualized. Individual client characteristics and the type of intervention approach used can affect the dosage required. Some findings have indicated, however, that it takes approximately 20 hours to teach a new skill.

There is variation from one district to another about how the dosage is indicated on the IEP. Some clinicians indicate number of minutes per week, others state number of minutes per month, and still others indicate amount of time per year. Some IEPs state the number of sessions students will receive per year, others get more granular and state number of sessions per week or month. Some specify that treatment should last the full school year (approximately 32–36 weeks), whereas others specify blocks of time such as 9 weeks, 15 weeks, 21 weeks, and so on. The amount of time, frequency, and duration specified on the IEP is considered a minimum, not a maximum.

There are benefits of writing plans that specify the amount of time in terms of monthly or yearly hours versus weekly minutes. Those benefits include: flexibility for providing the services, accommodating class schedules and requirements, increased opportunity to integrate services into the classroom, ability to make up missed sessions, ability to incorporate others into the treatment program, and scheduling options that fit complex students' schedules. Here is an example of the various options for accomplishing 4 hours or 240 minutes of services per month:

- 10 minutes, 6 times per week
- 15 minutes, 4 times per week
- 20 minutes, 3 times per week
- 30 minutes, 2 times per week
- 60 minutes, once per week
- 60 minutes, 2 times per week on alternating weeks

Children with greater severity need more support and assistance to succeed. Generally they require longer periods of intervention. The amount of services can be increased by expanding service delivery into multiple settings and incorporating other people as providers. Increasing the amount of services in this way is likely to lead to greater generalization of skills. Multiplying the amount of time and number of providers increases the potential for faster and more effective skill acquisition.

The location of services can and should be modified to meet goals and needs as well. Not all sessions need to take place in the therapy room. There can be a mix of classroom and therapy room or all services can be offered in the classroom.

Taking a Different Perspective for Planning Services: The PAC Framework for Determining Appropriate Models of Service Delivery

When devising a comprehensive service delivery model, there are four major concepts of service provision that should be considered. First, the model should recognize that communication impairments affect learning success. Second, the model should create an optimal environment for providing speech-language services. Third, the model should incorporate collaboration and sharing expertise to develop effective program goals, objectives, and intervention strategies for children. Fourth, the model should integrate speech-language goals, objectives, and techniques into the student's learning experiences.

Blosser and Kratcoski (1997) developed a conceptual framework for guiding decisions about selection of appropriate services to meet particular clients' needs. They define the process of selecting the appropriate service delivery model as determining the unique combinations of *providers, service activities, and contexts* (PACs) necessary to meet the specific needs of the individual with communication disorders.

The conceptual framework is based on three premises. First, there are essential characteristics that define good service delivery. Second, service delivery must be creative and flexible. Third, the provider, activity, and context must be clearly specified in the Individualized Education Plan (treatment plan), the Individualized Family Service Plan (IFSP), or the Individualized Transition Plan (ITP).

Premise One—Characteristics of Good Service Delivery Models

According to Flower (1984) the essential characteristics of good service delivery models fall under five headings: efficacy, coordination, continuity, participation and economy. Here are some simple questions to help determine if the service delivery model selected meets the student's needs.

1. *Does the service make a difference to the child?* The first obvious criterion, *efficacy*, is whether the service makes any difference to the student. Screening services can usually be judged in fairly objective terms; however, other services are often more difficult to assess. Evaluation by the clinician and the insights of families, clients, and other professionals all provide information of a subjective nature, but it is frequently difficult to determine whether achievements have, in fact, occurred.
2. *When multiple professional services are provided to the same individual, are all services coordinated and working toward the same end?* Several different types of professionals serve children with communication disorders. Some of these may provide services that are directly related to the communicative disorder, for example, the learning disabilities specialist working with a child with problems in language acquisition. Other professionals provide services with only peripheral relevance to the communicative disorder, for example, the occupational therapist in a classroom in which a child with autism is enrolled. Whenever multiple professional services are provided to the same student, the effectiveness of any of those services will often depend on the *coordination* with all other services.
3. *Is there an uninterrupted sequence of services, and is each phase staged and integrated?* Good care depends on the *continuity* of sequential services over a period of several months or sometimes several years. This often requires multiple professional services, that is, a total plan for services, with each phase staged and integrated into an uninterrupted sequence toward the ultimate goal.
4. *Are the individual's wishes, motivations, and interests considered by incorporating the individual and family members in the decision-making process?* Providing intervention services without regard for the child's understanding of the purpose of treatment or how therapy will help may seriously affect the effectiveness of those services. *Participation* by the client and the family in decision-making processes, to the greatest extent possible, ensures the opportunity for excellent services.
5. *Are the time, energy, funding, and other resources used most efficiently to accom-*

plish the goals? Economy does not only mean spending as little money as possible. It refers also to the conservation of time and energy. The conservation of financial resources, as well as the orderly management of services to avoid waste, and the achievement of efficiency through careful planning constitute the broader definition of economy.

Flower's five criteria are helpful in assessing service delivery models. Each school system is unique. The school clinician should strive to implement the service delivery options that best fit the organization of the school system, needs of the students, and professionals on staff. Many of the factors on the following list seem to influence the number and types of options some school districts offer. Although children are supposed to be provided with appropriate services that meet their needs, many clinicians report that factors such as these influence decision-making in their schools (whether they should be considered legitimate factors or not).

- Availability of qualified professionals;
- The geographic location of the schools, the clinician's "home" office, and the distance and travel time between these locations;
- The availability of working space in each of the school;
- The type and severity of the communication problems within the schools;
- The number and population of the schools;
- Time allotted for coordination activities, including: in-service training; supervision of paraprofessionals or aides, administration of diagnostic tests; preparation of records, parent conferences, placement team conferences, and collaborating (with classroom teachers, special education personnel, and administrators);
- School policies affecting transporting students from school to school to place them in locations where they may receive the appropriate services;
- Student enrollment in each grade level. It is entirely probable that the junior high schools and the senior high schools may have smaller population of students with communication impairments than elementary schools; and,
- The support of the school administration and teaching staff.

Premise Two—Service Delivery Must Be Creative and Flexible

The service delivery option selected must fit the needs and lifestyle of the student. In addition, it must be integrated into the school context. This means that various key aspects of service delivery must be manipulated to meet the student's unique needs. The aspects that can be tailored include:

- The provider who delivers the services (SLP, teacher, parent, OT, peer, assistant);

- The type of services provided;
- The amount of contact time the speech-language pathologist actually spends with the student;
- The location for providing services (resource room, therapy room, classroom, lunch room, etc.);
- The mode of service delivery (technology-assisted, written format, verbal interaction); and;
- The materials and techniques used for assessment and intervention (curricular, clinician made; commercial process-oriented, product-oriented).

Premise Three—The Provider, Activity, and Context (PAC) Must Be Clearly Specified

In most discussions of service delivery, collaboration is treated as a distinct and unique service delivery model. In the PAC model, collaboration is a required and necessary component for providing services for all students. In other words, unless significant others are integrated into the intervention process, treatment cannot be effective.

Providers (P)

In the PAC Model, communication partners who can foster meaningful change in a student's communication performance are referred to as "providers." They make changes by knowing how to implement appropriate procedures such as eliciting, modifying, and/or reinforcing communication responses. Traditionally, the SLP is viewed as the only person who can make changes and who has the ultimate responsibility for this role. However, in the PAC model the SLP is not assumed to be the only or even the best provider. To improve efficacy, both assessment and intervention require *shared responsibility* among all of the student's significant communication partners.

Numerous providers should be involved in the assessment and intervention process. They are determined by the student's needs at a given point in time, the activity to be completed, and the context in which the activity is to be conducted. Providers may change over time as the child's communication skills improve and intervention needs or goals change. Clearly, this model assumes that there should be multiple providers for each student.

When implementing any model of service delivery, the SLP's role includes guiding the team as they weigh the following decision: "Who are the most appropriate persons to conduct or provide specific communication-related activities with this student and in what context?" Several factors must be weighed when making the decision regarding who might be an effective provider. The person should have a meaningful relationship with the student (teacher, parent, sibling, or friend). The severity of the disability also makes a difference. Sometimes the problems are so severe that providers need to be introduced more slowly and over an extended period of time. The partner's general knowledge and understanding of the communication disability will also impact on the decision. Sometimes, they will need to be educated about the disability before being brought into a more active role. The individual's willingness to participate in the program, and situations and contexts of interactions also will help determine the involvement and the success of the involvement. In determining providers, the SLP and fellow team members should consider the following questions:

- Who are the key communication partner's in this youngster's life (parents, other caregivers, teachers, co-workers, tutors, peers)?
- Are there barriers that would prevent the person from delivering specific assessment and/or treatment procedures (time constraints, location, motivation, conflicting philosophies, fear, lack of information, inadequate skills)?
- Can these barriers be resolved through training and/or counseling (in-servicing, support groups, workshops, written materials, audio and video materials, observation, demonstration)?
- What is the most appropriate provider role for each communication partner considering the outcomes/goals for the client at the specific point in time? (observe and report behaviors, model, question, prompt, correct, reinforcing).

Examples of potential providers in addition to the SLP are parents, siblings, general educators, special educators, tutors, intervention specialists, psychologists, friends, administrators, occupational therapists, and physical therapists. Key roles played by individuals such as these will enable services to be carried out throughout the daily routine.

Activities (A)

The tasks that comprise the total case management for students with communication disorders are referred to as "activities" (A) in the PAC model. The primary tasks can be grouped into four major categories including:

1. planning to determine courses of action in all aspects of case management;
2. assessing to determine strengths and needs;
3. implementing treatment procedures; and,
4. evaluating services to determine the efficacy and to identify if modifications are necessary.

Clearly, the SLP is not the only person qualified to perform these activities. Through shared responsibility, the team can gain more valuable information and make more efficient use of shrinking resources. Each of the activities can be easily explained to fellow team members. Here are some examples of how to explain the activities.

Planning. A significant portion of the SLP's service delivery time involves planning. Teams must spend adequate time and effort to determine the appropriate course of action needed to meet each student's needs. Planning involves tasks such as discussing assessment findings, reviewing pertinent data, determining goals and objectives, selecting appropriate intervention procedures, and modifying intervention plans. This planning often takes the form of meetings where several participants from various disciplines come together to present their perspectives. Within the PAC model, the emphasis during planning efforts is on who the providers will be and what activities they will conduct and in what context.

Assessing. The purpose of assessment is to identify the student's communication strengths and needs as well as the extent of services necessary. Unless information is also gathered regarding the priorities and concerns of the student, his/her family, and other important individuals, an appropriate service plan cannot be developed. Within the assessment process, all individuals who can contribute information are considered Providers. In the PAC Model, the goal of the identification and assessment aspects of service delivery is *not* to identify *what is wrong*. Instead, the goal is to *identify what works for a particular client in a particular setting when assisted by particular people*. Thus, the SLP's role is to provide a framework for obtaining, organizing, and synthesizing the information.

Implementing Interventions. Perhaps the most primary activity in service delivery is providing intervention. As the intervention plan for a student is developed, different providers will inevitably assume different roles for implementing intervention. For example, one provider (such as the SLP) may introduce a new skill to the client, while a second provider (the parent) reinforces the targeted behavior and a third provider (the teacher) observes the child's performance to determine additional communication skill areas to be targeted in the future. Clinicians working within the school setting often express confusion about how to work collaboratively with teachers. Following the PAC model provides a useful way of understanding how to make collaboration work so that it is beneficial to all concerned.

In the PAC model, the SLP assumes the responsibility of preparing providers for the activities they will conduct. For example, to involve key communication partners in implementing intervention, the SLP must prepare them for the role by teaching them to:

1. identify when a communication breakdown has occurred;
2. recognize that it is related to the individual's communication disability; and
3. know the appropriate procedures to implement to bring about change at that time.

One way to help others understand the key roles they can play is to provide guidance and training. Consider this a service delivery option that is appropriate to the needs of the majority of children on the caseload. Providing in-service training, both formal and informal, is a functional way to reach teachers, parents and others. It can impact a great number of students without the SLP providing direct service. In addition, it would be helpful for the SLP to also participate in in-service training to learn more about the school curriculum and expectations for students.

There are many ways to provide training including providing information via 5-minute "quick-hits" at faculty meetings, distributing written handouts, and providing materials. Share ideas with teachers during informal conversations or in-service presentations. Place fact sheets on bulletin boards. Show others how to elicit correct responses or correct incorrect responses by demonstrating speech and language techniques. Lend useful materials to teachers and encourage them to try them out in the classroom. Volunteer to participate on curriculum selection committees. Provide routine updates about students' progress and suggest activities teachers might want to try.

Evaluating Efficacy and Outcomes. Intervention is effective when the student's communication performance is appropriate for the contexts in which he participates. In the school setting, this means he or she can perform the required tasks in the classroom setting. This can only be determined by reports provided by the astute providers in the client's various communication environments. The SLP's role is to solicit information, analyze it, and work with other providers to make appropriate modifications.

Identifying Appropriate Activities. In deciding those activities that are necessary to address the child's needs, teams should contemplate these "activity related" questions:

1. What tasks do the Providers need to complete for this student at this particular point in time (identify needs, design interventions, teach others to implement interventions, evaluate progress)?
2. What Providers would be most appropriate for performing each task (Consider such factors such as: the person's relationship to the student; the frequency of contact the provider and student have with one another; the provider's level of understanding, experience, and training relative to the disorder and the necessary intervention; and so on)?
3. What steps should be taken to prepare the Providers to perform these activities and who should take the steps? (Providing in-service training, demonstrations, written materials, audio or videotapes).
4. What materials do the Providers need to conduct the Activity? (Observation and data collection forms, assessment checklists and materials, surveys and questionnaires, resource lists, stimulus materials, augmentative or assistive devices.)

Contexts (C)

The situations, conditions, environments, or interactions where communication is required are referred to as the "contexts." During planning opportunities, providers should jointly determine the most appropriate contexts for conducting specific activities necessary for case management. The range of contexts and conditions for each student is extensive. In determining contexts, the SLP should consider demands and expectations for communication required in the context. Specifically, the team must consider:

1. What are the primary contexts in which the student communicates or must transfer newly learned behaviors

(home, school, learning activities, curriculum, community, work)?

2. What contexts provide natural opportunities for communication or for practicing the targeted behaviors (instruction, play, large group activities, recreation and leisure, routines, vocational settings)?
3. What contexts provide opportunities for observing and evaluating communication performance and progress?
4. Does the environment restrict or promote communication skills for this individual?

Appropriate contexts include the regular education classroom, resource room, curriculum, cafeteria, recess, home, community, vocational settings, and so on. Services can be delivered in numerous locations using a wide variety of treatment approaches. During planning, emphasis should be placed on determining the best context for implementing recommended interventions. Unfortunately too often clinicians place students into a particular context and do not consider if it is the most appropriate match for the child's needs.

Many creative clinicians have developed interesting and exciting programs to meet the needs of various populations they serve. It would be impossible to list all of them but an overview will help capture the essence of what can be accomplished when a team of SLPs and their education partners put their minds to the task. The following sections provide descriptions of contexts, in addition to the classroom or therapy room, that some clinicians establish for providing various types of services.

Table 8–1 presents a series of questions SLPs and their education team colleagues can consider to develop a comprehensive, efficient, and effective service plan for students.

Early Intervening Services

Not all children who exhibit problems communicating are eligible for speech-language intervention services. When teachers or others note that children exhibit delays or experience struggles within the learning situation, they should make others on the education team aware and seek their input on strategies for helping the student. They should also take steps to provide assistance to the student, including modifying the classroom environment or instructional practices, to see if changes will result in improved performance. In schools, this is referred to as "early intervening services." As a result of federal legislation, the responsibility for identifying children who struggle is described as a "general education initiative" within the school organization rather than a "special education initiative." This means that students are served within the general education setting rather than a special education setting such as a self-contained classroom or through enrollment in related services such as speech-language, occupational, or physical therapy. It also means that funding for early intervening services is supported through the general education funding sources rather than special education funding sources. A portion of IDEA funds can be allocated for supplemental instruction and teacher training.

Table 8–1. Key Variables to Consider When Planning Services

The range of speech-language services, including prevention, assessment, intervention, and collaboration, must be delivered in a way that most effectively and efficiently meets each student's needs and enables the student to reach his or her highest potential.

There are a number of variables that should be considered in developing the most appropriate service delivery plan for each student.

In this model, collaboration is not considered a unique model of service delivery. Collaboration should be an integral part of all therapy.

Key Variables	*Options*
What activities are to be delivered?	Observation Assessment Planning Intervention Evaluation
Who will provide the services?	Therapist Teacher Family member Other educators or specialists
What is the environment or location for intervention?	Away from the classroom (therapy room) Classroom (general education, special education, unique program) Other school contexts (lunch room, playground, extracurriculars) Community Home
What other students should be included?	No other students Students with similar disorders (2+) Peers/nondisabled (2+) Family members
How intense should the services be?	Frequency (how many times per week, month, year) Amount of time for each session (hours per week, month, year) Duration (amount of time the services should last—week, month, year) *Identify the intensity for each environment and provider. *Identify ways to vary the intensity based on student's needs and progress.

continues

Table 8–1. *continued*

Key Variables	*Options*
What is the context for the therapy?	Therapy treatment (different than classroom learning activities). Classroom curriculum or lesson (including teacher instructing lesson, joint instruction therapist/teacher, center activity, individual learning activity). Alternative Augmentative Communication or technology
What steps need to be taken to integrate services?	Identify additional providers (teacher, parent, aides). Train providers Coach providers

In order for early intervening services to help children in the best ways possible, general education teachers should collaborate closely with special educators, including SLPs. There are several formats that are considered early intervening including professional development, support services, and scientifically based literacy instruction to name a few.

Speech-language pathologists are in a great position to recommend assistance and strategies to teachers or support to students because of our understanding of the language skills necessary for literacy and learning. Some unique aspects of early intervening services include individualized instruction, collaborative approaches, and determining if learning improves by modifying the instructional approach. Thus, the instructional method is clearly defined and student's progress is tracked over time to observe changes.

Response-to-Intervention: A Prevention and Prereferral Model

Response-to-Intervention is an option that school districts employ to provide early intervening services to children who struggle in the learning situation. The National Association of State Directors of Special Education (NASDE) describe RTI as the practice of providing high quality instruction and intervention matched to students' needs, using learning progress over time and level of performance, to make important educational decisions (2011). RTI uses a problem solving methodology and research-based, scientifically validated interventions to support students. Educational decisions are guided by data. Assessments are used for three purposes: (1) screening to identify which children may have a problem that needs further assessment; (2) diagnostics to identify what interventions specific students need based on their performance in diagnostic assessments; and (3) progress monitoring to identify if the intervention and instructions methods are working.

The RTI model is a multitiered approach to providing assistance to struggling learners. The type and level of intensity of the assistance varies depending on the nature of the student's difficulty. RTI is considered a prevention and early prereferral educational intervention model, designed to prevent students from failing. It is also an identification model and can be used to help determine if students will respond to evidence-based interventions or if they are eligible for special education or related services. RTI supports students who are not performing at the same level and learning rate as their peers, especially those experiencing reading and learning problems. RTI is considered a "general education" rather than a "special education" model. Therefore, students who are experiencing difficulty in the general education classroom can receive help before they fail.

RtI incorporates many of the following key principles:

- Student progress is monitored.
- Data-based documentation must be kept on each student.
- Decisions should be made by education team members in collaboration with one another.
- High quality, evidence-based instructional and behavioral supports are provided.
- Interventions are matched to student's individual needs and at the appropriate level of intensity.

A hallmark of the Response-to-Intervention model is the use of a multitiered strategy for determining and providing the level of instruction and support needed to help students achieve their goals. The intent is to prevent learning and behavior problems and to more accurately identify students who may be eligible for special education services. Generally there are three tiers progressing from a low level of intensity to a high level of intensity of assistance. Here is a representative example of the students served and intensity levels for the three tiers.

Tier 1

Evidence-based instructional strategies are recommended by the team based on screening and referrals. Instructional activities are applicable to the whole general education classroom. Activities can be tailored to meet individual student's needs. The student's performance is monitored and documented to determine if the intervention is making a difference. Tier 1 is viewed as a preventive, proactive approach.

Tier 2

Students in this tier are considered at-risk and should benefit from supplemental services and additional support to successfully access the curriculum. Similar to Tier 1, they remain in the classroom. Activities are designed for instruction of small groups of students within the classroom setting. Instruction is differentiated. Parents are informed and included in the planning but are not required to provide written consent.

Tier 3

Students who don't make adequate progress are enrolled in special education classes to receive more intensive services with adapted content, instructional methodology or instructional delivery. The student receives comprehensive evaluation by multiple sources in order for the team to make their recommendations. Activities are differentiated and students receive instruction in small groups or individually. Tier 3 is more intense, more frequent, and individualized than Tiers 1 and 2.

RTI falls into the category of problem solving approaches. Fuchs (2003) projects that 80% of at-risk students can achieve their educational expectations through Tier 1; an additional 10 to 15% will attain their grade level performance through assistance at the Tier 2 level, and approximately 10 to 15% will require Tier 3 supports. Children at the Tier 3 level may need special education testing and instruction and remedial intervention, including speech-language services.

SLPs are uniquely positioned to contribute in the RTI process in their schools because of the strong link between communication and learning (Ehren, Montgomery, Rudebusch, & Whitmire, 2011; Ukrainetz, 2006) . Being able to communicate and interact effectively in the learning situation is essential for literacy acquisition. SLPs are skilled at identifying students in general education who are at risk due to their communication skills. They are also prepared to contribute to program design. The RTI process fosters a strong collaboration between teachers and SLPs so that they may jointly to develop and select instructional strategies that will resolve children's learning difficulties. When SLPs are involved in RTI approaches, they focus on communication and instructional strategies that teachers can use to support and improve student performance. Here are some tips that will lead to SLP's successful participation in the RtI process (Blosser, 2009):

- Acquire knowledge about the relationship among disabilities and reading problems, classroom instruction, and student performance.
- Become knowledgeable about the curriculum standards for each grade.
- Identify the impact of the disability on the skills necessary for reading.
- Understand the requirements for school accountability, especially IDEA and ESEA.
- Become familiar with test modification and accommodations and alternative assessments.
- Strive to be an active and effective member of the educational team.
- Observe and work with the student in the classroom setting to become familiar with expectations and instructional practices.

Unfortunately, some school districts and many SLPs have not yet fully clarified the SLP's role in the RTI process. Their participation may be limited because they may not be able to work with students unless they have an IEP. Others aren't able make time on their busy schedules for the problem-solving meetings and ongoing collaboration. Administrators limit some from participating because they are not sure that RTI fits within the scope of practice for the SLP. Roth, Dougherty, Paul, and Adamczyk (2010) provide an excellent synopsis of the role SLPs can play at each tier of instruction. Their book offers many suggestions of classroom modifications and oral language activities that can be used in the classroom. Tier 1 examples of the SLP's role include screening to identify students at risk for academic and social problems; interpreting screening results and reviewing student's performance on classroom and standardized assessments; and analyzing the communication expectations within the classroom. In addition, SLPs are well equipped to recommend ways to modify the learning environment, assist teachers in identifying causal factors, breaking down complex tasks, providing staff development programs, and providing practice materials. At the Tier 1 level, the SLP can assist the classroom teacher by conducting in depth screening, analyzing curricular materials, pre-teaching or re-teaching important curricular concepts, and providing short-term instruction in the classroom or as a pull-out service. At Tier 3, the SLP can provide more intense instruction, conduct more intense assessments, and identify factors that would lead to a full evaluation.

Blosser (2009) recommends establishing a plan describing the teacher's responsibilities for implementing the intervention strategies during classroom activities. To do so, the problem-solving team (SLP, teacher, and others) should discuss and agree on the following topics:

- A brief description of the student's communication or learning problem
- Examples of classroom performance that is resulting in the teacher's concern.
- Specific speech or language behaviors to be improved.
- Recommended intervention strategies that the teacher should try.
- Time during the day when the teacher should use the strategy.
- Number of times during the day, week, or month it is to be used.
- Type of probe test that will be used to determine if progress is occurring (curriculum-based tasks).
- Methods for administering the probe (observing, testing, interviewing).
- Schedule for administering the probes (weekly, monthly, every 9 weeks).
- Preparation the team needs in order to implement the strategy.
- Appointment for the team to reconvene to discuss progress and next steps.

Service Coordination

Children with disabilities and their families frequently require a broad range of intervention services. Physical and mental health care may be necessary as well as financial assistance and therapy services. Therapies might include speech-language intervention, aural habilitation, physical therapy, occupational therapy, visual training, counseling, and the like. Numerous professionals representing multiple agencies are charged with delivering the services. As a result, goals, treatment programs, and services are often fragmented and/or duplicated. In addition, complications arise for reimbursement for services because the agencies each may have different funding streams.

Coordination of services is essential to improve the quality of services offered to children and their families. The central question asked is, "What help does the family of a child with disabilities need to function well?" Emphasis is placed on collaborative planning and efficient, effective service delivery. To achieve this service coordination, professionals from a variety of disciplines and agencies must strive to understand one another's disciplines. Through this model, the family is involved meaningfully in all aspects of planning, implementing, and monitoring their child's programs.

One of the agencies involved in service delivery for children is the educational system. School clinicians have opportunities to coordinate their services with professionals both inside and outside of the school system. The clinician can contribute much to the service coordination process. For example, she can share information about the services available in the schools. Many health care professionals are unaware of services that are available and how they can be accessed. In addition, he or she can explain the child's communication impairments and their impact on the child's ability to function. The speech-language program and educational program planned for the child can be explained in terms that are understandable. Redundancy and assistance with facilitating multiple goals can be accomplished through collaboration with other professionals.

Specialized Services

Many school districts create specialized program services to meet the needs of specific populations. These programs may evolve because a particular expertise is needed or for economical or geographical reasons. Following are some examples of specialized services.

Diagnostic Therapy

Some school districts and regional resource centers offer comprehensive diagnostic services at diagnostic centers. Students are enrolled in these programs for only a short period of time. After evaluations are completed, results and recommendations are shared with the parents and school personnel. Individualized educational plans are formulated and implemented in different contexts.

Hospital or Home-Based Intervention

In the home and/or hospital-based context, educators and clinicians travel to serve students who are unable to attend school because of confinement to their homes or to a hospital setting. This context is employed when providing services to school-age children who have physical or mental disabilities that prohibit them from participating in the school environment. For example, children with brain injury may receive educational services in the medial setting and then at home prior to returning to school full time.

Parent Training

Instruction is often provided to parents with children who have communication disorders, developmental disabilities or who are at risk. The clinician provides guidance and instruction in techniques for assisting infants and preschoolers in developing appropriate communicative behaviors and skills. The services may be provided in the school, a center, the child's home, or other approved facilities.

Residential Placement

The residential context is usually reserved for children with severe and profound impairments who have medical, behavioral, judicial, or education needs beyond that which can be provided at school or in the home. Education and specialized services are provided in addition to daily care.

Self-Contained Classroom

Some school districts establish special education classrooms for children who present a particular type of disability, such as autism, vision impairment, or hearing impairment. Teachers and other team members are responsible for providing academic as well as curriculum instruction and therapy or other instructional support interventions. Children may receive intervention both inside and outside of the self-contained classroom.

Resource Room

Many schools identify educators and classrooms where support services are provided, including focused tutoring for specific academic subjects. There may also be equipment and electronic devices to enhance concept learning.

Articulation Resource Center

Clinicians in the San Diego School District established a resource center for serving students with articulation delays. Rather than enroll students in a traditional special education based speech and language therapy program, they receive intensive intervention in a resource center setting. Results are promising. Some students' articulation errors are corrected in approximately 20 hours. This demonstrates that intensive services provided within a condensed time period can yield good results. Students don't attend therapy throughout the entire school year, missing valuable class time (Taps, 2008).

Academic Credit Classes for Middle School and High School

Providing services for high school students can be challenging but very rewarding. Current trends in service delivery for adolescents encourage practitioners to focus on preparing students for graduation and successful participation in postsecondary education and future careers. Larson (2011) provides some very interesting strategies for motivating adolescents with language disorders. Among her recommendations are: offer a course for credit, assign grades to performance, use existing school time blocks, group students in creative ways, use classrooms in "acceptable" parts of the building, work with education colleagues, and call the intervention program a "communication skills class" or "club."

Receiving grades and academic credit for participating in the speech-language intervention program often motivates middle and high school students. The credit is usually one-quarter or one-half as much as a typical academic course and enrollment and may be repeated. Clinicians wishing to use this model must work with administrators, teachers, the curriculum team, and counselors to determine where the course best fits in the school curriculum. Some districts offer courses of this nature as an elective in the language arts area. Others structure the class for developing students' functional or social-vocational communication skills. Still others offer courses as personal enhancement classes. In this type of program, one class period of the student's schedule is devoted to work on language skills. The course might be titled "Communication Skills." During the class period, the speech/language pathologist services several students whose language learning and remedial needs would benefit from this type of scheduling. Course content may include vocabulary development, problem-solving techniques, listening skills, social and conversational speech, question-asking and answering strategies, nonverbal communication skills, study skills related to language, and survival pragmatic language. Service is provided in a more natural environment than is possible in a separate speech therapy room. Examples of language interactions, language modeling, and cueing may enhance the teacher's interaction with students. Language skills are incorporated into the academic curriculum, thus enhancing opportunities for generalization and carryover of language skills into everyday life.

In order to be considered a legitimate course, there must be a defined course content, learning objectives, learning activities, and grading criteria commensurate with other courses offered. For example, students can be objectively evaluated on factors such as attendance, level of involvement and participation in class activities, completion of assignments, and efforts made toward reaching identified targets and goals. The course can be listed as an elective course option in the student's school handbook and scheduling can be done through the school computer along with all other academic scheduling. If the scheduling system is refined, groups of students with similar communication disabilities can be formed.

Organizing the program in this manner makes it more acceptable to students who may be sensitive about their speech or language difficulties. It also promotes interaction of students with similar concerns. This enables practice of functional speech and language skills. Another advantage to this scheduling plan is that students begin the year with the speech-language therapy program as a part of their schedule rather than an addition to it.

After School and Summer Programs

One way in which many school clinicians have extended their services is to offer after school or summer programs. Most school districts refer to the summer programs as Extended School Year (ESY). They establish specific criteria for determining which students can participate in the ESY program. Reasons for carrying out a summer program might include providing intensive therapy for children with severe disabilities or providing make-up services for students who missed large amounts of service during the school year. Many of the after school and summer programs are financed by the local education system. Some have been underwritten by foundations, grants, or local service clubs. Many times the program is offered as a joint effort of both the school system and a voluntary organization. In this sort of program, usually the building, facilities, supplies, and so on are furnished by the school, whereas the clinician's salary is paid by the community group. The clinician in charge of the program is charged with establishing criteria for accepting children and will need to carry out the necessary diagnostic or therapy procedures. Often, only a limited number of children can be accepted, depending on the number of staff members available. Summer programs are usually well received in a community, and once started are often repeated during subsequent summers.

Telepractice

Technology influences every aspect of our life. Through technology, speech-language services can be provided synchronously or asynchronously. Therapists can work in remote locations away from the school or home. This provides great opportunity as well as challenges for school practitioners. Remote and underserved school districts consider telepractice as an option to meet the communication needs of their students.

Telepractice is defined as "the application of telecommunications technology to delivery of professional services at a distance by linking clinician to client or clinician to clinician for assessment, intervention, and/or consultation." (ASHA Position statement, 2005; Brown, Juenger, & Forducey, 2007). ASHA's position is that, "the quality of services delivered via telepractice must be consistent with the quality of services delivered face-to-face" (ASHA, 2004).

Over the past several years, therapists, organizations, and universities have researched the effectiveness of live, interactive video conferencing to provide speech-language services to people who could not otherwise access them. The literature in the field of communication disorders reports several studies that demonstrate the efficacy and benefits of telepractice as a viable method for delivering speech-language services to children and adults in medical, home, and school settings. Telepractice is seen as one of the solutions to the shortage of speech-language pathologists, especially in rural school districts and districts that have difficulty attracting SLPs to their area.

Teams of ASHA members are leading the way to provide representative examples of effective telepractice services. There are recommendations regarding the knowledge, skills, and competencies needed by professionals who provide telepractice (Grogan-Johnson, 2010; Grogan-Johnson et al., 2010). Official policies have evolved that support and provide standards and guidance for the delivery of services via telepractice. In 2010 a new ASHA Special Interest Group was formed to provide a forum for the telepractice community, SIG 18.

School-based telepractice incorporates data sharing and the use of interactive online activities during therapy. Therapy sessions generally include individual students or small groups. Therapy goals are consistent with those established for face-to-face therapy. Some limitations have been identified including limited ability to collaborate with education team members, practice in the classroom environment, and involving the telepractice SLP in the activities of the school. These problems are not insurmountable and will likely be resolved in future phases of telepractice development.

Scheduling Services

In Chapter 7, systems for identification children who are eligible for services were discussed. One aspect dealt with the identification and further diagnosis of children who were possible candidates for intervention. Let us now turn our attention to the scheduling of children for services. In implementing a program based on the expanded service delivery concept, the SLP allocates the amount of time to be spent providing assistance to the child and the type of intervention approach relative to their functional communication performance. For example, children who are functioning at fairly high level and need only minimal assistance receive services less frequently, at a lesser intensity, and for a shorter period of time than those who are functioning at a lower level and need more assistance and greater intensity and frequency of services. In both instances, additional providers can be incorporated into various aspects of intervention services. All children identified as needing services would receive them, but the decisions for how the services are delivered, when and where they would be delivered, and who would deliver them is dependent on the child's need versus traditional scheduling routines.

Service plans that are based on the needs of the child meet the letter and the spirit of federal legislation. Rather than servicing "schools" the SLP is servicing children. Too often, administrators expect the SLP's time to be divided equally among school buildings and children on the caseload without consideration of the individual needs of the children. This puts the quality of the program at risk.

Guidelines for developing the caseload should be flexible and adaptable for large, small, or medium-sized school populations and a wide variety of communication disabilities. They also can be applied to pupils from preschool through high school. The most basic consideration in planning the therapy program is to make the best use of the time allotted. This is not much help to the beginning clinician, however, who must decide whether to schedule children for 15-minute or 30-minute sessions or longer; to work in the classroom or use pullout; to group or not to group. Perhaps the most efficient approach is to take a careful look at the schedule of classes in the school and then determine a therapy caseload and workload schedule that coincides with the school's class schedule. This does not necessarily mean that therapy sessions should be the same length as classes, but it would be helpful to both teachers and students if there were some coordination between the two. Nor does it mean that all the sessions should be planned for the same amount of time. Some sessions may be 20 minutes in length, and some may be 45 minutes. Some would be once per week, others would be three times per week. The decision about the amount of time should be made by the clinician on the basis of the child's needs. More time may be needed for group sessions or children with severe impairments. The child in the generalization stages of therapy may require ten or 15 minutes several times a week. High school students who may be able to assume more responsibility for their own progress may need only one one-hour session per month. The amount of time scheduled for each child may change as the child progresses. Classroom teachers should be informed of the fact that change will occur during the year and that their input would be valuable in considering any changes in the time. The key word in planning the amount of time per therapy session is flexibility and the criterion is what is in the best interest of the child. The responsibility for making good use of the time is the clinician's. In recent years, SLPs have developed many interesting scheduling models that reflect the variables discussed above.

Itinerant Scheduling

Traditionally, speech and language services have been provided on an itinerant basis. Scheduling has been based on state and district regulations that define eligibility, caseload, number of child-contact hours per week, and ratio of clinicians to school populations. By providing more options for delivery of services instead of relying solely on the itinerant model, more children who need help can be reached. This does not imply that the itinerant model is not a good model when it is used in the appropriate circumstances. However, it does mean the speech-language pathology professional must break the habit of thinking of it as the only option.

Many of the children with severe communication disorders, as well as those with mild-to- moderate deviations, will be in general education classrooms with speech-language intervention services provided by the school clinician on a itinerant basis. The itinerant model has been used from the time it was originally offered in 1910 by Ella Flagg Young, who felt that it protected the young teacher from "depression of spirit and low physical conditions resulting from confinement in one room for several successive hours while working with abnormal conditions." Not until recent years have other systems of service delivery and scheduling been developed. These have come about as a result of mandatory legislation, emphasis on reserving time during the day for focusing on subjects such as reading, more sophisticated tools, larger numbers of children needing services, and the recognized need for a multidisciplinary approach.

The itinerant model may be effective in situations where schools are within a few miles of each other or where school populations and caseloads are low. It may also provide continuous therapy for children who need more frequent intervention over a longer period of time, such as children with language impairments, fluency problems, hearing loss, or learning disabilities. The itinerant (or traditional) model may take several forms. The school clinician may serve one, two, or three schools, working with children in small groups or individual children on an intermittent basis once or twice a week. However, it should not be implied that all itinerant services are restricted to pullout scheduling.

Intensive Scheduling

Another model of scheduling services is the intensive cycle, sometimes called the block system. In this model the child is seen four or five times a week for a specified and concentrated block of time, usually four, six, or eight weeks. The intensive scheduling model enables the clinician to provide a greater number of hours of treatment within a condensed amount of time. Some clinicians use intensive scheduling to provide a high number of services to children with severe communication impairments who will benefit from more frequent services. Others elect to use an intensive scheduling model for children with minor communication impairments. For example, they provide services daily, for short amounts of time for six to nine weeks. Children can then exit the therapy program in a shorter amount of time rather then attend for the entire school year.

Specialization

Another possible option is to appoint a clinician to provide specialized services to a designated population of students. In a variation of this model in a large school system, part of the staff might provide a traditional itinerant schedule while one or more clinicians would serve as "specialists," matching their strengths and/or specific training to the students' needs. By focusing on a particular population or disability group, the clinician can strengthen his or her knowledge of the disability and develop an expertise at assessing student's problems and delivering appropriate treatment strategies. Generally, when this model is implemented, a schedule plan and routine is followed. For example, the SLP may move from school to school in a district providing services only to students in the life skills class or those with autism spectrum disorders or high school students working on vocational skills. Other examples of specialty services are the assessment team or providing instruction to teachers who are teaching reading skills to middle school students. He or she would visit three schools and see only those children in the designated population group, some in small groups and others in the classroom setting. This format provides opportunities for observing in the classroom, meeting with teachers, modeling appropriate communication behaviors, introducing different intervention methods, creating specialized materials, and more.

Flexible Scheduling

Flexible scheduling models enable SLPs to schedule and provide services that are truly matched to student's needs instead of arranged on a homogeneous schedule that is the same for all students. By varying the schedule and location of services, the clinician can provide services in the therapy room as well as the natural environment of the classroom. Progress in the general education classroom can be monitored. Opportunities are presented for sharing expertise, training, and recommendations with other colleagues. Flexible scheduling plans are more in line with federal laws (Carlin, 2011). Perhaps the most important benefit of flexible scheduling is that therapists can allot time in their day for completing other mandatory workload duties including paperwork and documentation, evaluations, student related meetings, and collaboration. There is also room in the schedule for providing make-up services.

The 3:1 scheduling model of service delivery is an example of a flexible scheduling model. It has received great attention by SLPs across the country in the past several years. Many clinicians refer to the 3:1 model as a "caseload/workload" model. Proponents of the model indicate that it enables clinicians to effectively provide intervention, manage their workload, collaborate with teachers, and align the speech-language program with the curriculum (Annett, 2004; Soliday, 2001). The 3:1 schedule model designates three weeks out of each month for direct intervention with students and one week for indirect intervention and workload activities that are performed "on behalf of the child" (Carlin, 2011). Activities that are generally performed are meeting with teachers and parents, modeling and teaching strategies, conducting assessments, developing therapy materials, modifying the student's environment, programming AAC devices, completing paperwork, participating in building level activities, conducting home visits, and problem-solving. Some districts have modified the 3:1 model to meet their unique administrative and scheduling needs. For example, some districts use an 8:1 model that parallels a nine week grading period.

The 3:1 model is exemplary of the type of creativity and innovation that our profession has been seeking to enable clinicians to complete the important tasks that are required to provide the breadth and depth of services necessary to meet the complex needs of the children we serve. Guided by the leadership of SLP Sharon Soliday, clinicians in the Portland, Oregon School District initiated the 3:1 model during the 2001 to 2002 school year. They initially began with a pilot project modeled after a school system in Wisconsin that had been implementing the model for years. To gain approval and buy-in for trying a different model, the Portland SLPs held discussions with school administrators. They made a compelling argument by reinforcing the need for SLPs to support students in their general education classrooms and sharing data that demonstrated how the new model would impact caseload size. They also ensured district administrators that they would collect data and be accountable for the clinicians' time and activities. As the Portland SLPs approached the implementation as a project, they were able to report their successes as follows. There were increases in third-party Medicaid reimbursement, fewer session cancellations, increased collaboration efforts, and better morale among the SLPs (Annett, 2004).

Clinicians who successfully implement the 3:1 model recommend that it is imperative to be transparent about how time is spent. For example, avoid explaining the model by saying, "I do therapy for three weeks and have one week off." The fourth week isn't "off." Rather, what is accomplished that week is considered an important part of the SLP's workload. The activities are necessary in order to provide the breadth and depth of services necessary to ensure that treatment is successful and students achieve their goals. Following the example of the Portland School District SLPs, it is smart to provide sample calendars that demonstrate how time is used during the intervention weeks as well as during the indirect week. It is recommended that SLPs document time spent collaborating with teachers and parents, the nature of those interactions, and the results.

Combining Scheduling Models

Another option for scheduling services is to institute a combination of models. For example, the clinician may decide to combine the itinerant model with the intensive cycle scheduling system. Obviously, this would be easier to arrange if there were more than one SLP on the staff, if Speech-Language Pathology Assistants (SLPAs) were available, if the program were carefully coordinated, and if the clinicians and the school administrators all agreed on the program.

Scheduling Groups of Children

Although some therapy in the public schools is carried on in individual sessions, most services are provided in group sessions. Initially, the clinician is faced with the task of deciding which children should be placed in a group. The answer would depend on the needs of the child at any given stage of therapy. Some children may need an intensive approach to master some skills, and this may best be accomplished by working alone with the clinician for a short period of time. Later, that same child may be ready to use these skills in a social context, and a group experience would best fit this need. The makeup of the group is an important factor in planning for optimal therapy results. Some clinicians find it more productive to work with a group of children who have similar problems, whereas for other clinicians the homogeneity of problems is not as important as grouping children of the same age level.

There are several factors to consider when setting up therapy groups. First, understand that there are no correct or incorrect ways of grouping children. Groups must be flexible and must meet the needs of each child enrolled. Second, grouping is done to control the factors that enhance learning. Third, groups should not become static. As children learn and as needs change the composition of the group should change. Fourth, groups should be structured but not rigid. A structure assists learning and if learning is not taking place there is no purpose for the existence of the group. Fifth, the size of the group should depend on its major purposes; however, a group of more than five or six students to one instructor tends to lose its instructional effect, especially when therapy sessions are scheduled only for 30 minutes. Often, several children from a single classroom are recommended for therapy. Depending on their disabilities and needs, they may or may not be able to be accommodated in the same group and scheduled for the same therapy time. The teacher's input in scheduling is essential so consideration can be given to academic subjects the children will miss and disruptions that will occur as they enter and leave the classroom.

Students with speech, language, or hearing disorders should not be put in therapy groups simply to accommodate more students in the SLP's caseload or because there is a time slot available. The rationale for placing a student in a group should depend on the needs of the student and the purpose of the group.

Working with Teachers and Administrators to Plan Schedules

SLPs may encounter difficulty with scheduling because everyone is competing for the student's learning time. Required or fun learning activities may take place while the student is out of the classroom, resulting in missed information if the student must routinely miss the same subject. By considering the classroom schedule, it may be possible to schedule around important subjects or special activities.

Constructing a daily, weekly, monthly, or yearly schedule is not an easy task. Clinicians go about the complex process in many different ways. Some use hand designed schedule forms, others use excel charts, and others assemble their schedule as they would a puzzle. Help is available in the form of scheduling software. One company in particular, Caselite Software (http://www.Caselitesoftware.com) has led the way in designing a simple-to-use, efficient system for creating and maintaining the SLP's schedule. The speech-language pathologist simply inputs key information about his or her workload and about the children to be served such as: their grade or school placement; their teacher's name and classroom schedules; their speech-language disorder; the amount of services they are to receive; the frequency for the services, and whether they are served individually or in a group. Time is allocated on the schedule for activities such as lunch, assessments, AAC preparation, team meetings, and documentation. A schedule is then produced through the wonders of technology.

DISCUSSION QUESTIONS AND PROJECTS

1. Why is it important to have definitions of service delivery models that are uniform and agreed on by professionals in the field?

2. You are the school SLP. How would you explain the range of service delivery options to a group of elementary teachers in your building?

3. Interview some SLPs presently working in programs where the various service delivery options are employed. What questions will you ask them?

4. Using Flower's list of essential characteristics of good service-delivery models, devise a list of questions under each of the five headings. The purpose of the questions would be to evaluate the service delivery models found in a typical school.

5. Think of one therapy session you have observed or conducted. What really made that session stand out in your mind as being excellent or not so excellent? Use Flower's list of essential characteristics of good service delivery models to summarize your observations.

6. Familiarize yourself with numerous contexts within the educational system where services can be provided and identify ways to conduct services in those contexts.

7. Meet with a small group of practicing speech-language pathologists. Ask them to describe the various programs and contexts they utilize for delivering services.

8. Obtain an hour by hour description of an SLP's schedule. Find out the ages, grades, and disorders served; the service delivery models employed; and the intervention providers, activities, and contexts for each child on any one given day of the week. Now describe that SLP's caseload and workload. If you are a practicing SLP, exchange the above information with a colleague.

9. Would you schedule children for intervention during recess? Art class? Physical education? Reading? Social studies? Explain the rationale for your answers.

10. Does the severity of the problem have any influence on the time of day you would provide service to a youngster?

9

Developing a Relevant Intervention Program

Does a child's disability impact his or her performance in the classroom? If yes, would speech-language services make a difference in the student's classroom performance, ability to access the curriculum, ability to communicate with others, and/or ability to reach his or her potential? These are huge questions that administrators, educators, therapists, and parents ponder every day. When school teams evaluate a student, they seek to determine how the disability the child presents may be interfering with the student's learning. Key educational areas that may be affected are academic, social-emotional, and vocational performance. If everyone agrees that there is an adverse effect upon educational performance, the student's eligibility for services is confirmed. Regardless of the type, amount, frequency, location, or intensity of services offered, it is important that the services are educationally relevant. In other words, they must make a difference in educational performance. Focusing on educationally relevant skills helps the student pay attention to teacher's instructions, participate in a wide range of learning activities, answer questions, seek assistance, follow directions, demonstrate appropriate social and emotional skills, and recall facts. School team members must join forces to determine how to best structure intervention so that it is educationally relevant. The SLP plays a very valuable role in the decision-making process. In this chapter planning, implementing, and evaluating intervention services are discussed.

Educational Relevance— What an Important Concept!

Collaboration is needed to achieve educational relevance. Hanft and Shephard (2008) describe the school-based collaboration as, "an interactive team process that focuses student, family, education, and related services partners on enhancing the academic achievement and functional performance of all students in school." Teachers can provide insights into the demands and expectations for performance in their classroom. They have the best knowledge of the learning objectives, curriculum, and instructional methods. They also can contribute information about distractions, rules, pace, and the general classroom environment. The school SLP spends most of the working day involved in some aspect of service delivery. Development of the intervention plan is guided by input and decisions made by the clinician in collaboration with teachers, parents, and others. The service delivery plan and intervention must be appropriate and relevant to the student's communication disability and educational needs. It is not necessary at this time, nor would space permit, to discuss the various philosophies and treatment approaches for each specific disorder. It is sufficient to say that the school clinician should be well versed in the current treatment practices as well as the school curriculum. There are a number of approaches available, and the choice will depend on what best serves each child. Each therapist and educator has a responsibility to keep up with current trends and practices in the field. Family members can provide insights about the home situation and factors that may be contributing to the student's attitude or motivation. SLPs can discuss the nature and characteristics of the disability and help their education teammates understand how these characteristics interfere with a student's ability to succeed. They can also offer positive recommendations for modifying the classroom environment, adapting learning materials, utilizing specific instructional or intervention strategies, or developing key skills to promote success. Sound planning is necessary for any educational or therapy program to be successful, regardless of the disability. Planning and collaborative strategies can lead to powerful outcomes!

Planning Individualized Programs

Effective intervention requires a comprehensive planning process. Planning begins with the referral and team decisions of next steps. Many questions follow the referral. Should the student be monitored for a period of time? Can the student be helped if the classroom environment is modified or if the teacher implements specific intervention strategies during instruction in the classroom? Does the student need further assessment? If therapy is advisable, what intervention approaches make most sense? What options for delivering the services should be recommended? What outcomes should be expected? How can performance in school be improved as a result of intervention?

When an evaluation is completed, one or more team planning conferences are held. At that time, the SLP works with the student's parents, a representative of the school district, the student's teachers, and other appropriate professionals to plan the special education and intervention program. During the conference, decisions made are based on data gathered during the multifactored assessment and evaluation. The nature and degree of the student's disability is determined. Eligibility for special education services and the potential benefits of instructional support is determined. The mode for service delivery is considered and the goals, objectives, and procedures for intervention are identified. The SLP and other team members should come to the meeting prepared to discuss the nature of the student's communication impairment, its impact on educational performance, recommendations for treatment, ideas for integrating treatment into educational activities, the roles and responsibilities of each team member, and training necessary to prepare people to help and support the student. In cases where only speech and language problems are the primary concern, fewer individuals may be involved in the planning. However, the need to meaningfully incorporate others does not change.

An *Individualized Education Program (IEP)* is developed for children ages 3 or older. The *Individualized Family Service Plan (IFSP)* is used for infants and toddlers 0 to 3 years old. In addition to the IEP, an *Individualized Transition Plan (ITP)* is prepared for older students.

SLPs are valuable members on the planning team. The following assessment strategies are recommended prior to planning a service delivery and intervention program for students:

- Conduct an environmental assessment to determine communication climate or situations that may pose difficulty for the student.
- Determine the communication needs required for accomplishing classroom objectives and daily classroom requirements.
- Analyze the communication behaviors of key persons with whom the student will be interacting.
- Based on the information gathered, work with the student's family and teachers to restructure the environment and modify communication interactions in order to strengthen communication skills.

An Approach to the Planning Process

Sound planning and program management are necessary for any educational or treatment program to be successful regardless of the disability. Planning treatment programs poses substantial challenges for education teams. Careful thought, organized, imaginative planning, coordinated actions, and skillful management are required to achieve desired outcomes. Treatment plans must meet expectations and requirements imposed by many different entities including parents, teachers, funding agencies, and federal legislation. Although these challenges seem to be insurmountable, they also offer planners opportunities for developing excellent programs if time and care are taken.

According to IDEA, the education plan must be tailored to meet the unique needs presented by each individual child in accordance with recommendations from significant educators and family members.

Unfortunately, plans sometimes focus on correction of specific behaviors, development of particular skills, or completion of tasks. They fail to reflect a comprehensive, integrated view of the student. Taking this approach limits the effectiveness of all educational efforts. A more meaningful approach is to design a service delivery and intervention program that is more student-centered by also modifying and strengthening the environment in which the student learns, lives, works, and plays.

Blosser and DePompei (2002) recommend implementing an *ongoing planning process* (Figure 9–1). A useful framework for understanding this type of planning process is to approach it as though planning a trip. Figure 9–2 presents the ques-

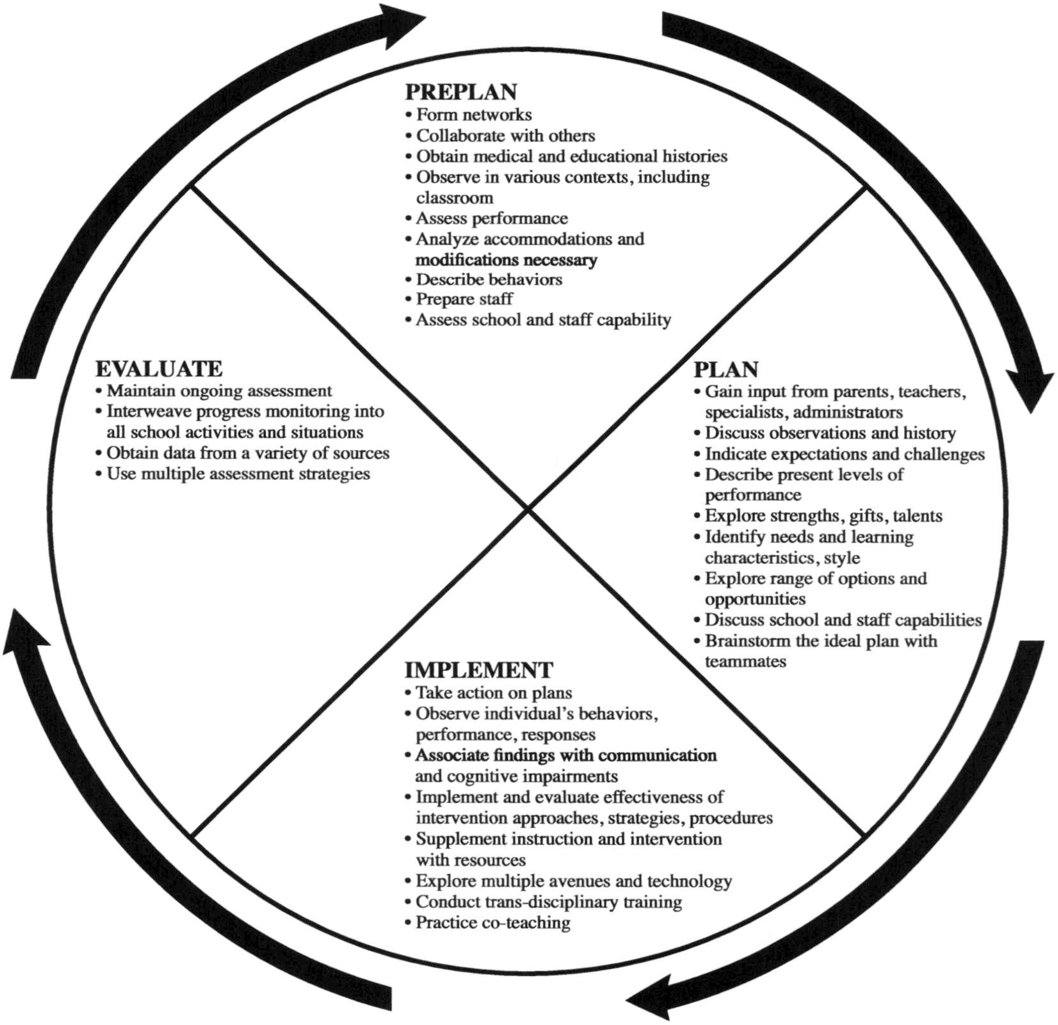

Figure 9–1. Ongoing planning process.

1. *"Where is the individual now?"* What is the nature and extent of the student's communication impairment? From a number of perspectives, what are the resulting impairments, strengths, and needs? How do the communication problems impact on the student's overall performance in a variety of situations?
2. *"Where do we want him or her to go?"* The long-term outcomes we want the student to achieve should be determined. Consider this question especially in relation to the general education curriculum and participation in school-related activities. We want students to achieve their maximum potential. Treatment planners need to decide if the services and programs they are offering for the student will help him or her participate maximally in educational, work, and social activities.
3. *"When do we want the student to get there?"* What is the time line for implementing the program and achieving the desired outcomes? Treatment for communication impairments generally occurs over several months and in some cases, over several years. Evaluation of the student's performance must be continuous with ongoing review of the modifications and strategies that are implemented and how they are working.
4. *"Who do we want and need to take with us?"* In order to plan and implement the program effectively, who must be involved? The individuals that have a real stake in the student's success should be at the table when plans are made. Time should be spent improving understanding of the student's strengths and needs, considering the policies that guide service delivery, the challenges that are likely to be faced, and the resources that will be available for support.
5. *"How do we want to go?"* What approaches to intervention are most effective for meeting the needs of the student? Any mode of treatment that will bring about the desired outcomes should be tried. Clinicians and educators should be willing to try creative approaches to meet the student's needs. There is not a "one size fits all" to therapy. Team members need to be a part of the learning process: gaining a better understanding of the communication impairment, learning to work together as a team, identifying opportunities to promote the student's successes, and striving to continually improve the quality of the student's performance.
6. *"How much will the trip cost? What resources will be necessary to implement the plan?"* The team must decide what resources it will commit to achieve the desired outcomes they decide upon. It takes a lot to provide assistance to children. Resources include finances as well as personnel, time, and service options.
7. *"How will we know when we have arrived?"* What are the benchmarks against which the team will measure the student's success? We must know if the modifications we make and the strategies we implement are making a difference. The intervention program and student's progress should be evaluated in an ongoing manner to determine the appropriateness and suitability for meeting the student's needs.

Figure 9–2. Questions for the planning team for planning the intervention plan.

tions the planning team needs to ask when formulating an individualized plan for the student. Implementing the ongoing planning process and addressing each of the elements in the process will yield a plan that addresses skill development for the student, support and coaching for educators so they can implement intervention strategies, and system support to build a school culture that promotes a climate of support for children with disabilities.

There are four phases to the ongoing planning process. Phase I is the *Preplanning Phase* where groundwork is laid and the design for services and treatment is developed. The team is formed and each team member begins to gather pertinent data including: the student's history and current status; the environments in which learning will take place; and the skills, needs, and potential contributions people in the learning environment can make on the student's success. A wide variety of assessment procedures are administered during the preplanning phase. This enables planners to gain a comprehensive perspective about the student's strengths and needs. Also, importantly, the team can begin to gain understanding of what the school and people in the school have to offer to support the student as well as the modifications needed to enable success. At the end of Phase I, the team should be able to identify the obstacles that will interfere with the student's success.

In Phase II, the *Planning Phase*, the team begins to work collaboratively to analyze information gleaned during the pre-planning phase. Then together, the team determines the student's needs, goals, objectives, and workable strategies for preparing the child to function effectively in school and other environments. Meeting time is devoted to deciding the "who," "what," "where," "when," "why," and "how" aspects of the plan. Team members collate information from family, teachers, specialists, health care providers and others. The anticipated demands and expectations the student will confront in the classroom are identified. Thus, the student's strengths and needs are explored in the context of changes that might occur if modifications are made. The roles and responsibilities of team members (providers) are identified and clarified.

In Phase III, the *Implementation Phase*, action is taken on the plan. The climate for effective intervention and teaching is established and opportunities for learning are provided. This includes learning by the student as well as learning by educators, through in-service and other forms of training. Modification strategies are tried, with careful observation to see if the child responds positively.

During Phase IV, the *Evaluation and Improvement Phase*, the plan is reviewed to determine how well it is or is not working. The degree of success at achieving desired outcomes is determined. The team determines if further modifications are necessary and discusses next steps. Thus, the planning process, including information gathering and observation, begins again.

Developing the Individualized Education Program

The cornerstone of IDEA is the student's Individualized Education Program (IEP). IDEA includes requirements or standards for IEPs. The IEP provides documentation of why and how the student with disabilities will receive special education and related services, including speech-language services. The IEP is written collaboratively by the IEP team, including the parents or caregivers, and includes pertinent descriptions of the student's strengths and needs, goals based on those needs, and the educational services necessary to meet those goals. The goals must relate to the general education curriculum, address the student's participation in the educational process, consider expectations and demands in the educational setting, and be measurable. Although this process seems relatively straightforward, unfortunately, schools and education teams continue to struggle with how to prepare and execute IEPs that are relevant, effective, and developed in an efficient manner. If team members do not collaborate to develop IEPs, goals will not be understood by fellow team members, they will not address school performance or participation in the general education setting, nor will they be measurable.

The IEP is the vehicle that directs and guides the development of meaningful learning experiences, helping each child achieve the goal of becoming contributing and valued members of the community. The standards indicate that IEPs must include parent involvement, a focus on the general education curriculum, verification that team members are qualified and prepared to serve the student, accommodations, statewide and district-wide assessments, and progress reports. Interventions must be evidence-based. SLPs are required to adhere to specific timelines for conducting assessments, holding the IEP meeting and implementing services if indicated.

Speech-language pathologists and the educators with whom they work must consider all of these elements when they develop the IEP. The school district is responsible for training staff on the components of IEPs. Although these standards are intended to improve the education of children with special needs, it is anticipated that school districts will struggle with how to implement some of the requirements, especially with how they can enable students with disabilities greater access to the general education curriculum and how they can ensure that educators are prepared for the teaching challenges.

Figure 9–3 provides a format for conducting an interview with the teacher to determine the impact of communication disability on the student's performance. Table 9–1 presents the specific steps that should be followed by the SLP in partnership with education teammates to identify the student's needs and to recommend modifications.

TEACHER INTERVIEW
OBSERVATION OF COMMUNICATION AND PERFORMANCE IN THE CLASSROOM

Date ______________________ **Student** ______________________

Interviewer ______________________ **Teacher** ______________________

School ______________________ **Grade** ______________________

INSTRUCTIONS: Through conversations with teachers, develop a profile of the student's communication skills and performance within the classroom setting. Highlight strengths as well as problem areas. Use the questions listed below to guide the discussion. Analyze the information gathered and use it to formulate recommendations and strategies for services.

INTERACTIVE COMMUNICATION SKILLS/PERFORMANCE	**TARGET FOR SERVICE?**
How would you describe the student's overall performance in your class at this time? *Recommendations:*	
What are three successes the student has experienced recently in your classroom? *Recommendations:*	
Now describe three problems and talk about how you handle them. *Recommendations:*	
Tell me about the student's ability to tell stories, relate events, or convey information. *Recommendations:*	
Describe the way the student begins, ends, and maintains conversations. Is it appropriate for the situation? *Recommendations:*	
Explain how the student responds to humor, sarcasm, and figures of speech. *Recommendations:*	

Figure 9–3. Conducting a teacher interview. *continues*

INTERACTIVE COMMUNICATION SKILLS/PERFORMANCE	TARGET FOR SERVICE?
Do you feel the student recognizes and uses appropriate vocabulary considering the age and situation? *Recommendations*:	
Is the student's voice and intonation level appropriately suited to the situation, place, and intent? *Recommendations*:	
Can the student locate details and facts to answer questions and draw conclusions? How does he or she go about trying to do so? *Recommendations*:	
Is the student able to comprehend written material from a variety of sources (newspaper, magazine, content area texts, reference materials)? Is this skill demonstrated through summarizing and recalling main ideas? *Recommendations*:	
Describe the student's performance when following written direction to complete a task (worksheet, recipes, problems, directions for building models). *Recommendations*:	
Characterize the student's written work (grammar, word choice, sentence structure, organization, appearance). *Recommendations*:	
Does the student's response time permit him or her to respond to question when asked, participate in classroom discussions, complete assigned tasks? *Recommendations*:	
What motivates the student to change or improve performance efforts? *Recommendations*:	

Figure 9–3. *continues*

INTERACTIVE COMMUNICATION SKILLS/PERFORMANCE	TARGET FOR SERVICE?
Identify behaviors that might be helping this student do well. *Recommendations*:	
Now, identify behaviors that might be interfering with the student's success. *Recommendations*:	
Based on your knowledge of children and your experience in teaching, what steps do you think are necessary for helping this student at this time? *Recommendations*:	
What are three specific strategies you have tried to use to help this student? Why did they work or not work? *Recommendations*:	
PROFILE OF STUDENT'S INTERACTIVE COMMUNICATION AND ACADEMIC PERFOMANCE: **RECOMMENDED TARGETS FOR SERVICE AND SUMMARY OF RECOMMENDATIONS:**	**RESPONSIBLE PROVIDERS**

Figure 9–3. *continued*

Table 9–1. Steps to Assessing and Planning Modifications

Determine Tasks/Activities to Be Accomplished	*Date Completed*
Identify the student's communication characteristics and needs. • Meet with the planning team • Profile the student's performance	
Adhere to established policies and procedures for evaluating, exchanging the student, obtaining information, and communicating with potential providers.	
Obtain a concise statement of the student's communication problem as it appears in school-related situations from teachers and parents.	
Confirm adverse effect on performance.	
Identify the providers who will evaluate the student's strengths, problems, characteristics, learning styles and needs. Make recommendations based on findings. The student's parents must be included at this time. ***Family members are considered to be equal providers and the home is an equal context.***	
Select a mutually agreeable meeting time that is sufficient in length to avoid having to rush discussions.	
Compile descriptive information about the students' communication skills and performance in academic and social situations. Include samples of work. Compile a portfolio and profile of performance. **TOOLS: Formal tests; observations; teacher/parent interviews; educationally relevant assessment procedures (portfolio, work samples, etc.)** Include a student interview to determine the student's perspective of problems he/she is experiencing and ways he/she thinks other people can help or hinder. **TOOLS: Student interview**	
Construct a performance history and generate a report characterizing the student's skills, capabilities, and needs.	

continues

Table 9–1. *continued*

Determine Tasks/Activities to Be Accomplished	*Date Completed*
Conduct the meeting and exchange information, taking care to relate findings to academic and social performance.	
Ask yourself and team members: "Do we have all the information necessary to develop a data-based description of this student's current level of performance that can be used to drive the formulation of intervention outcomes and strategies?" You will know the answer to this question if you can answer these two questions: **Where is the student now?** **Where does the student need to go?**	
If you can answer these two questions, you are ready to begin seeking the answer to this question: **How will we get him or her there?**	
Identify environmental characteristics and needs • Meet with the planning team • Design appropriate interventions	
Analyze the communication manner and style of important communication partners (Teachers, family, peers). **TOOLS: Communication Style Identification Chart** Help the student's important communication partners analyze their own communication behaviors (manner, style, etc.) to determine if specific characteristics help or hinder the student's communicative performance. Discuss the match and/or mismatch between the partner's communicator's manner and style and the student's problems and needs. Jointly select the communicative intervention strategies that will reduce the mismatch between the partner's manner and style and the student's communication needs. **TOOLS: Recommend strategies for modifying communication styles to accommodate the needs of students with communication disabilities.**	

Table 9–1. *continued*

Determine Tasks/Activities to Be Accomplished	*Date Completed*
Analyze the classroom climate and teacher's instruction style and format. **TOOLS: Classroom Observation Guide** Help analyze the style and format of the classroom instruction to determine if specific modes of instruction help or hinder the student's communication performance. Discuss the match and/or mismatch between the classroom instruction style and format and the student's problems and needs. Consider key aspects of teaching instruction such as planning instruction, managing instruction, and delivering instruction. Jointly select the teaching instruction strategies that will reduce the mismatch between the teaching instruction style and format and the student's communication needs. **TOOLS: Teacher-to-student instruction strategies; classroom adaptations and modifications; student-to-student instructions strategies; student learning strategies.**	
Analyze the environmental factors that might influence performance. **TOOLS: Classroom Observation Guide** Helps analyze key physical, social psychological aspects of the learning environment to determine if specific components help or hinder the student's learning and communicative performance. Consider components such as noise level, visual stimuli, seating arrangements, student's location in relation to typical instructional position, location of learning and work material, attitudes of teachers and peers, teacher expectations, opportunities for social-communicative interactions, etc. Jointly select the environmental components that can be manipulated to reduce the mismatch between the environmental factors and student's learning and communication needs. **TOOLS: Teacher-to-student instruction strategies; classroom adaptations and modifications; student-to-student instruction strategies student learning strategies.**	

The IEP Team

The IEP Team determines the impact of the disability on the student's progress in general education. Education is broadly interpreted to include academic achievement as well as social, emotional, and vocational components. Team members should ideally be familiar with the core curriculum standards as well as the state assessments used to calculate adequate yearly progress (AYP).

Presumably, the team will consist of people who know the student very well and who can provide information based on their knowledge of the child or the situation. The participants should be decided on a case-by-case basis based on the child's needs and best interests. The team composition most likely would include some combination of the following individuals: the child's parents, at least one regular education teacher, at least one special education teacher or special education provider, a local education representative, and an individual who can interpret the instructional implications of the evaluation results. When appropriate, the child should also be present; especially if he or she is 14 years or older. The team members may change yearly depending on the student's grade level and academic/vocational program.

Team members may perform more than one of the above roles. The local education agency (LEA) representative should be qualified to supervise specially designed instruction, know the general curriculum, and be aware of the availability of resources. The SLP would be considered a special education provider if a communication disorder were the primary disability.

The parents are expected to be treated as equal participants and to play an active role in the planning and intervention process. They can provide critical information about the child's strengths and needs. They should be given opportunities to express their concerns and thoughts about the impact of the disability on the child's ability to progress in the general curriculum and participate in assessments. They should be included in decisions about the services that the student is provided. The child will be best served if the parents' expertise is sought and valued and if they are incorporated into the intervention plan. Chapter 10 provides information about how to mentor parents and teachers to be effective participants in that role.

All participants should contribute to developing, reviewing, and revising the plan. This includes proposing behavioral interventions and strategies. Dependent on the student's needs, it may also include accommodations, supplementary aids and services, adaptation of learning materials, program modifications, or support for school personnel so that they will be able to deliver the required services. Many must be involved in implementing the plan if it is to succeed.

Some school districts have had to send students out of the district to obtain a particular type of services that have been deemed necessary to meet the student's unique needs. When external services are contracted by the local board of education for a specific child, the IEP is written by the district personnel involved and contains the information regarding the nature of the service provided. Whenever possible, the external professional should be included in the preparation of the IEP.

IEP Forms and Content

States and school systems have flexibility to design their own IEP forms. Therefore, IEP forms may look different from one school system or state to another. Even though there may be variation, the IEP content must include certain types of information according to federal regulations. The requirements can be found on the Office of Special Education and Related Services Web site (2011).

The IEP must be specific for each child who receives either special education or related services or both. A single IEP is written for a child enrolled in regular or special education and receiving both special education and related services. The instructional support (or related) service may be speech-language intervention services, physical therapy, occupational therapy, adaptive behavior, counseling, or many other services that would support the student's success in school. Many students receive more than one instructional support service in addition to their classroom placement.

The Individualized Education Program

An Individualized Education Program must be developed for each school-age student identified as having a disability and needing special education placement or instructional support services. The plan should include a description of the student including demographic information, the disability, and the educational level and functional status. The IEP also presents a plan of future goals. The IEP (or IFSP and ITP) should provide a cohesive picture of who the child is, where the child has been, where the child is currently, and where the child is going. For younger children, the emphasis is placed on education, whereas with older children, the emphasis is placed on postsecondary goals including higher education and work.

Components of the IEP

Each of the major components necessary for the IEP is described in the following section. The components conform to the IEP requirements contained in the public law. Creativity and flexibility should be used when developing the IEP so that the student's needs can be properly addressed. The suggested components are designed to provide speech-language pathologists, educators, administrators, and family with information about the child and the educational demands, needs, and environment. As a secondary benefit, the information can lead to improvements in the program and case management procedures. The complexity of the IEP content will vary from student to student. Table 9–2 illustrates the required components of the IEP. These components may be revised when federal laws change. Examples of forms used in the IEP planning process are included in Appendix C.

Table 9–2. Components of the Individualized Education Program (IEP)

Vision	Explore the hopes and dreams that are held for the student for the future. Solicit the family's and student's preferences and interests.
Present level of educational performance	Review and document relevant data on the student including progress on current IEP, evaluation team report, family and student input, interventions, assessments, observations, and special factors. Provide a picture on how the student's disability affects involvement and performance on the general curriculum. Include information about strengths and needs.
Annual goals and short-term objectives	Develop annual measureable goals and objectives or benchmarks/milestones which enable the student, to the extent that is appropriate, to be involved with the general curriculum. Determine the services necessary to meet the student's needs.
Amount of special education or related services	Indicate the projected beginning date, frequency, and duration of services to be provided.
Supplementary aids and services	Determine the accommodations, modifications, or assistive devices and program modifications or supports for school personnel that will be needed for the student to progress in the general curriculum and to participate in extracurricular and other nonacademic activities.
Participation with students without disabilities	Decide the extent of participation that is possible with students who do not present disabilities in regular classes or in extracurricular activities.
Accommodations or modifications	Indicate the modifications that should be provided in the administration of state or district assessments of student achievement in order for the student to participate in the assessment project.
Transition service	Focus on the student's courses of study by age 14. Focus on interagency responsibilities or needed community supports by age 16.
Notification of transfer of rights	Document that the student has been informed of the rights that will transfer to the student upon reaching the age of majority.
Evaluation procedures and methods of measurement	Specify how the student's progress will be evaluated (e.g., criterion-referenced test, standardized test, student product, teacher observation, or peer evaluation). Indicate how often the evaluation will take place (e.g., daily, weekly, monthly, each grading period/semester, or annually). Report progress as often as progress is reported for general education students.
IEP team members	Record signatures of all members of the IEP team that developed the IEP.

Demographic Information

Identification information is provided about the child and his or her family or caregivers. Key information about the student includes: name, address, gender, grade, contact information, and parents or guardian information. The school district the student is assigned to is listed. In addition, information about the language spoken in the home is included.

Meeting Information

The date of meetings and purpose of the meeting are indicated. For example, the meeting may be to determine eligibility, to establish the initial IEP or to conduct an annual review, review the IEP, or make amendments. IEP timelines are also documented. It should be noted that the meeting to determine eligibility and the meetings to develop the IEP are two separate events. The evaluation report with all the details about assessment procedures and findings are discussed to determine eligibility and included in the eligibility document. The IEP refers to the evaluation and eligibility reports, summarizing the conclusions and recommendations.

Child's Profile

In this section, information that will help the team understand the student is captured. The student's strengths and needs are summarized. Background information and parental concerns are included. Results of state or district wide assessments are indicated. The academic, developmental, and functional needs of the student are explained. This includes information about behavioral issues, communication, hearing, vision, sensory and motor functioning, social emotional, and preacademic or academic skills. Information about assistive technology needs and how assistive technology is used is included as well. There also may be statements about needs that have been identified by team members but that are not addressed on the IEP. In this case, the reasons for not addressing those issues must also be stated.

Assessment Information

As discussed previously, informal and formal assessment procedures used to determine the child's needs and eligibility for special education should be included. No child can be placed in special education based on a single assessment procedure. The goal of assessment is to determine the student's ability to function and perform required learning tasks. Standardized and nonstandardized assessment methods should be used. Teacher interviews and classroom observations are especially important tools for determining how the student performs in the learning environment. Eligibility is based on both identification of a disability and demonstration of need for specially designed instruction.

The team is responsible for reviewing the results of the multi-factored evaluation. If an IEP is already in place for the student, the team reviews that document during annual or triennial reviews. Team members must explain the student's present levels of educational performance including progress, strengths, capabilities, interests, and needs displayed at home, school or in the community (Rudebusch, 2011). The results of the assessments should be described and interpreted in a manner that facilitates understanding by participants.

The evaluation report should include complete names of all assessment instruments should be used. The date of assessment and the name and title of the examiner also should be included. It is very important to administer and score the assessment according to prescribed instructions and protocols. Assessment results are not valid or useful unless scored and interpreted according to the recommended procedures. Sometimes it is necessary to modify the administration procedures to accommodate the needs of the child. The evaluator should make notations of adaptations or modifications made during the administration of the test. It would be unethical to enroll a student in an intervention program based on a test that is incorrectly administered or scored. Based on the evaluation information presented, the team determines the student's areas of need.

Current Levels of Development, Academic Achievement, and Functional Performance

Data based statements of the present level of academic achievement and functional performance must be developed from the assessment information collected. These statements are referred to as Present Level of Education Performance and indicate the performance level for specific academic and functional tasks or behaviors. Preferably, each statement will include a quantitative (numerical) and qualitative (descriptive) reference to the child's performance level. Performance levels can be indicated for academic performance or communication skills such as language, speech production, voice, reading, hearing, or other communication skill areas. The team can obtain an understanding of how the student is performing in comparison to peers and how the student's disability affects involvement and progress in the regular education curriculum from this section. Special factors including strengths, parental and teacher concerns, and current assessment data are included. The description of the student's Present Level of Education Performance provides a profile from which to launch discussion about the student including strengths, capabilities, interests, and needs displayed in school, in the community, or at home. In addition, scores achieved on state standardized tests are included, especially scores on language arts, social science, history, listening, speaking, reading, and writing.

Need Statements

Need statements show the direction of change that is to occur as the present level of educational performance is modified. Need statements indicate that a behavior should be changed (increased or decreased).

Measurable Annual Goals

Goals indicate the projected level of performance for the child as a result of receiving the special education and related services indicated in the IEP. There are several key aspects that should be included in the Measurable Annual Goals: the goals can reasonably be expected to be accomplished within 12 months; how the goals are aligned to academic content standards; a clearly defined behavior or action; an explanation of the conditions (situation, setting, materials) in which the behavior is to be performed; the criteria for mastery; and the direct relationship between goals and the student's Present Level of Educational Performance. The goals are measurable targets for achievement. Goals should allow the student to participate in the general curriculum as well as in social, emotional, extracurricular, and vocational areas. Some districts have developed goal banks that can be accessed electronically.

Methods for Measuring the Student's Progress Toward Annual Goals

There is great flexibility in the methods that education teams may use in order to measure progress. It is very important for the team to agree on the methods and clearly determine the process to be used for implementing and reporting the measures. Some examples of methods include:

Anecdotal records

Checklists

Curriculum-based assessments

Inventories

Performance assessments

Portfolios

Observation

Rubrics

Running records

Short-cycle assessments

Work samples

Short-Term Measurable Instructional Objectives

The Annual Goals are broken down into short-term objectives or benchmarks. The specific performance skills to which the instructional objectives relate; for example, language or articulation, must be delineated. "Instructional Objectives" indicate the intermediate steps leading to the goal. In the legislation they are also referred to as benchmarks. They include specific behaviors that will be acquired as the child moves toward accomplishment of the annual goal. Each annual goal may have a number of instructional objectives depending on the intermediate steps needed to accomplish the goal. A significant component to the IEP is the determination of how and when each objective (and goal) will be evaluated to determine the student's progress and success. Each objective should include the components such as the procedures to be used to measure the objective, the criteria, the schedule for review, the person responsible for that objective, a review of progress, the special education services to be delivered, the length and duration of the service, and the context (or setting) in which the behavior is to occur.

The objectives should be written using terminology that links the goal to the curriculum. This will ensure that the educators are all addressing the objectives and that the effect of the disability on the student's performance is the focus of the special education services. Progress on objectives is reported.

Extent of Participation in the General Educational Environment

The IEP identifies the special education and related services to be provided to the student. Incorporating services into the educational setting implies that the treatment will occur within educational environments such as the classroom. For that to happen effectively, there are a number of modifications or supports that schools usually consider. The accommodations and special services that are necessary to ensure that the student can access the general curriculum are included. Some examples include reducing the amount of work, adapting the work in some way, assessing learning in different ways, assigning preferential seating, and other similar modifications. Educators should be creative as they explore modifications that might help the student perform better to meet learning outcomes. Materials, presentation format, task requirements, grading practices, delivery of instructions, content, and physical or environmental modifications are all examples of those aspects of the instructional process that can be modified.

Assistive technology based on the child's identified needs must be discussed by the IEP team. This includes modern technology as well as monitoring hearing aids and ensuring that devices are made available if required. Assistive devices are those items of equipment that is used to support a student's functional capabilities (Gillette, 2011).

Primary or unique methods and materials that are needed to complete the instructional objectives are included under the recommendations section of the IEP. Recommendations should include the following components: what, how many, and how often.

The explanation of modifications also includes an indication of who will provide the service. Options include individual therapists and educators or teams of educators. Parents are also given responsibilities for implementing specific aspects of the plan.

Amount, Frequency, and Duration of Services

The IEP must include a statement of the amount of services, date the services will convene, and how long they are likely to be provided. This demonstrates the school's commitment of resources. The amount of time to be committed must be appropriate to the specific service and stated clearly in the IEP. The discussion of the amount and duration of services should be managed carefully. Some parents believe that "more services are better." School districts have many different approaches to determining and committing to the amount and duration of services. Some districts indicate total number of hours or minutes of services to be delivered during the entire school year. Others designate a number of sessions. Some specify an amount of services per week. It is also important to explain the options for the location of services as well (therapy room, resource room, general education classroom, other locations on the school campus or community). Taking the time to discuss the value of conducting therapy in different locations during the development of the IEP will provide greater opportunities to meet the students' needs as his or her skills change throughout the year. For example, a recommendation could be made to initiate therapy outside the classroom until new skills are stabilized and then move intervention into the classroom to assist the student with generalizing the newly learned skills.

Parents must be notified if changes to the IEP are recommended. If the IEP team and the parents can agree to a change in services (such as frequency and duration) via a telephone call or other means of contact, that change can be documented and included in an existing IEP. If, however, a team member, especially the parent, requests it, a formal meeting of the IEP team must be held. The procedures for advance notice must be followed.

Accommodations or Modifications

The IEP should also include an explanation of the accommodations or modifications that are recommended in order to enable the student to access the curriculum as well as participate in statewide and district-wide testing. Accommodations do not alter the amount or complexity of the curricular material. Examples of accommodations include steps such as allocating extra time, and providing a scribe to assist with writing lengthy papers. Modifications do alter the content by decreasing the amount or complexity. In order to provide the level of support students need, school personnel may need to participate in specialized training or be assigned an aide to assist them in the classroom. They may also need to learn to use equipment or resources. In addition, students may need assistance to meet their medical needs. These accommodations, modifications and support are listed on the IEP with indications of whether they are optional or required.

Progress and Status Reports

There is a requirement for reporting progress and a method for maintaining ongoing contact with the parents and others about the student's achievements. Federal legislation mandates that schools implement a process for evaluating and reporting progress to parents on regularly scheduled basis. Many methods can be used for accomplishing this task including face-to-face meetings, written notes, E-mail, phone calls, journal entries, or report cards.

On the date the instructional objective is to be accomplished, or on any other regularly scheduled review date, the evaluation component in the instructional objective can be executed. Using a status code or descriptive statement can indicate progress the child has made in completing the objective. By describing the student's mastery of a particular skill, staff will be able to indicate the amount of progress made by the child. Revisions and comments that provide insights about the student's performance should be included to provide information that can be used in developing future IEPs. Some standards against which performance is measured are school standards and instructional benchmarks, peer performance, and professional judgment based on educators' assessment and observation. Many districts require that SLPs report the child's progress to parents at the same time that report cards are issued.

Verification and Documentation

Schools are bound by law to inform and include parents in the planning and intervention process. The IEP form contains space for documenting the parents' address and signatures indicating their understanding of the proceedings.

Special Education and Related Services Needed

The special education and related or instructional support services the child needs in order to receive an appropriate education and participate in the general curriculum should be described. Statements should include descriptions of the specific educational alternatives, the types of services to be provided, who will provide them, the location, the amount and duration of services to be provided, and the frequency with which the service will be provided. The reason these topics are so important is because they represent the level of commitment of resources (including personnel qualifications and time). The amount of time to be committed to each of the services a child needs must be appropriate and clearly stated in the IEP in a manner that can be understood by everyone involved in the development and implementation of the IEP.

The parents' or guardians' signatures must be secured to indicate they approve of the services that will be provided to the child. A summary statement is included indicating the recommendations and the rationale for the decisions. The IEP team meeting may be convened and the plan developed without the parental attendance if the school district makes reasonable attempts to get them to attend and they refuse. The school district must maintain complete records of attempts to arrange meetings at mutually agreeable times and places. This includes the speech-language program. If the SLP is having difficulty connecting with the parent, the school administration should be notified so that correct procedures are followed.

Creating IEPs for a large caseload can be a very time-consuming task. Some clinicians have made the job more efficient by using computers and word processors. They create data banks to store statements of intervention goals and objectives and templates of explanations of information that is typically provided in reports. They then can efficiently prepare a report by selecting appropriate comments and inserted information that is relevant for the particular student such as test scores, characteristic behaviors etc. Many publishers of speech-language pathology resource materials have created comprehensive sample resources containing functional, relevant IEP goals and objectives that are educationally appropriate for school-age children. Most school districts invest in commercial IEP writing programs.

Other Elements

Other issues that are generally discussed and considered are nonacademic and extracurricular activities.

An example of an IEP form can be found in Appendix C (Ohio Department of Education, 2011).

Individualized Family Service Plan (IFSP)

The public education laws specify guidelines for serving the needs of infants and toddlers presenting developmental delays. The laws assign responsibility to the states to establish criteria for eligibility. Consequently, criteria may vary from state to state. The law requires that the services be multidisciplinary and that service delivery plans reflect coordination of services among local agencies. Provision of services to the child's family is an integral component of the law. Federal regulations mandate that a systematic service plan be developed. This is referred to as the Individualized Family Service Plan (IFSP). An IFSP documents and guides the early intervention process for children with disabilities and their families. Similar to the IEP, family members and service providers work as a team to plan, implement, and evaluate services. The plan must span one year with a 6-month review, specify outcomes for the child and family, and name a service coordinator from the profession most relevant to the child or family's needs. Collaboration is reinforced as a service delivery model for this population. Services may be provided in the home, at a local school location, or in a center.

With the exception of services provided to the family and the emphasis on the child's health-related needs, several components in the IFSP are similar to those of the IEP. A meeting is held with the family and professionals who can provide services to the child. The goal of the meeting is to establish a plan for achieving the desired outcomes. Gillette and Robinson (1992) describe a process for developing an IFSP. They include a sample meeting agenda, time schedule for discussing pertinent topics, and sample planning forms. Prior to the meeting, the coordinator should gather pertinent background information about the child and family to facilitate greater understanding of the needs and possible ways to meet the needs.

The IFSP format can be used to focus the attention of meeting attendees and guide the discussion. The components of the IFSP are similar to the IEP. The topics listed below should be addressed in writing and face to face during discussions:

- Introductions and background information including identifying information about the child, family, and disciplines/agencies represented;
- An overview of current medical, health, and rehabilitation services being provided to the child;
- A summary of the child's current health, development and family functioning including the child's strengths and needs and the family's strengths and needs in relation to the child;
- The child's health outcome, providers, and methods of service delivery including identifying the providers, the location, duration, frequency, and intensity of each service;
- The child's development outcome, providers, and methods; again determining professional providers, service schedules (numbers of contacts, length of contacts, and location of service), family involvement and measures of child development to be used;
- The family's life outcome, providers and methods; determining services that may be needed in the following areas: support, child care, education, family life

planning, financial resources, and community resources; and

- As the meeting draws to a close, a service coordinator should be identified.

Individualized Transition Plan (ITP)

When IDEA was re-authorized, it included a mandate that schools should plan for students' transitions from school to work and/or postsecondary activities. Transitions are considered "the life changes, adjustments, and cumulative experiences that occur in the lives of young adults as they move from school environments to more independent living and work environments" (Wehman, 1992). Transition can also include changes in self-awareness, body, sexuality, work, financial needs, and mobility.

Blosser and DePompei (2002) believe that this is a rather limited interpretation of transition because it focuses only on transition from school to work. It does not take into account transition into school from health care settings by students with health care needs. Nor does it consider transition into the school setting for preschoolers with disabilities. Planning for transition from preschool to school enables teachers and clinicians to work together to identify critical skills needed to enter school and participate in daily learning activities. More importantly for children with communication disabilities, the limited interpretation of transition does not account for the many transitions students experience as they progress through school from grade to grade, subject to subject, or teacher to teacher. This is especially notable as children enter middle school. An expanded definition of transition gives perspective to the problems students often experience in school throughout the day or from year to year. This explanation of transition illustrates the daily stress that is placed on students' communication performance. Transition into each situation carries with it unique and different demands and expectation for communication performance.

The law requires that a statement of needed transition services be included as part of the IEP for students with disabilities beginning no later than age 16, and when appropriate age 14 or younger, and annually thereafter. The intent was to ensure that students with disabilities have the opportunity to lead rewarding and productive lives after leaving school. The goal is to provide opportunities for work or study, independent living, and community participation.

There are four essential components of transition planning as defined by IDEA: planning and services should be based on student needs and preferences; transition planning should be oriented to postsecondary outcomes; transition planning should include a coordinated set of activities; and services should promote movement from school to postschool settings.

Speech-language pathologists can serve as significant members on the transition planning team in school districts by helping other team members understand the difficulty students encounter as they transition from one situation to another. The success of the student's transition from one situation to another (including high school to the world of work) is influenced by the following factors:

1. The nature and extent of the student's communication impairment;
2. The demands and expectations of the specific situation;
3. The level of understanding of the people in the student's environment;
4. The quality of treatment and services the student receives;
5. Opportunities for success; and
6. The student's readiness and preparation for the situation he or she is about to enter.

Transition planning differs from the IEP because it focuses on the types of services needed to achieve long-term postsecondary goals such as postsecondary education, vocational training, supported employment, continuing education, adult services, independent living, community participation, and the like. The composition of the transition team is important to the development of an effective transition plan. At a minimum, the student, parents, teacher, and other relevant staff members should be present when the ITP is developed. Speech-language pathologists can be significant members on the transition planning team in school districts.

A review of the professional literature on planning transitions for students (deFur & Patton, 1999; Clark et al., 1991; Wehman, 1992) indicated that the guiding principles listed below make the transition proceed smoothly.

Transition Efforts Should Start Early

The 1997 reauthorization the Individuals with Disabilities Education Act (IDEA) recommends that educators and parents begin the transition planning process at as early an age as possible. Schools should establish a systematic K to 12 transition education program where elementary students gain a strong foundational base that will help them as they transition through school and after they leave school (Clark et al., 1991). Transition activities should be initiated early to ensure a seamless transition to postschool settings. Most school districts initiate transition planning when the child reaches age 14. At that time, vocational assessment is added as part of the multifactored evaluation process. The information obtained can be used to develop an Individualized Transition Plan (ITP).

Planning Must Be Comprehensive

Students must be looked at from a comprehensive point of view to determine their needs as they progress through school. Comprehensive transition planning includes periodic review of where the student is with regard to the following aspects: employment, further education and training, leisure activities, community participation, health (physical, emotional, and spiritual), self-determination/self-advocacy, communication, interpersonal relationships/social skills, and transportation/mobility. The speech-language pathologist has much to contribute about the dynamics of communication related to each of these areas. In some cases, the SLP will help prepare the student for the next step; in other cases, the SLP will make recommendations for the transition plan. Prerequisite skills that will be necessary for success should be the focus of treatment and intervention.

The Planning Process Must Balance What Is Ideal with What Is Possible

Special educators are often troubled and frustrated because they cannot do everything that it takes to help their students. We must learn to be satisfied with our contribution when we do what we consider to be our absolute best effort. Given that students will experience many different transitions, the individualized transition plan should be reviewed and updated on an ongoing basis.

Student Empowerment Is Essential

Students must be at the table when plans for their future are being discussed. This may be uncomfortable for the student as well as for the professional but plans will be much more effective if the student's interests and motivation are considered. Enabling the student to participate will also foster greater independence and self-advocacy. These skills may be necessary as students progress to higher education settings. The earlier we begin inviting students to participate in the discussions of their educational program, the more likely they will gain skills that will help them as they progress throughout life. Students will flourish if they are provided with options and opportunities to participate in many different experiences.

Family Involvement Is Critical

It is valuable to have families involved in all aspects of the student's education. This is even more crucial for families of youngsters with severe disabilities. They will be the ones who must ensure ongoing services for their youngster, especially after the student leaves school. Seek their input and value their contributions, whatever they may be. Some families are not capable and others are not interested in participating, whereas others want to be a part of every decision that is made about the student's education. Professionals must learn to deal with each type of parent, providing the information that is needed when it is needed. It will be useful to gain good understanding of the family dynamics and involve them in crucial transition planning activities as much as possible.

Transition Planning Must Be Sensitive to Diversity

Transition planners must demonstrate sensitivity to diversity issues including dimensions such as: cultural diversity, race, ethnicity, religious beliefs, gender, and sexual orientation. It is especially important to make recommendations to the student and family with these aspects in mind.

Transition Planning Should Help Students and Their Family or Caregivers Access Supports and Services

Youth with special needs and their families should be informed of the extensive variety of supports and services available in the community. This will help them understand that they are not alone when they encounter difficult situations. There are numerous people in every community and work situation that have knowledge that can be helpful to the success of individuals with disabilities.

Transition Planning Should Include Preparing the Environment

Preparing the environment where the student will be going and the people in that environment to support the youngster can help facilitate success. Each situation the student enters poses a different set of demands and expectations for the student's communication skills. SLPs can help identify and modify those features of the environment that might pose challenges or obstacles for the student. Family members, friends, teachers, and others can play very active roles in ensuring smooth and successful transitions. The Individualized Transition Plan should specify the persons who will be involved in the transition including describing their role, ways they can help, and skills they need to develop to provide assistance.

Community-Based Activities Are Important

Assessment and training should be carried out in real-life situations. That way, the student can be prepared for situations that are likely to be encountered. It will also help the student generalize practiced skills to everyday occurrences.

Interagency Commitment, Cooperation, and Coordination Are Critical to Successful Transition

It is likely that students with disabilities will need to access many different types of services. This can be made easier if personnel in various agencies form positive relationships with one another and coordinate their services. In this way, movement from one service provider to another will be smooth and will not create undue stress or duplication of services for the student and their family.

School Administrators Should Be Involved in Planning Transitions

In order to implement successful transitions for students, administrative support is often necessary. Therefore, it is helpful to have administrators present when ITPs are being formulated and written.

Transition Plans Should Be Evaluated Periodically to Be Sure They Are Current and Relevant

Writing the transition plan is only the beginning. Similar to IEPs, the transition plan should be re-visited periodically to be sure that the priorities, goals, objectives, and decisions that have been made are still suited to the student's needs and capabilities.

Core Curriculum Standards

Education reformers suggest that schools should prepare students to meet specific education standards. The belief is based on the premise that by raising the standards, school achievement will also increase and students will be better prepared to enter college and the world of work. In addition, they will participate as citizens in a democratic and global society. The Common Core Curriculum Standards explicitly state the knowledge and skills that all students are expected to master. The standards describe what students should know and be able to do. What are those standards and where does speech-language intervention fit? The standards provide clarity about the content and skills that should be taught at each grade.

Each state may organize its standards in different ways. However, since there are many similarities from state to state, in 2010 the National Governors Association and the Council of Chief State School Officers recommended that a national Common Core of academic standards be adopted. The goal is to clearly define and articulate learning expectations for all students, teachers, and schools.

Efforts have been underway across the nation for years to define "exit expectations" for high school seniors in English language arts including reading, writing, listening, speaking and language. It is imperative that our nation's schools make strides in making sure that students graduate ready to pursue higher education and employment—or college and career ready. Educational standards also define the "benchmarks" or key points along the learning path from kindergarten through twelfth grade. The intent is for the curriculum and formal instruction to consistently line up with the expectations for learning indicated by the standards. This national agenda will most likely impact the way speech-language services are delivered in the future and the interpretation that students are eligible for services. The SLP should be familiar with the Common Core Curriculum standards, expectations, and curricula for each of the content areas but especially for the Language Arts, Literacy, Math, and Science areas. Knowing the standards enables SLPs to align speech-language intervention with the educational expectations and to identify and measure what students know and are able to do. It also enables us to determine if our intervention and support services are improving performance.

The standards for English/Language Arts generally recommend that the teaching of reading and writing should be integrated. Students should learn to read a variety of texts: fictional, non-fictional, informational, historical, political, and social/cultural. Students should learn to read visual texts such as film, television, photographs, graphics (charts and illustrations), and technologic texts, such as via the Internet. Students are expected to learn to write for a variety of purposes and audiences. They should know the various purposes of writing as well as the technical and mechanical aspects. Thus, students are expected to be able to speak, listen, view, and visually represent language to self-reflect, communicate with others, and learn. Of all the areas of the curriculum, the greatest link between the standards and the services SLPs offer are within the English/Language Arts standards. The standards expect that students will increase their vocabulary, be prepared for 21st century careers, and use formal English in writing and speaking. A compelling argument can be made for the need for speech-language intervention for a student who is unable to perform to the highest expectations of the standards due to communication impairment.

Regarding the mathematics standards, students are expected to value mathematics, become problem solvers, and learn to reason mathematically. They should be able to communicate about mathematics and using math-related terminology. Students are supposed to learn math so they will be able to function in society and be able to compute, estimate, and use technology. Many students with communication disabilities have difficulty learning mathematics because of the abstract nature of the concepts presented. In fact, even students in the general education setting who do not present communication impairments may struggle with the language of mathematics. In other words, they may be able to do the required mathematical calculations but struggle with understanding the problem as it is presented in writing. Teachers should be advised of the impact of language on understanding and communicating about mathematics.

Science, like math, has become the focus of much discussion regarding the needs for educational reform. Critics do not believe that students are being adequately prepared in the area of science in order to perform effectively in society after leaving school. Scientific literacy is considered necessary for everyone. Students must be able to make informed decisions, discuss scientific and technical issues, and understand the natural world. There is an expectation that they will be able to understand science as inquiry, physical science, life science, earth and space science, technology, and other concepts and processes. Like math, learning science implies that the student will understand abstract concepts. In addition, students must learn difficult vocabulary and be able to manipulate complex information and sequences. Again, the SLP can contribute much to teachers' understanding of why students experience difficulty with the math curriculum by explaining the link between language and learning.

The social sciences include history, geography, civics, government, and economics. The social science standards state an expectation that the student will become a responsible citizen, understanding the responsibility that is entailed. Through these content areas, students learn to respect the institutions and laws of government. In addition, they are to learn about diversity and other cultures. Students who have difficulty comprehending language in the written form and recalling facts will likely have difficulty meeting the expectations of the standards.

School SLPs must have a good understanding of the structure, scope, and sequence of the general education curriculum followed for each grade and subject area in their school district. All school districts have manuals available describing these components and the competencies students are expected to gain as they progress through school. The manuals may be referred to by a number of names including "scope and sequence," "course of study," "school curricula," or "competency guidelines."

The wise clinician will obtain a copy of the school curriculum and state academic content standards from the curriculum director in the school district and coordinate the speech-language program with the curriculum. An example of the elements included in the scope and sequence for a Language Arts curriculum is provided in Appendix D to demonstrate how valuable these materials can be for program planning. It is the SLP's responsibility to understand the curriculum. There are many resources available. Perhaps one of the most comprehensive resources is provided by Education World which includes every state's curricular grade by grade standards for fine arts, language arts, mathematics, physical education and health, science, social studies, and technology (http://www.education-world.com).

Modifying the Instructional Environment

SLPs have a responsibility to provide teachers with specific suggestions for creating a "communication positive" climate in their classroom. This can be done by jointly arranging classroom materials, space, and activities so that communication exchanges will occur. With guidance from the SLP, teachers can learn to use several interactive communication strategies to elicit correct speech-language production, reinforce children's attempts to practice what they are learning in the therapy program, and facilitate correct productions when communication errors are observed. Accommodations, instructional strategies and modifications must be incorporated into the IEP. Some examples of modifications are illustrated on Figure 9–4. Several specific communication strategies teachers can implement are presented in Chapter 10.

Making Speech-Language Intervention Relevant to the Students' Educational Needs

School is a communication-based environment. Therefore, students who exhibit communication impairments are at risk for academic failure. This means they will not be able to progress in the general education curriculum without assistance. Success in the school setting depends on the ability to communicate effectively in classroom and social situations where functional communication skills are necessary. For example, children must respond appropriately when asked questions. They must understand the meaning of vocabulary words and concepts unique to numerous subject areas. They are expected to interact socially with adults and peers. In order to gain information, they must be able to formulate questions and use appropriate phonology, syntax, semantics, and pragmatics so others can understand them. They have to understand relationships between sounds and symbols. It is essential for them to follow written and verbal instructions; organize thoughts in verbal and written expression; and comprehend large amounts of information presented by the teacher.

The school speech-language clinician can increase students' potential for success by making the intervention program relevant to students' academic needs. When developing goals for speech-language intervention, the SLP must describe the relationship between the student's IEP goals and the impact they will have on classroom success. Haskill describes two approaches for developing relevant goals.

X	TEACHER-TO-STUDENT INSTRUCTION STRATEGIES
	Determine your expectations for successful communicative performance in your classroom (work) environment.
	State and clarify expectations for communicative performance to the student.
	Analyze the communicative demand made of the student by classroom activities and assigned tasks.
	Help student prioritize learning goals and tasks.
	Guide student to recognize reasons why communication attempts are inaccurate or inappropriate.
	Introduce important information at a level that is commensurate with the youngster's developmental, mental, and communicative capabilities.
	Individualize assignments and tests to accommodate special communicative needs (reduce the number of questions; alternative modes of response).
	Avoid abrupt changes in topic during class discussions (use transitions from topic to topic).
	Provide listening guides and outlines for lectures.
	Connect "who," "what," and "where" questions to information desired from student when asking questions.
	Cue the student with words such as: "first," "second," and "next."
	Introduce stories and curricular units with visual cues such as pictures, outlines, etc.
	Permit alternative response modes such as drawing, pantomime, selecting answers from choices.
	Ask probing questions to see if student comprehends important information.
	Use sentence completion strategies when you don't understand the student.
	Arrange opportunities for practice.
	Provide feedback and guidance to increase understanding of successful and unsuccessful attempts.
	Observe and evaluate performance routinely and systematically. Modify teaching strategies based on information gained.
	Provide incentives to stimulate communicative interaction.
	Teach the student to recognize and measure components of successful performance.
	Encourage the discussion and sharing of problems the child may be experiencing. Help the child understand the relationship between the communication problems and the difficulties being experienced.
	Implement teaching approaches that actively involve the student in learning activities.
	Be observant of stressors placed on the child by others (teachers, peers, family, administrators). Reduce stressors as much as possible.
	Use additional ideas based on your knowledge of effective instructional strategies.

Figure 9–4. Instructional accommodations and modifications. *continues*

X	**STUDENT-TO-STUDENT INSTRUCTION STRATEGIES**
	Use cooperative learning strategies.
	Pair the student with a buddy to use reciprocal teaching strategies.
	Provide small group activities to facilitate peer tutoring and modeling.
	Select a fellow student to act as a "buddy" to help the youngster participate meaningfully in class and school related activities.
	Select a "fellow student coach" to help the child stay aware of instructions, transitions from activity to activity, assignments, and so on.
	Directly teach peers to implement specific interactive communication strategies so they are prepared to provide models and facilitate positive responses when the student has difficulty communicating or learning.
	Encourage friendships and sharing through social and extracurricular activities based on the child's capabilities and interests.
X	**CLASSROOM MODIFICATION TECHNIQUES TO PROMOTE EFFECTIVE COMMUNICATION**
	Permit and encourage the use of assistive devices including calculators, computers, tape recorders, assistive listening devices, and more.
	Formulate a system to help the child maintain organization (such as schedule books, assignment notebooks, "to do" lists).
	Accompany textbooks and work pages with supportive materials (pictures, written cues, graphic illustrations).
X	**STUDENT LEARNING STRATEGIES**
	Encourage the student to reread instructions more than one time, exercising care to underline, highlight, and note important elements.
	Ask the student to repeat instructions verbatim before initiating a learning task.
	Verify the student's comprehension of directions by requesting that the instructions be restated using different terminology.
	Have the student review the work after completing it. Encourage proofreading of assignments before submitting them, looking for completeness and accuracy.
	Provide the student with opportunities to repeat assignments at another time to see if performance can be improved.
	Invite the student to ask questions and to clarify information not understood.
	Have the student write instructions on a separate sheet of paper.
	Have the student self-evaluate work to see if it is appropriate, verbalizing correct and incorrect aspects of the work.
	Teach the student to use specific graphic organizers such as: flow charts, comparison/ contrast charts, story map, sequence maps.

Figure 9–4. *continued*

In a "standards-referenced" approach, the team develops the student's goals and then identifies the standard that best reflects that goal. In a "standards-based approach," the team starts with the content standards and generates the IEP goals and objectives. In practice, the SLP can incorporate objectives and materials from the classroom into the therapy program. The teacher can reinforce communication skills and use intervention strategies during classroom activities.

The creative clinician needs only to look to the school curriculum and classroom to obtain materials and resources for the intervention program. Textbooks, workbooks, and teaching kits provide materials and activities that are age appropriate, interesting, and motivating to students. By developing speech-language therapy goals around the curriculum, the clinician can increase the student's chances of using appropriate communication skills while responding in the classroom. Following are examples of educationally relevant treatment objectives that would prepare a student to perform better within the classroom learning situation:

- To appropriately respond to questions *from the end of the social studies chapter.*
- To correctly produce target phonemes taken *from the student's weekly spelling list.*
- To generate and combine sentences *about life's events to create an autobiography.*
- To verbally recall details *from a story assigned in reading group.*
- To verbally describe (in sequence) four steps *to a science experiment.*
- To correctly explain *the rules to a sport being taught in gym class*
- To comprehend mathematical concepts *stressed in math class.*
- To produce syntactically correct sentences *using the weekly vocabulary list from language arts class.*
- To use appropriate pragmatic skills *during a small group craft activity.*
- To use fluent speech to recite an *oral book report for English class.*
- To explain orally and in writing *the steps to solve a math problem.*

The next steps for preparing these objectives would be to identify the condition(s) that must be met for the student to master the desired behavior and the standard or criterion that the team will use to determine whether the intervention strategies have been effective and the desired level of student performance has been met. Some conditions might include "with verbal cues" or "in response to the teacher's questions." Examples of criterion for goal mastery could include the district educational standards or instructional level for a given grade level, developmental norms, or professional judgment.

Thompson and Thompson (2002) encourage SLPs to teach in "units of study" rather than teaching isolated word lists, random worksheets, or discussing unrelated topics in therapy. By using vocabulary and concepts that relate to units of study that are presented in the class will increase the student's chances of performing better during classroom instruction.

Universal Design for Learning

As general education teachers, special educators, speech-language pathologists, and other professionals strive to provide students with access to the best education and intervention possible, frameworks for designing effective education are necessary and helpful. Universal Design for Learning (UDL) is a recent concept that captures key principles for providing an educational environment and instructional practices that enable learners to gain knowledge, skills, and enthusiasm for learning. UDL is viewed as an excellent mechanism for ensuring that all individuals have an equal opportunity to learn. This has been the pillar for American education for decades.

An organization called CAST (The Center for Applied Special Technology) has led the way in developing the UDL concept and exploring ways of using newer technologies to provide better educational experiences for students with disabilities. CAST's National Universal Design for Learning Task Force explains that UDL simultaneously enables educators to use flexible teaching methods and materials to remove barriers to the curriculum and provide the supports that students need to succeed (CAST, 2011; National Universal Design for Learning Task Force, 2011). Numerous education-related organizations that serve the needs of children and educators, including ASHA and CEC, are working together to promote the use of UDL to improve students' achievements.

UDL provides a framework and guidelines for modifying the educational environment, collaboration among professionals, and co-teaching. These concepts have been reinforced throughout this text. Although the term UDL may be new to many SLPs, the key elements of UDL have been recommended for years. A key premise about UDL is that teachers (both general education and special education) and related services professions (including SLPs) plan together to create a curriculum that meets the needs of students from the start of their education. Through collaboration and co-teaching educators, special educators, and therapists jointly ensure that instruction is connected to the academic standards and that students receive consistent instruction and intervention throughout the educational environment. Through UDL, speech-language pathologists can ensure that therapy intervention is educationally relevant and that strategies are carried out throughout the day.

The UDL Guidelines prepared by CAST can be used as a blueprint by education professionals and therapists to plan lessons or units of study or to develop the curricula. This includes goals, methods, materials, and assessments that work for all children. It also means considering how to remove barriers and optimize levels of challenge and support. Flexibility, creativity, and customization are the underpinnings to UDL.

Universal Design for Learning focuses on three primary brain networks (National Center on Universal Design of Learning, 2011) that humans use in the learning process. They are the Recognition Networks, the Strategic Networks, and the Affective Networks. Each is briefly explained below.

Recognition Networks— The "What" of Learning

This network incorporates the way we gather facts and categorize what we see, hear, and learn. Examples are recognition tasks such as recognizing letters, words, people, writing style, and so on. Instruction and intervention strategies include varying the way in which content and information is presented.

Strategic Networks— The "How" of Learning

This network is reflected in planning and performing tasks. It is how we organize and express ideas. Learners demonstrate their Strategic Network when they write an essay, solve a math problem, or conduct a science experiment. Instruction and intervention strategies include providing multiple ways for students to express themselves or let others know that they understand a concept or can answer a question.

Affective Networks— The "Why" of Learning

This network addresses how learners get engaged and stay motivated. The Affective Network involves how learners get excited, challenged, and interested. We need to consider multiple ways for getting students engaged and motivated in the learning situation.

Three primary principles guide UDL and form the underlying framework for the UDL guidelines. The principles are based on the neuroscience research presented above. The three principles follow.

Principle I: Provide Multiple Means of Representations

This recommendation is based on the premise that learners differ in the ways that they perceive and comprehend information. The differing perceptions may be due to learning differences, cultural differences, linguistic differences, sensory disabilities, and more. Some children learn faster or slower than others. Therefore, presenting information in different ways will increase the potential for the student learning the information.

Principle II: Provide Multiple Means of Action and Expression

Learners differ in the way they access knowledge and demonstrate what they know. Children who cannot express themselves verbally or complete a written test or maneuver around the classroom cannot demonstrate what they know. Therefore, providing students with multiple ways of expressing what they have learned enables educators to verify that learning has taken place and that knowledge has been gained. Alternative and augmentative modes of communication can open many doors for conveying knowledge for children with severe communication disorders.

Principle III: Provide Multiple Means of Engagement

Affect is a crucial element in the learning process. Children who are excited about learning and fully engaged in the learning situation will gain more information. Some students like to learn in large groups, others learn better alone. Some are spontaneous, others more structured. Educators who understand these dynamics and take steps to give each child an opportunity to engage at a level that is most comfortable for them will result in greater motivation to perform classroom assignments.

The CAST Web site offers extensive examples of these principles and sample lesson plans that are created with the principles and strategies in mind (http://www.CAST.org).

Planning and Evaluating the Treatment Session

Four key components comprise the UDL curriculum. They are the goals, methods, materials and assessments. These components are not new to educators or SLPs. However, the difference between considering these components in a traditional way and considering them in a UDL framework is that UDL considers learner variability and creativity. Therefore, more options and flexibility are incorporated into the lesson.

There are considerations the school SLP needs to make when planning instructional objectives for individual lesson plans. First to be considered are the goals for a particular lesson. What does the clinician hope the student will accomplish? What knowledge, skills and concepts is the student expected to master? Are the aims reasonable? Is the student aware of the goals for that lesson? Has he or she helped formulate them? Do the clinician and student agree on the goals? Will these goals bring the student closer to the final goal? Along with the specific goals for each treatment session, the clinician and student must be in agreement on the general, or long-range, goals. In other words, what are the outcomes? What is finally to be accomplished in the way of improving communication? In the UDL curriculum, more pathways for learning, tools for teaching, strategies, and options are incorporated.

After the goals are established, the team determines the methods or approaches for intervention. Evidence-based methods are required. UDL guidelines recommend basing the method on the learner's methods, the context, the classroom climate, and the student's social/emotional state. Progress is continually monitored to determine the student's acquisition of knowledge and response to instructional and intervention methods.

The next component is the materials to be used to present the content and determine the learner's knowledge. Multiple media are recommended for constructing materials. In UDL there should be variation in choice of content and options for providing supports.

Assessment is described as the process for gathering information about a student's performance. Multiple types of materials and methods are used to make educational decisions about the knowledge or skills the student has gained. In the UDL framework, assessment information is used to guide instruction.

Instructional and intervention lessons should be based on the child's needs, the general and specific goals of therapy, and the evaluated results of previous lessons. The clinician may wish to consult with the parents concerning home assignments or with the classroom teacher on generalization activities.

Motivation

Much has been written about motivating students. There is general agreement that student engagement and motivation are necessary to produce good and lasting results. It is not uncommon to hear clinicians comment that they wish they could motivate their students. This would imply that motivating is something one does to another person. However, motivation is something that is within the person, driving him or her to achieve. It is not realistic to think that clinicians are able to motivate clients. Rather, the recipients of our services will make a change in communication behavior only if personal values and attitudes compel them to do so.

SLPs who use games, negative reinforcement, positive reinforcement, rewards, punishment, shaping behavior, and so on provide incentives and inducements that may bring about changes in behavior. If the inner drive, or the motivation, is absent, however, there may be regression or lack of what is commonly referred to as carryover or generalization; or there may be no change in behavior.

Although the clinician is highly eager to change the child's speech-language behavior, it does not necessarily follow that the child will share that feeling. In some cases the child may be highly motivated to hang on to an immature speech and language pattern because it may be a way of controlling, satisfying, or coping with other members of the family. Or a child may enjoy the attention that immature speech and language bring.

What are the implications for the clinician in regard to motivating students? Much can be accomplished by shifting from a teacher-centered orientation of motivation to an understanding of the attitudes and values present in the child's motivation for learning. Therefore, a child-centered approach is suggested. In this approach, the SLP focuses on the child's interests and needs when designing the session. Developing a sense of the child's emotional state of being and the meaning of his or her nonverbal responses helps the astute clinician shape the tone of treatment. It is desirable for the clinician to have a foundation in developmental psychology, a sensitivity to the nuances of the therapeutic relationship, and a willingness to learn as much as possible about an individual child's emotional functioning. Understanding the feelings of the child may be as important as any diagnostic information that is gathered.

Evaluating the Effectiveness of the Therapy Session

Following each intervention session, the clinician and/or teacher should evaluate the effectiveness of the session. What should the evaluation include? In order to decide, let us look at the goals. Did this treatment session accomplish the specific goals set forth in the therapy plan? Did the methods, techniques, and materials employed bring about the desired results, or could the same results be accomplished by simpler, more direct methods? Did the student understand why he or she was asked to perform specific tasks? In other words, did this intervention session make sense to the student? Did it include an opportunity for new learning or generalization? For practice? For review? Did the instruction have any relationship to the student's specific communication and academic needs? Were the techniques and materials adapted to the appropriate age level, gender, interests, level of understanding? Were barriers to learning removed? Paradoxically, it is possible for a therapy session to be well taught and interesting to the student yet still not have any bearing on the communication problem and its eventual solution!

Was the clinician able to establish an excitement by the student? Was the clinician genuinely interested in both the student and plans for the session? Did the clinician talk too much, or too little? Did both clinician and student seem to feel at ease? Was the clinician in charge of the session or did the student take over?

All of these questions need to be answered concerning every lesson. The questions are appropriate for group sessions as well. Too often the criteria for a treatment session are based on whether or not the student enjoyed it and whether or not good rapport existed between the student and the clinician. Although both are valuable components, there is much more to a successful lesson. Careful preparation, execution, and retrospective evaluation of therapy sessions, both group and individual, are essential ingredients of good therapy.

Therapy plans may serve still another purpose. When progress reports, case closure summaries, periodic evaluation reports, and written communication are required, the treatment plan may serve as a source of reference and an evaluation of progress of therapy. The contents can be used to prepare communications and reports. In addition, the therapy plans can be employed by a substitute SLP should there be a need.

Considerations for Special Populations

Since the early 1970s the role of the SLP in the schools has continued to evolve. Much of the terminology has changed, research has added new dimensions, and service delivery methods are more flexible and diverse. In the early days programs known as "speech improvement" were designed to help preschool and early primary children improve speaking and listening "habits."

Interestingly, programs for special populations today have their roots in the concerns of the early practitioners. Today's SLP must be interested in an ever expanding list is communication disorders and issues related to treating special populations. Attention must be directed toward prevention of speech, language, and hearing problems in infants and preschool children. School districts are wrestling with ways to handle the communication difficulties of bilingual and nonstandard speakers of English. Language disorders in children and adolescents constitute the major focus of the SLP's time and interest.

There are many options for the delivery of educational services. The individual needs of the children determine the amount and type of supplemental services required. The speech-language clinician may be working with teachers of children who present with autism spectrum disorder or are developmentally delayed, emotionally disturbed, hearing impaired, or learning disabled. The children in these groups may also require the help of the reading specialist, physical therapist, occupational therapist, academic tutor, psychologist, and others. This means that the school clinician will be working closely with the child's classroom teacher as well as with other specialists and the parents of the child. All personnel must keep in mind that instruction should be student-centered and child-oriented. The specialists involved work as a team, and each team member has specific responsibilities that are known to themselves and other team members.

The literature in the field of communication disorders provides professionals with extensive discussion of approaches for treating children with communication impairments. It is not the intent or purpose of this book to suggest specific intervention approaches. There are many books and resources available that discuss specific communication impairments. However, there are considerations that need to be made for developing an intervention program that meets the needs of special populations.

As mentioned earlier, SLPs must be prepared to continually review the literature about new EBP intervention approaches that might have promise. Then, they need to be discriminating in their use with students while determining if the approach has promise for their population or not.

Literacy (Reading and Written Language Disorders)

The National Education Goals (U.S. Department of Education, America Reads Challenge, 1997) stated that all children in the United States will start school ready to learn and that every adult American will be literate. The National Literacy Act of 1991 (Public Law 102-73) defined literacy as "an individual's ability to read, write, and speak and compute and solve problems at levels of proficiency necessary to function on the job and in society, to achieve one's goals and to develop one's knowledge and potential." The Core Curriculum Standards (2010) address preparing students for work and college. Understanding these issues is important for all educators including speech-language pathologists. As language is the foundation for learning and there is a relationship between spoken and written language, speech-language pathologists have an important role to play in developing children's literacy skills. In 1999, ASHA established an Ad Hoc Committee on Reading and Written Language Disorders to develop a technical paper and position statement describing the roles and responsibilities of speech-language pathologists related to reading and writing in children and youth (ASHA Ad Hoc Committee on Reading and Written Language Disorders, 2000). The position statement provides an understanding of why speech-language pathologists should plan an active role in this initiative. The technical paper clarifies how this can be done. Speech-language pathologists who are striving to link their programs with the educational curriculum should refer to these valuable resources.

Many of the same children who exhibit communication impairments also demonstrate reading and writing difficulties (Blachman, 1998; Catts & Kamhi, 1999). It is imperative, therefore, for SLPs and other educators to understand the relationship between spoken and written language. The ASHA position includes the following statements: Language is the foundation for the development of listening, speaking, reading, and writing skills. Spoken and written language build upon one another; thus, there is a reciprocal relationship. Youngsters who present spoken language impairments frequently have difficulty learning to read and write. Instruction in spoken language can result in gains in written language. SLPs can and should contribute to the reading component of the language arts curricula through the following actions (ASHA Ad Hoc Committee on Reading and Written Language Disorders, 2000):

- Implementing prevention programs designed to foster language acquisition and emergent literacy;
- Identifying language behaviors that place children at risk for later reading problems;
- Assessing children's literacy abilities;
- Providing intervention that builds on and encourages the relationships between spoken and written language;
- Collaborating with other educators to shape or modify the curriculum to strengthen understanding of the link between language and learning;
- Documenting and monitoring outcomes of language intervention; and,
- Advocating for effective literacy practices in schools.

The speech-language pathologist may be the first to recognize that a child is at risk for reading and written language problems. If the following characteristics are present, the SLP should begin to alert other educators and the family of potential problems: difficulties in phonological processing, including phonological awareness; multiple articulation problems; word retrieval difficulties; language compre-hension problems; delayed discourse abilities; verbal memory difficulties; and limited meta-linguistic or meta-cognitive awareness (ASHA Ad Hoc Committee on Reading and Written Language Disorders, 2000).

Current research supports using language based approaches to develop spoken as well as written language skills. This recommendation is based on the philosophy that language learning should be an integrated process involving interactive and naturalistic intervention practices. Emphasis is placed on teaching language and reading skills using real conversational contexts and situations. The components of language and reading are not fragmented into separate components (such as phonology, morphology, syntax, semantics, and pragmatics). Rather, communication is presented as a whole process to be used to understand and transmit meaning. Clinicians who are involved in working with students' literacy suggest that the SLP work closely with the classroom teacher to plan meaningful learning activities, provide realistic and functional opportunities for facilitating communication, and encourage the student to actively participate during the learning activities.

A valuable role for SLPs is to work with classroom teachers to improve reading proficiency in the classroom. SLPs have much to contribute to educators' overall understanding of how language skills relate to the learning process, especially reading, writing, and language arts. The SLP should share information on the "language-reading connection" with the teacher, and together they plan ways of structuring and achieving goals for the language-delayed child at risk for reading problems.

To avoid fragmented learning experiences, the child's language program in areas such as writing, spelling, reading, speech, and auditory processing should be coordinated and based on concepts of language acquisition. Following are several language procedures that can be recommended to improve students' reading skills:

- Teach phonological awareness concepts such as rhyming, segmenting, and synthesizing;
- Teach the correspondence between graphemes and phonemes;
- Establish phonemic awareness of speech sounds;
- Help children learn to identify how speech sounds relate to the written alphabetic symbol;
- Teach students to discriminate various stress patterns across words;
- Help students learn to recognize when one word stops and another begins;
- Develop semantic awareness of word labels and functions;
- Help build reading accuracy and encourage rhythm and melody during oral reading;
- Acknowledge and permit the student to read in his or her native dialect;
- Write stories composed by the children using their language patterns;
- Recommend that adults read various types of materials to children;
- Involve children as active participants in meaningful language and reading activities;
- Explain how stories are typically organized;
- Demonstrate how to ask questions to obtain additional information;
- Stress comprehension skills;
- Incorporate vocabulary and reading material from the child's classroom reader into therapy activities; and
- Present the reading words in the context of a phrase using a modifier or verb, not in isolation.

Children who demonstrate reading difficulties are generally referred for a thorough reading analysis, which may be done by the reading specialist. The speech-language clinician and the reading specialist should strive to learn one another's professional terminology. Often they are talking about the same things but using different terms. The reading specialist and the SLP have much in common and much to offer one another. Duplicating services can be avoided by establishing a close working relationship with reading instructors as well as curriculum specialists and teachers.

Cultural and Linguistically Diverse Populations

The issue of providing speech and language intervention services to children whose native language is not English or who speak different dialects has been a topic of intense discussion among professionals. Public Laws do not permit federal funds to be designated for services that are elective or for children who do not demonstrate disabilities. The United States is a multicultural population. There is an increase in the percentage of the school-age population from ethnically diverse backgrounds.

School districts vary greatly in the type of services they offer to youngsters who are from diverse cultures. Some districts employ a cadre of specialists who provide English-as-a-second-language (ESL) services. Some SLPs perform that role. Unfortunately, in some areas of the country no one particular discipline has claimed this population group. Therefore, students may be served inadequately or not at all.

Much of the intervention process for English Language Learners is dependent upon the relationship established between the individual with a communication difference or impairment and the clinician. Therefore, the relationship is affected when the client and clinician speak different languages or come from different cultural backgrounds. Clinicians need to have an understanding of the various cultures they will encounter in their communities. Acceptance of speech-language services may be affected by cultural variables such as traditions, customs, values, beliefs, and practices. It is important to know about the speech, language, and behavioral characteristics associated with specific cultures. It is essential to have knowledge of the unique aspects of a language in order to assess or remediate the phonemic, syntactic, morphological, semantic, lexical, or pragmatic characteristics. SLPs should increase their awareness and understanding of specific assessment materials and treatment strategies known to be effective for particular ethnic populations. Caution must be taken to avoid making stereotypical generalizations and formulating erroneous expectations. It is necessary for clinicians to modify intervention paradigms to incorporate alternate strategies and culturally distinct styles of learning.

With so much blending occurring in the world, it is hoped that future professionals demonstrate a high degree of cultural sensitivity. Clinicians can increase their awareness of the cultures they serve by gathering the following information about the ethnic groups in their communities (Cheng, 2011; Hanson, Lynch, & Wayman, 1990):

- The countries of origin, languages spoken, and numbers of individuals from the ethnic group living in the community;
- The social organization of the ethnic group and resources available within the community;
- The prevailing belief system within the community including the values, ceremonies, and symbols important to that culture;
- The history of the ethnic group and current events directly and indirectly affecting the culture;

- The methods used by the members of the community to gain access to social services; and
- The attitudes of the group toward seeking assistance.

Various degrees of English proficiency may be observed in speakers from diverse populations including those who are bilingual English proficient, limited English proficient, and limited in both English and their native language. Assessment and intervention should be conducted in the student's primary language for those who are limited in English.

Dialectal differences cannot be construed as speech or language disorders; however, we must make sure that the student does not present a disorder in the native language. Experts in second language suggest that dialectal differences are differences from Standard American English that are based on the rules of the dialect, not on the speaker's ability to understand or speak. They reflect the internalization of the language rules of a primary culture or subculture.

To consider these children speech-language disordered would be improper. Their difficulty with English is not due to a language disorder but to a language difference. Differences may be found in the linguistic structure, the phonological system, and the inflectional use of voice. Differences also exist in the cultural background at verbal and nonverbal levels.

There is little doubt that speech, language, and hearing deviations and disorders do exist among minority populations, including Hispanics, blacks, Asians (including Pacific Islanders), and American Indians (including Alaskan natives). In identifying communication disorders and deviations in diverse populations, the SLP must be careful not to confuse a dialect with a communication disorder. According to a paper drafted by the Committee on the Status of Racial Minorities (1985), "It is apparent that the assessment and remediation of many aspects of speech, language, and hearing minority language speakers require specific background and skills. This is not only logical and sound clinical practice, but it is the consensus set forth by federal mandates . . . " The report further indicated that state regulations are being developed to acknowledge the need for specific competencies to serve minority language populations. In California, for example, school districts are being encouraged by the education agency to require resource specialists, speech-language pathologists, and school psychologists to pass a state-administered oral and written examination on Hispanic culture, the Spanish language, and assessment methodology before they conduct assessments for Spanish-speaking children with limited English proficiency.

Harris (1985) discussed the importance of the clinician's investing time and effort to learn about the culture of the population that he or she serves. Harris, who was co-director of the Native American Research and Training Center, University of Arizona, stated, "To appropriately measure and evaluate the English performance of minority language children on measures of speech and language, the examiner must be familiar with the behavioral characteristics of that group as they relate to language learning and language use. The level to which the particular child employs the traditional linguistic/cultural practices of his ethnic/minority group must be determined in order to assess his performance in an appropriate manner."

For example, requesting an Apache child to answer incessant questions, especially to answer in English, may put the child into a cultural conflict in which his or her resulting behavior (silence) may not be indicative of potential or knowledge but rather of cultural integrity.

This is not to say that school SLPs should not evaluate and provide services to children who have limited English proficiency and who have speech, language, or hearing impairments. Interim strategies may be employed, such as utilizing interpreters or translators; establishing interdisciplinary teams, including a bilingual professional (for example, special education teacher or psychologist); or hiring a bilingual SLP or audiologist.

In regard to social dialects (Black English, Standard English, Appalachian English, Southern English, New York dialect, Spanish-influenced English), it is the position of the American Speech-Language-Hearing Association (1983) that " . . . no dialectal variety of English is a disorder or a pathological form of speech or language . . . [however] it is indeed possible for dialect speakers to have linguistic disorders within the dialect." An essential step toward making accurate assessments of communicative disorders is to distinguish between those aspects of linguistic variation that represent the diversity of the English language from those that represent speech, language and hearing disorders.

Roth et al. (2010) recommend several classroom accommodation strategies to help English Language Learners in the classroom including the following:

- Preteach key words and concepts
- Provide dictionaries in the student's native language
- Use classroom materials that show various cultures.
- Provide material in the parents' preferred language to increase their understanding of their child's education and needs.

Attention Deficit and Central Auditory Processing Disorders

In order to benefit fully from the classroom situation, children have to be able to hear the teacher's message and understand what it means. Children who exhibit problems related to attention deficit and central auditory processing disorders are at risk for failure due to their inability to effectively process the information that is presented to them. They may have difficulty discriminating sounds, attending to spoken messages, making associations, recalling sequences of information, and processing the information they hear. Determining the existence of problems related to an auditory processing disorder is a complex task. There are several assessment and diagnostic tools that can be used to assess auditory processing skills. The speech-language pathologist should be key members of the evaluation and planning team for this student.

The SLP can stress the importance of listening skills for the learning situation. In addition to providing direct instruction, clinicians can provide teachers with valuable information about techniques they can use to help students with these problems function more effectively in the classroom. Clark (1980) recommends a number of strategies that teachers can use for increasing listener potential. First and foremost, they must gain the student's attention and reduce distractions. It is advisable to provide preferential seating so that the student has the advantage of hearing the teacher's instructions and comments. Teachers must monitor their speaking delivery style and provide instructional transitions, giving students the opportunity to benefit from their awareness of the teaching moment. Environmental assessment should consider the quality of the listening or acoustic environment. Efforts should be made to minimize noise and other distractions in the classroom. Recommend that teachers use visual and written teaching aids and avoid auditory exhaustion. Frequent checks should be made of the student's concentration and comprehension. Teachers should take steps to encourage participation and provide support or reinforcement during learning activities. By taking steps such as these, teachers may soon realize that strategies such as these benefit all students, not just those with listening or learning disorders.

Severe Communication Disabilities

Millions of Americans demonstrate severe communication disabilities. The federal laws have mandated the provision of services to children with severe and profound disabilities. Children with severe disabilities must be educated to the extent that their limitations allow. There is wide variation in the degree of disabilities demonstrated and capabilities of children who are impaired. Therefore, SLPs, teachers, and other school personnel must evaluate each child and plan an intervention program specific to that child's strengths and needs.

Some children with severe developmental delays do not begin to use words until the age of five or six, whereas others may learn to communicate by pointing and gesturing. Those with severe and profound deficits may never learn to communicate meaningfully. Early intervention, parent education, and interdisciplinary collaboration are important factors in a program for children with severe and profound mental retardation and developmental disabilities.

Some students have neuromuscular, neurologic, or physical disabilities that are so severe that they are unable to use speech as a primary method of communication. They may even be unable to use standard augmentative communication techniques such as gestures, facial expressions, and writing. The disabilities may be the result of congenital conditions, acquired disabilities, or progressive neurologic diseases. These students may have been diagnosed as having cerebral palsy, multiple sclerosis, oral or facial deformities, developmental verbal apraxia, autism, or dysarthria. They also may have central processing disorders or severe expressive aphasia. Children who acquire traumatic brain injuries or spinal cord injuries may have reduced communication skills. Many students who are unable to communicate verbally or vocally have normal or near normal receptive language abilities and normal nonverbal intelligence.

To treat children such as these, the SLP works closely with the family, regular and special education teachers, physical and occupational therapists, psychologists, and health professionals. The National Joint Committee for the Communicative Needs of Persons with Severe Disabilities developed a number of recommendations for serving individuals with severe disabilities. The Committee was composed of professionals representing a wide variety of disciplines including speech-language pathologists, special educators, occupational therapists, and physical therapists. Their recommendations included several principal tenets clinicians might use to guide their decision making for facilitating and enhancing communication among persons with severe disabilities: (a) communication is a social behavior; (b) effective communicative acts can be produced in a variety of modes; (c) appropriate communicative functions are those that are useful in enabling individuals with disabilities to participate productively in interactions with other people; (d) effective intervention must also include efforts to modify the physical and social elements of environments in ways that ensure that these environments will invite, accept, and respond to the communicative acts of persons with severe disabilities; (e) effective intervention must fully utilize the naturally occurring interactive contexts (e.g., educational, living, leisure, and work) that are experienced by persons with severe disabilities; and (f) service delivery must involve family members or guardians and professional and paraprofessional personnel (National Joint Committee for the Communicative Needs of Persons with Severe Disabilities, 1992).

Intervention goals generally emphasize development of self-help skills and social and adaptive behavior. It is important to select activities that are representative of common situations that may occur in the pupil's experiences.

The speech and language services provided depend on the needs of each child. Following is a list of numerous responsibilities SLPs may undertake when treating persons with severe expressive communication disorders:

- Assessing, describing, documenting, and evaluating the communication needs;
- Evaluating the learning environment and recommending appropriate modifications;
- Evaluating and assisting in the selection communication aids and techniques;
- Developing speech and vocal communication to the fullest extent possible;
- Evaluating and selecting the symbols for use with the selected techniques;
- Developing and evaluating the effectiveness of intervention procedures to teach skills and strategies necessary to utilize augmentative communication in an optimal manner;
- Integrating assessment and program procedures with family members and other professional team members;

- Training persons who interact with the individual; and
- Coordinating augmentative communication services.

The speech and language services provided depend on the diagnosis of each child. The most advantageous method or methods of communication are determined and may include gestural systems if appropriate, symbol systems, and orthographic or pictorial systems. Depending on the mode of communication selected, the process may include augmentative communication devices such as communication boards, computerized devices, speech output devices, synthetic voice instruments, word processors, and other electronic and mechanical apparatus.

Intervention for children with severe disabilities should focus on improving communication competence and functioning within the student's home, school, and community environments. Gillette (2011) provides comprehensive recommendations for helping students with severe disabilities achieve communication competence. She discusses the importance of two primary components: *Environmental planning* and *communication skill planning*. She recommends collaborating with education team and parent partners to establish and implement a communication intervention plan. Gillette's Communication Opportunity Inventory and Essential Communication Skills Inventory provide a systematic method to survey environments, opportunities, and partners available to implement interventions. Completing the inventories enables the clinician to determine appropriate goals for intervention for the student, managing the environment, and preparing the communication partners.

Autism Spectrum Disorders (ASD)

ASD is a disability that interferes with the normal development of effective reasoning, social interaction, and communication skills. Some refer to autism as "the ultimate learning disability." Persons with ASD experience difficulty understanding what they see, hear, and sense. They are unable to communicate effectively with others and relate to the world outside the self (Autism Speaks, 2010).

IDEA required that school districts take steps to identify and serve students with ASD. Because communication skills are so greatly affected by this disability, the SLP plays an important role in assessing and planning intervention for students with ASD. Clinicians should be familiar with the characteristics of ASD and accepted procedures for evaluating students. Several complex characteristics are associated with this devastating disability. Children exhibit severe delays in development of communication skills and understanding of social relationships. They are unable to recognize and respond to the behavior and communication of others. They experience problems with judgment and recognition of simple cause and effect. Their responses to sensations of touch, sight, and sound may be inconsistent response (oversensitivity or undersensitivity). Students demonstrate variable patterns of intellectual functioning; individuals may show high level skills in one domain and low performance in another. Activities and interests are restricted and they may repeat body movements and routines. Many of these characteristics are also symptomatic of other severe disabilities. Therefore, it is important that the diagnosis of autism be made by a team of health care and special education professionals who are familiar with the characteristics of ASD.

Development of effective treatment strategies for this group of individuals is still in its infancy. Although the literature about intervention is growing rapidly, a definitive set of answers regarding the most effective methodologies has not yet been generated. It generally is recommended that intervention stress the development of functional communication and learning skills to encourage safety and independence. Clinicians should use intervention techniques that emphasize development of pragmatic language skills, work within a highly structured format, stress generalization of skills to various situations outside of the therapy or classroom context, use augmentative communication strategies, and incorporate the family into treatment planning and implementation.

Hearing Impairments

The educational audiologist should oversee management of hearing loss. Most school districts do not employ audiologists. They must rely on services provided on a shared or contractual basis. In the absence of a staff audiologist, the speech-language pathologist has greater understanding of hearing loss than any other professionals in the school setting. There are several aspects of care for these children for which the SLP may be responsible including making medical and audiological referrals when indicated, facilitating acquisition and use of assistive listening strategies and devices, developing teachers' awareness and understanding of hearing loss, making recommendations for general education programming, developing speech and language skills, and monitoring the student's hearing aids.

It is important for educators and parents to understand the problems children will experience if their hearing is impaired. Even mild hearing loss can greatly impact upon school success. Flexer (1999) states that, "all hearing losses involve educational issues and some also involve medical issues." In the absence of the educational audiologist, the SLP is the most appropriate person for conveying this information to other educational staff members and the family.

Flexer, Wray, and Ireland (1989) suggest that speech-language pathologists need to be aware of three areas that are critical to classroom success for children with hearing impairments: hearing and the impact of hearing loss on classroom performance; the use of sound enhancement technology for habilitation and environmental access for persons who are hearing impaired; and the use of educational management strategies which emphasize hearing rather than minimize it. They offer the following list of hearing-oriented topics to assist the speech-language pathologist in delivering adequate services and answering pertinent questions posed by teachers who have children who are hearing impaired in their classrooms.

Hearing

- Classrooms are auditory-verbal environments with "listening" serving as the basis for classroom performance.
- Hearing loss occurs along a broad continuum ranging from a mild hearing loss to profoundly hearing-impaired; not as two discrete groupings of normally hearing or deaf. In fact, about 92 to 94% of hearing-impaired persons are functionally hard-of-hearing and not deaf.
- Hearing loss, whether mild or profound in nature, negatively impacts on verbal language, reading, writing, and academic performance.
- Speech may be audible to someone with a hearing loss, but not necessarily intelligible enough to hear one word as distinct from another.
- Persons with hearing losses need the signal of choice to be 10 times more intense than background sounds in order for speech to be intelligible; an impossible classroom listening situation.
- Appropriately fit sound enhancement equipment, typically FM units (in addition to wearable hearing aids), are necessary for any hearing impaired child with any degree of hearing loss to function in a mainstreamed classroom because this equipment improves the signal-to-noise ratio.
- FM equipment must be fit by an audiologist who is mindful of: (a) The acoustic characteristics of the equipment; (b) Methods of coupling equipment to personal hearing aids; (c) Psychosocial issues of visual deviance; and (d) Multiple equipment settings to allow flexibility in various listening environments.
- FM equipment must be functioning and teachers must be comfortable with its use, or it is of no value. Teachers should be made aware of how amplification systems work and understand that even the best sound amplification systems can be compromised by poor room acoustics, especially too much reverberation.
- The Ling 6-Sound Test is one method by which the classroom teacher can screen equipment function.

Educational Management Strategies That Focus on Hearing

- Auditory skills training and development should be implemented during all therapy and classroom activities.
- "Listen," as a cue word used by all staff, can alert the hearing-impaired child to upcoming instructions.
- Teachers are encouraged to repeat or rephrase comments from other students in the classroom.
- Pre- and Post-tutoring programs can provide necessary redundancy of instructional information.

Children with long-term hearing loss may demonstrate psychosocial and educational needs. Special education programming may be appropriate to meet the needs of individuals with any and all degrees of hearing loss. When making educational decisions, the special education placement team should consider the full range of service delivery options. This would include integrating the child into the regular education classroom and providing teacher in-service and supportive services. With adequate training and comprehensive support services, the regular education classroom teacher can have increased awareness of the impact of hearing impairment on a student's classroom function, and learn to adequately meet the student's needs.

In some school districts, SLPs take responsibility for teaching students with hearing impairments to communicate. The Listen Foundation (2010) describes five approaches that are frequently used: (1) The *auditory-verbal* method teaches children to use their residual hearing to learn spoken language. Integration into the hearing world is stressed. Appropriately fitted hearing aids and assistive listening devices are essential; (2) The *auditory-oral* approach is similar. It also uses aided hearing. Intervention is usually presented individually or in small groups and also teaches lip reading; (3) The *oral* approach introduces hearing during specific auditory lessons, and places emphasis on lip reading and written communication; (4) *Total communication* provides the child with a variety of communication methods simultaneously including signs, finger spelling, lip reading, speech, and use of residual hearing; and (5) *Manual communication* does not consider spoken language as a necessary component for communication. It considers sign language as the natural language of all deaf persons.

Parents should be provided with a clear explanation of all of these methods and invited to participate in the selection of a teaching method. Of course, before the SLP undertakes implementing a particular method, he or she should understand the philosophical basis and implementation techniques.

Children with hearing impairments should be monitored by an audiologist to ensure that they see a physician when necessary and that they are properly fitted for hearing aids and assistive listening devices.

Traumatic Brain Injury (TBI)

Each year, over one million American children and youths sustain a traumatic brain injury (TBI) as a result of motor vehicle accidents, falls, sports injuries, and abuse. Years ago, many of these children would have died. However, due to decreased emergency response time and improved medical treatment, lives are now being saved. Thousands of children injured will have to be hospitalized and will suffer from severe or moderate symptoms as a result of their injuries (Brain Injury Association, 2011). Individuals who sustain a brain injury may enter, exit, and re-enter treatment at any point along a broad continuum of care that includes: medical settings, rehabilitation settings, residential or transitional programs, long-term care settings, and special classes in school.

Traumatic brain injury may affect children's capabilities in a broad number of areas including physical, cognitive, communicative, behavioral, and social skills. Although many problems exist with this population following injury, the cognitive-communicative impairments experienced appear to be the main barriers to successful reintegration into home, school, and community.

Treatment after brain injury may be ongoing for years. Students' behaviors may change drastically in that time period. Consequently, more frequent evaluations and revisions of the IEP are required. During the team planning meeting, the SLP can provide a few representative examples of the deficits the student brain injury may exhibit, the resulting behaviors teachers might observe in the classroom situation, and the cognitive-communicative intervention strategies which would be effective for developing communicative skills. Information such as this can be helpful when jointly planning the treatment plan for the student.

Table 9–3 illustrates a few representative examples of the deficits students with TBI may exhibit, the resulting behaviors teachers might observe in the classroom situation, and the cognitive-communication intervention strategies which would be effective for developing communication skills (Blosser & DePompei, 2002). Information such as this can be helpful when collaborating with teachers and parents or planning the IEP.

Behavior Problems and Disorders

Research shows that one-third of students fail to learn because of behavior problems that interfere with their ability to fully attend to and engage in the classroom. Schools have been wrestling with their role in the education and treatment of students with behavior disorders. In fact, the most recent reauthorization of IDEA provides schools with mandates for evaluating and providing services to this group of students. The SLP should be a member of the evaluation team. Oftentimes behavior disorders are manifested by problems with communication—either understanding the language of others or effectively communicating emotions, needs, wants, and positions. Many times students with socioemotional or behavior disabilities exhibit intelligible communication but have complex comprehension or pragmatic difficulties. Their performance may be affected by medication they are taking. The SLP can play a very meaningful role in helping student, teachers, and parents understand how to improve communication interactions. Townsend (2011) reports evidence that one of the best ways to manage challenging behaviors is to foster social-emotional competence (such as the ability follow directions, control emotions, get along with peers and adults, and stay on task), which research shows leads to academic achievement. The Mariposa Student Success Program (Townsend, 2011) is designed to prepare educators, special educators, related services providers, and families with training in how to implement relationship-building and problem-solving skills to use with children who demonstrate behavioral issues. The Mariposa programs presents methods to support specific students and manage challenging behaviors. It offers insights into how to maximize instructional and intervention time with students by learning to identify obstacles that prevent children from focusing and concentrating.

Table 9–3. Cognitive-Communicative Impairments, Representative Classroom Behaviors, and Recommended Cognitive-Communicative Intervention Strategies

Cognitive-Communicative Impairments	*Behavior*	*Cognitive-Communicative Strategy*
Word-retrieval errors	Answers contain a high use of "this,""that," "those things," "whatchamacallits." Difficulty providing answers on fill-in-the-blank tests.	*Word Recall:* Teach the student association skills and to give definitions of words he or she cannot recall. Teach memory strategies (rehearsal, association, visualizations, etc.).
Verbal problem-solving ability is reduced	In algebra class, the student may arrive at a correct answer, but not be able to recite the steps followed to solve the problem.	*Problem-Solving:* Teach inductive and deductive reasoning at appropriate age levels.
Poor reasoning skills	After behaving inappropriately, the student is unable to discuss actions with teacher.	*Reasoning:* Privately (not during classroom situations or in front of peers) ask the student to explain answers and provide reasons.
Reduced ability to use abstractness in conversation (ambiguity, satire, inferences, drawing conclusions.)	Says things that classmates interpret as satirical, funny, or bizarre although they were not intended to be that way.	*Semantics:* Teach the student common phrases used for satire, idioms, puns, etc.
Delayed responses	When called upon to give the answer, the student will not answer immediately, appearing not to know the answer.	*Processing:* Allow extra time for the student to discuss and explain. Avoid asking too many questions.
Unable to describe events in appropriate detail and sequence.	When relating an experience, details are out of order, confused or overlapping.	*Sequencing:* Teach sequencing skills. Direct the context of the student's responses.
Inadequate labeling or vocabulary to convey clear messages.	Inappropriately labels tools in industrial arts class.	*Semantics:* Teach the student vocabulary associated with specific areas and classroom activities.

Source: From Blosser & DePompei (2002).

Abused and Neglected Children

An unfortunate condition that seems to be more widespread is that of the battered or neglected child, who may also have communication problems. The maltreatment of children usually falls into one or more four general areas: physical abuse, neglect, emotional maltreatment, and sexual abuse.

Some forms of abuse and neglect are easily recognized, such as beatings that leave facial bruises or being repeatedly locked out of the home for long periods of time. The more subtle forms of abuse may include verbal abuse, poor supervision, or overly strict discipline. What is the school clinician's role in regard to abused and neglected children? First, the SLP should be alert to the signs of abuse. It is important to keep in mind that abuse occurs among the rich and well educated as well as the impoverished. The next step is to report suspicions to the principal, backed up with as much evidence as possible. Although suspicions may be wrong, a life could also be saved. Children who are maltreated often exhibit learning disabilities. They show symptoms such as distractibility, inappropriate behaviors, poor memory skills, and inattentiveness. These symptoms are often blamed on the emotional distress the child may be experiencing due to the abuse. When symptoms such as these are noticed, the child should be referred for a multifactored evaluation, including speech-language and hearing testing. The behaviors may actually be related to brain damage caused by physical abuse.

Working with Adolescents

The interest in preparing adolescents in high schools and vocational high schools for jobs in the outside world provides a unique challenge to SLPs. It is essential that adolescents who struggle with language skills be provided with intervention and support. SLPs can contribute to students' academic success. Ehren and Murza (2011) present a compelling case for SLPs to orient intervention toward workforce readiness, especially in light of the Common Core Standards and our national goal to prepare students for college and work.

The number of SLPs providing services in high schools and vocational schools is not known at this time; however, the number is smaller than those in elementary and middle school. By the same token, it is not known how many adolescents with speech, language, and hearing problems are in high school or vocational schools.

Awareness of the psychology of the adolescent age group is important to the school SLP. A strong desire to be accepted by peers and not to be different from them sometimes underlies a resistance to therapy. A good working relationship with the teachers can do much to encourage students enrolled in therapy to maintain good attendance in sessions. Regardless of how severe the communication deficit may be, it is of secondary importance to the student at this age level. The intervention program should be based on the student's personal and workforce related communication. Intervention can be developed around such topics as workforce language, computing, getting a job, preparing applications for college, and other subjects of interest. Students preparing for graduation can be introduced to the following topics: (1) selecting correct word choices, (2) eliminating slang, (3) speaking clearly with the appropriate volume and rate, and (4) eliminating syntactical errors.

High schools may have transitional programs. In this type of program the student moves from school to the work force, with activities focused on exploring employment opportunities, assessing vocational potentials, vocational training, and job placement. For students in the secondary transitional programs who have communication handicaps or limited communication skills, the services of the SLP are utilized. The school staff often carries out the programs with the cooperation of the vocational education staff or potential employers.

Working with Groups of Children

In a sense all therapy is group therapy. A dyadic group (group of two) in speech, language, and hearing consists of the clinician and the student. Therapy groups in the schools consist of the clinician and from two to five students, or in special instances, more students. The purpose of a therapy group is to help the student in such a way that in the future he or she becomes independent of the relationship. The clinician is a facilitator who is aware of the feelings, values, and tensions of the participants. The clinician may play the role of an impartial judge in the event of friction. He or she keeps the group members moving toward the completion of the tasks at hand. Group therapy provides opportunity for peer modeling and support, socialization, and the development of interactive, social communication skills. Groups also enable students to use their new skills in a social situation. Practice and drill routines do not give children the same type of practice for using new communication skills readily in social and interpersonal situations.

The SLP must be able to create the kind of environment in which the student is able to learn to use new skills and change existing behaviors. A group situation provides a greater possibility for this than does a one-on-one relationship between the SLP and the student. Dynamic group interaction can provide the forum for children learning to support one another in therapy. Children can learn to elicit responses from one another and provide modeling, corrections, and feedback. They can learn to judge each other's productions as correct or incorrect and apply reinforcements to shape appropriate productions. In this model, constant interaction and learning is a positive experience.

Care must be taken that group therapy doesn't become individual therapy with one child speaking and the other children in the group simply listening, watching, and waiting for their turn. Passive participation has no therapeutic value. In groups structured like this, group interaction is limited if it exists at all.

There is no rule that says all therapy sessions must take place around a table. Working in front of a mirror, a flannel board, or a chalkboard will help group members to become better participants. It has been said that learning is movement. If this is true, the clinician who sits on a chair without ever moving, and the children who remain in their places during the entire session day after day, may not be making the best possible use of therapy time.

Counseling

Counseling is an important factor in a holistic approach to therapy. The SLP in the school system counsels both students and parents in communication problems. Some of the counseling is geared toward the prevention of problems. For example, the SLP may give a talk to families on the nature of speech, language, and hearing problems or the development of speech and language in infants and children. Or the counseling may be directly with the student, entailing self-perception, acceptance of the problem, understanding of the problem, relationship to peers, information about the specific disorder, reluctance to talk, and feelings about the problem.

The school clinician should be alert to any signs that would indicate that the student may require psychological or psychiatric treatment. Even the faintest doubt about seeking further professional help should be pursued.

Many school clinicians have found that fears and apprehensions surrounding many types of speech disorders are based on misinformation or no information. Much of the anxiety for both students and their parents can be alleviated by factual and general information. The student's negative feelings about the problem may also be allayed by the attitude of the clinician, who says, not only by words but also by actions, "I'm here to help you; we can work on this together."

Although SLPs are not trained as counselors, there is no question about their knowledge of their professional field and the fact that they have been doing counseling. Without counseling, therapy alone would be ineffective. Recognizing that there are some children whose emotional problems may go beyond the communication problem, the school SLP seeks consultation and possible referrals of such children to other agencies and services specifically designed to deal with them.

Prevention of Communication Problems

Professionals have a responsibility to include not only treatment but also the prevention of communication disorders. This includes early detection and treatment of young children. As discussed previously, services for children birth to 5 may be provided by a number of disciplines and should be coordinated. Family involvement is essential.

What does this mean to the school SLP? Essentially, it means that if you are employed as a school clinician in a state that includes in its laws the detection and treatment of young children, the responsibility of servicing these children will be with the local health care or education agencies. Because of financial restraints few school systems have this type of program; however, the detection and treatment of young children with disabilities are often being provided by local community voluntary agencies and by private agencies and health care programs.

The school SLP has a stake in encouraging and assisting these agencies in early detection and remediation. The earlier that handicapping conditions are identified, the better chance there is of remediation. And eventually fewer of these children will turn up in the caseload of the school clinician. Communication deviations that go untreated may develop into communication disorders and cause these children difficulties with the acquisition of such academic skills as reading, spelling, writing, and mathematics.

The SLP may intervene by providing information about speech and language development, environmental factors that influence development, and techniques to facilitate and stimulate speech and language development. Talks to groups of parents, early childhood educators such as daycare workers, preschool and nursery school teachers, members of the health professions, elementary school teachers and administrators, student groups, community organizations, and other professional groups, will help individuals understand how they may prevent and ameliorate speech, hearing, and language problems in children. Information may also be disseminated through newspaper articles, radio and television appearances, and other media. In a school or preschool the SLP may provide demonstration lessons for the teachers.

DISCUSSION QUESTIONS AND PROJECTS

1. Collect samples of Individualized Education Programs and Individualized Family Service Intervention Plans used in various school systems. Compare and contrast IEPs and IFSPs. How are they alike? How are they different?

2. If you are a student who is working with a child in your university-based clinic, develop an IEP or IFSP for that child.

3. Prepare a lesson plan for two of the students listed below. Be sure to show how you will incorporate information and materials from the school curriculum into your plan. Each speech-language goal should be related to some aspect of the classroom or a school subject. Students: an

8-year-old girl from Vietnam with limited English proficiency; a 3-year-old child with autism; a fifth grader with severe dysfluency; a third grader with a language-learning disability that affects reading comprehension; a 5-year-old with delayed articulation; and a high school junior with cognitive-communicative impairments as a result of a TBI.

4. Describe steps you could take to motivate a high school student who is not interested in participating in your therapy program any longer.

5. With a colleague, role-play a discussion you might carry on with a classroom teacher to explain a student's communication impairment, the impact of the impairment on the learning process, and recommendations of how the two of you might work collaboratively to facilitate generalization of communication skills within the classroom. Role-play your discussion for your classmates (one person assume the role of the SLP).

6. Prepare an in-service presentation for the teachers of a student with an emotional disability.

7. Plan a lesson for the fourth grade students on your caseload with multiple articulation problems. Base your lesson on a social studies unit.

8. What behavioral signs would alert you to the possibility that a student is being physically abused? What steps are required of the educators in your state if they discover abuse?

9. Plan a presentation for high school students who have had children. What might you tell them to encourage them to help their children develop appropriate communication skills?

10. Survey your classmates to determine the existence of various learning styles.

10

Collaboration: Creating Meaningful Relationships With Others

In Chapter 8 we described the importance of collaboration to achieve goals. Collaboration reinforces the need for SLPs to work closely with other individuals who are involved in the lives, education, and care of children. To implement collaboration effectively, it is necessary to understand those who interact directly with the SLP in order to help children with communication impairments. In other words, what can we expect from various individuals and what can they expect from us?

Speech-language pathologists are not the only professionals responsible for helping children develop or improve their communication abilities. Other individuals who are significant in a child's life can and should share that responsibility. SLPs are in a unique position to foster understanding of the nature of a child's communication challenges and what can be done to build communication competence. We can increase a child's chance of success by enabling those who know the child to play a critical role in the intervention process. Collaborating with important individuals in a child's life is an integral component of service delivery. To collaborate effectively, it is necessary to establish meaningful relationships with key individuals and take the time and effort that is required to help them understand the key roles they can play.

Parents and/or guardians are encouraged to take leading roles in planning the speech, language, and hearing services for their children. We can guide them on how and when they can help their children and the strategies they can use. Interactions with parents are not new for school-based clinicians. However, the importance of establishing meaningful relationships that can contribute to successful results cannot be emphasized enough. It is helpful to understand problems that interfere with interactions with families and strategies for forming meaningful relationships with them. The school speech-language pathologist is also a consultant to the community and a source of information on speech, language, and hearing disorders and services.

In this chapter, we examine the SLP's roles and responsibilities. We especially discuss the wonderful working relationships we can establish with other individuals who are involved with educating, caring for, or treating school children.

The Importance of Collaborating and Consulting with Others

In each situation and environment a child enters, there are demands for communication. Therefore, it is critical for individuals with whom children interact to learn the importance of communication for success, to recognize communication delays and disorders, and to play important roles in facilitating speech-language development and modification if problems exist.

Creating effective collaborative partnerships represents a philosophical approach to service delivery that ensures that the clinician, family members, and other professionals work together as a team to develop plans and strategies for helping children with communication impairments. They may also join forces to prevent communication problems from occurring. The child is the central focus of planning and problem-solving and each team member brings to the situation their own unique expertise and contributions.

There are three terms that are typically used to describe working relationships between colleagues and teammates. These are transdisciplinary, multidisciplinary, and interdisciplinary. In a transdisciplinary approach team members share roles and systematically cross discipline boundaries. The *transdisciplinary approach* is the most collaborative of the three. Professionals pool and integrate their expertise so more efficient and comprehensive assessment and intervention services may be provided. There is give and take between all members (especially with the parents) on a regular, planned basis. Professionals from different disciplines teach, learn, and work together to accomplish a common set of intervention goals for a child and her family. An *interdisciplinary approach* refers to connecting methods and concepts from many disciplines and perspectives in the pursuit of a common task. *Multidisciplinary* in the context of school service delivery means that professionals from different disciplines work together collaboratively to provide diagnoses, assessments, and treatment within the scope of practice and areas of competence of each discipline.

Idol, Paolucci-Whitcomb, and Nevin (1986) define collaborative-consultation as "an interactive process that enables teams of people with diverse expertise to generate creative solutions to mutually defined problems. The outcome is enhanced and altered from the original solutions that any team member would produce independently." Pershey (1998) reviewed numerous sources of information on collaborative models of speech-language service delivery. Several articles focused on the coordination of language intervention with reading and language arts instruction. Collaboration enables team members to:

- Determine the severity of the communication impairment;

- Assess the impact the communication impairment has on the student's academic and social performance;
- Define a student's communicative needs for various educational and social situations;
- Observe a student's communicative abilities under specific circumstances;
- Develop strategies for stabilizing the new skills the student is learning in therapy; and
- Monitor the student's progress after dismissal from a direct service program.

Several professionals (Blosser & Kratcoski, 1997; Damico & Nye, 1990; Marvin, 1990; Nelson, 1990; Wiig & Secord, 1990) have described the role of the speech-language pathologist as a collaborative-consultant for children with various communication disorders. To be successful in a collaborative-consultant role, the SLP must have a solid theoretical foundation in communication development and disorders; must be able to identify children's strengths and needs; must be able to develop prescriptive techniques; must understand the school curriculum and the learning process; and should be able to relate these aspects of communication to oral and written language.

The essentials of collaborative relationships that are successful involve cooperation, communication, joint planning and programming. Professionals focus on how they can effectively combine their talents, expertise, and schedules to facilitate a comprehensive program for children. To accomplish a collaborative model of service delivery, SLPs and their school partners must jointly identify goals that will help prepare the student to function effectively in the varied environments in which he or she lives and learns. People who have significant relationships should be involved and recommendations made that will enable others to try the intervention strategies that work best in real life situations such as the classroom, lunchroom, playground, reading group etc. Collaborative relationships can maximize our ability to:

- Define and clarify problems
- Generate solutions
- Determine strengths and weaknesses for learning
- Share responsibility
- Define communicative needs
- Observe communication performance in specific circumstances
- Develop strategies for stabilizing newly taught skills
- Monitor progress.

School Culture

The culture of the school organization influences the extent and quality of collaboration that goes on among the education team. Culture is the beliefs, attitudes, and behaviors that characterize a school. In a healthy school culture there is a sense of community as well as common goals and shared practices. There is agreement on curriculum and instruction. Most importantly, there is open and honest communication.

Seven important conditions that are essential to a positive school culture are as follows: (1) leadership buy-in; (2) open to new ideas and innovations; (3) a climate that encourages relationships and collaboration among educators; (4) systems in place that facilitate ongoing communication; (5) time allocated for planning and meeting; (6) a staff that is well prepared; and (7) goal alignment, with teachers and therapists coordinating around goals. If these conditions are in place, there is a greater likelihood that the education team will work together to ensure that students have success in therapy and classroom.

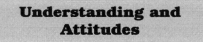

Understanding and Attitudes

The functions of the school SLP are ideally carried out as an equal member of the educational team. To provide the best possible treatment for students with communication impairments, the school speech-language pathologist must work cooperatively with students' families and with other professionals in the education community. Sometimes, this involves providing information and support. Often, it means receiving information and support. But most often, it entails both.

The attitudes others have toward the speech-language program are crucial to its success. Equally important are the attitudes SLPs display in relation to working cooperatively with other individuals to improve students' communication skills. In most situations, the reactions and quality of cooperation of individuals are determined by previous experiences or what the situation signifies to them. People possess varying degrees of difference in their understanding and attitude toward children with communication difficulties and toward the services of the speech-language-hearing pathologist. Parents, educators and therapists may differ in their beliefs about the need or goals for therapy. There may be divergent opinions about the seriousness of the communication behaviors or the recommended intervention methods. There may be a lack of clarity about the roles and responsibilities of the SLP leading to confusion and misinterpretation. This confusion may limit the effectiveness with which the SLP can function in school districts or individual school buildings. A concerted effort must be made to ensure that parents and other professionals are informed of and clearly recognize the functions of the speech-language pathologist within the school setting.

Although educators may be favorable toward the speech and language program, they may not have a thorough understanding that will enable them to provide assistance for children within the classroom setting. They may not understand the nature of communication disorders or the impact of communication impairments on academic performance. They may be unclear about the role and responsibility of the SLP or how to work in collaboration with the clinician. More importantly, they may be unaware of how to create favorable conditions for reinforcing speech and language skills or facilitating change and carryover.

Many school clinicians are doing a good job of collaborating and consulting with other individuals to build support and understanding of their school therapy programs. Their interactions lead to more comprehensive and effective services for students. Successful clinicians generally have good communication and interaction with parents and school professionals.

Figure 10–1 is a simple survey that SLPs can distribute to teachers in their schools to assess the depth of teachers' understanding of communication impairments, the SLP's role within the school setting, the goals of the speech and language program, and intervention strategies they can implement during their instruction and communicative interactions. There may be a wide range of understanding within one school building or throughout a school district. Understanding what teachers know and what they need to know can lead to a plan for providing training and establishing meaningful relationships with fellow educators.

Fostering Effective Involvement Through Mentoring

Current "best practice" philosophies for service delivery in health care and education settings support increased inclusion and involvement of families and teachers in the planning and carrying out assessment and treatment of individuals with disabilities. Federal legislation has consistently supported these philosophies by mandating equal responsibility for family and professionals in planning programs. As a result of these important steps, service providers in all types of settings are called on to have more frequent and regular contacts with families and educators of individuals they serve. They are seeking methods for working with families that are proven to be effective. They are looking for strategies that will result in the clarification of the roles and responsibilities others can play in intervention and education.

Family and teachers require support services and guidance in order to play meaningful roles. Everyone involved in the student's education should learn to interact effectively to obtain appropriate services and optimal opportunities for the student. It would be especially helpful for family especially to learn about the legal rights of students with disabilities and how to access financial assistance when needed. To accomplish these difficult feats, family and educators must first have a good understanding of communication disabilities. They must gain skills at interacting with service providers and other professionals at all levels. And, most importantly, they have to feel positive about their role and efforts.

Mentoring offers as a viable approach for preparing families and educators to play an important role in communication development and intervention of youngsters with speech and language disabilities. What is a mentor?

The origin of the term "mentor" dates to the time of Homer, specifically to *The Odyssey*. Homer describes his hero, Odysseus, preparing to set out on an epic voyage, though his son, Telemachus, must remain behind. Odysseus asks a trusted friend, Mentor, to guide and counsel Telemachus in his absence. From this ancient literary figure, mentor has come to mean one who helps guide a protege through a developmental process, whether that process is the transition from childhood to adulthood or from student to professional. Because of the complexity of this task, mentors are variously considered to be teachers, counselors, friends, role models, and more.

SURVEY OF TEACHERS' AWARENESS AND UNDERSTANDING OF SPEECH-LANGUAGE SERVICES

This brief questionnaire seeks to determine your awareness and understanding of the speech-language program in your school. Your responses will help us understand how to create meaningful partnerships between teachers and SLPs to ensure effective service for our students.

A Little About You

Grade or subject you teach ________________________________

Number of years you have been teaching ________________________________

Your Understanding of SLP Services

Indicate the number of students from your class who have or are receiving those services this school year. ________

Please rate your overall understanding of the speech-language services in your school. Consider aspects such as students' disabilities, the impact on students' performance in your classroom, therapy goals, therapy assessment and intervention approaches.

Great understanding	
Good understanding	
Fair understanding	
Don't understand	

Please rate your awareness of the range of options for delivering speech-language services (examples include: pull-out, classroom-based, integrated, monitoring, flexible scheduling, consultations, and combined models).

Very Aware	
Somewhat Aware	
Not Aware	

Rate the frequency with which you and your school's SLP communicate about the progress and status of students from your class who are currently enrolled in the speech-language program?

Frequently	
Sometimes	
Rarely	
Never	

Figure 10–1. Survey of teachers' awareness and understanding of speech-language programs.
continues

Rate your overall understanding of the following aspects related to the speech-language intervention services for students with disabilities.

My understanding of impairments and the need for services

Thoroughly understand	
Somewhat understand	
Don't understand at all	

My understanding of the impact of the communication disability on classroom performance

Thoroughly understand	
Somewhat understand	
Don't understand at all	

My understanding of goals of speech-language services

Thoroughly understand	
Somewhat understand	
Don't understand at all	

My understanding of speech-language intervention approaches

Thoroughly understand	
Somewhat understand	
Don't understand at all	

My understanding of service delivery options

Thoroughly understand	
Somewhat understand	
Don't understand at all	

My understanding of the role I can play

Thoroughly understand	
Somewhat understand	
Don't understand at all	

How did you gain your understanding of the speech-language services?

Service providers have provided information	
Discussions during student-related meetings	
Observations during therapy (in the therapy room or my classroom)	
Coursework or in-service	

Figure 10–1. *continues*

Rate the extent your collaboration with the SLP.

Extensive collaboration	
Some collaboration	
Very little collaboration	
No collaboration	

Rate the extent to which you participate in the assessment process to determine eligibility for speech-language services.

Always participate	
Occasionally participate	
Rarely participate	
Never participate	

Rate the extent to which you participate in the implementation of intervention strategies and techniques for speech-language services.

Always participate	
Occasionally participate	
Rarely participate	
Never participate	

Rate your perception of the impact of speech-language services on students' performance in your classroom.

Great impact	
Good impact	
Minimal impact	
No impact	

How would you rate your overall satisfaction with the speech-language program in your school?

Very satisfied	
Satisfied	
Somewhat Satisfied	
Not Satisfied	

What questions do you have about speech-language services in your school?

What recommendations do you have for increasing the level and quality of collaboration between teachers and SLPs?

What changes would you recommend to improve the speech-language program?

Figure 10–1. *continued*

The mentoring process can be described as a relationship in which a person of greater rank or expertise takes a personal interest in the professional and personal development of a newer person and provides experiences for the mentee (protégé) that have an unusually beneficial impact on the mentee's performance. Mentors have been described as advocates, teachers, counselors, role models, guides, facilitators, friends, and critics. Research has shown that mentors have a significant and positive impact of professional development and achievement. Mentoring has been used successfully in business and educational settings to assist teachers, professors, students and employees so they succeed and make effective contributions.

Mentees have derived many benefits from participating in mentoring relationships in these settings. Mentors can help mentees avoid obstacles, develop contacts, and gain insight into organizational systems. Mentees show learning at a faster pace and more thoroughly than their non-mentored counterparts. Newcomers understand the norms and rituals associated with being in a particular environment. They develop insights into acceptable and appropriate behavior for specific situations. Mentees gain understanding of expectations and patterns of interaction. Feelings of isolation are mitigated. They learn to access restricted information and key persons. They learn about important facts and operational policies and procedures. Perhaps most importantly, individuals who have been mentored report higher levels of satisfaction and enjoyment. To summarize, persons who are mentored develop those skills, forms of knowledge, attitudes, and values necessary to successfully and effectively carry out their occupational role.

Why Mentor Families and Educators?

Mentoring offers promise as an effective technique for developing the competencies and skills of people who are significant in the student's life. Creating mentor relationships can provide potential solutions to the needs, problems, and concerns families and educators experience. Just as employees in the work setting or professors in academe stand to make greater gains by being mentored, so do others stand a better chance of developing the skills they need for living with and effectively helping their child.

Similar to employee mentees in work settings, many benefits can be derived by implementing a mentoring approach for preparing families and teachers. The presentation of important information can be timed to parallel the needs to adapt to difficult and ever-changing situations. Family members can be introduced to the norms, rituals, policies, and procedures associated with medical, rehabilitation, or educational settings. Opportunities can be seized for developing the insights into acceptable and appropriate behavior for interacting with particular service providers in difficult situations. Others can gain familiarity with terminology, expectations, and patterns of interaction necessary for various situations. Feelings of isolation can be reduced because closer relationships generally form between mentees and mentors. One hopes that those who are mentored will assume leadership roles providing guidance to other families and professionals.

How Mentoring Differs from Other Types of Education and Counseling

Working with families of persons with disabilities is not new. Service providers have always held conferences with family members to explain students' disabilities and the treatment program. They have conducted in-service programs to improve family members' understanding of the treatment process. Many have invited family members to observe treatment and be a part of therapy. In response to federal mandates and accreditation standards, programs have established formal family education and counseling programs designed to provide information and improve the skills of family members and educators.

These efforts tend to be "generic" in nature. Often, the actual interaction time with family members is somewhat restricted. The explanation and exploration of important topics is limited. Service providers often "talk to" or "teach information to" their audiences. Efforts may range from providing brief introductory explanations to supplying written materials. The information disseminated is not always tailored to meet the family's individual needs and situation. Although efforts of this type are a good beginning, they may not always go far enough in preparing family to independently meet the challenges that lie ahead. Brief interactions such as these are good beginnings; but, they are not sufficient preparation to enable the family to make a real contribution in the intervention process.

Mentoring is different because the mentor and mentee form a different type of relationship with one another, one that is much closer and much more interactive. The mentor-mentee relationship is dynamic and changes overtime as the mentee gains confidence, skill, and independence.

Mentoring Activities

There are a number of mentoring activities that can be used with families and educators. These include informal contact, interactive dialogue, role modeling, direct assistance, demonstration, observation and feedback, and assistance with long-term planning. The activities are discussed in the following section. Brief examples of when these activities can be implemented are provided.

Informal Contact

This strategy can be implemented with family when they come to the school or participate in school activities. Educators can be reached at different times throughout the daily routine. Consider it an opportunity to impart important information whenever you engage in brief conversations with others.

Situations such as these are good opportunities for initiating and developing mentoring relationships. Mentors can use comments and questions to initiate relationships and discussions with those they identify as candidates to be mentees. Comments such as, "Call me if you need anything" and "Let me know if I can give you any information" can open the door to dynamic interaction and communication if conveyed with sincerity. Following are several questions framed to elicit discussion: "What would you like to know about Asa's speech problem?"

"What do you understand about Zoey's disability and needs?" "What do you understand about her capabilities and strengths?" "Is there anything bothering you right now about your son's program or your responsibilities" "Do you need help or assistance?" "How does Sam's dysfluency interfere with his relationship with other family members?" "Are you interested in learning the techniques and strategies we use in therapy?"

The family should be advised about the best times and means of making contact so that calls are not perceived as interruptions. Otherwise, communication breakdowns may occur if requests for assistance are made during busy or inappropriate times. Even though encounters of this nature may be brief, they afford mentors opportunities for developing the family's awareness of the environment, promoting confidence in the staff's skills, offering words of encouragement, passing along critical information, and providing general suggestions to increase understanding. Examples of information that can be conveyed during initial informal contacts are listed below:

- Information about the speech and language disorder;
- Medical aspects associated with the problem;
- The stages of physical and behavioral development of communication skills;
- How treatment will progress;
- The potential impact of the communication disorder on the student's learning, behavioral, physical, and emotional skills;
- Qualifications, roles and responsibilities of various staff personnel;
- Procedures for developing the IEP;
- Services available and procedures for accessing additional services; and
- Support organizations and resource centers available in the community.

Interactive Dialogue

Every contact with the family and teachers should be viewed as important and an opportunity for developing their awareness and skills. Mentors need to make special efforts to reduce anxieties and increase confidence and capabilities. Strive to make each contact and interaction meaningful. Seek others' ideas, opinions, and feedback. Involve them in planning treatment activities.

After treatment sessions, service providers often make general comments such as, "He did really well today" or "She was really trying hard." In mentoring relationships, comments would also be directed toward the performance or involvement of the educator or family member. For example, "Today we read stories in therapy. I'd like you to try reading these two stories at home (provide specific verbal and written instructions) and let me know how he does for you."

Mentors can help family adjust to their responsibilities and develop a more positive outlook by discussing concerns with them as they arise. Be sure to let them know how a particular activity relates to a class activity or household chore. Discuss their impressions of the reasons the student successful or not. Invite them to make suggestions or recommendations for improving or changing an activity.

Interactive dialogue can be used to promote understanding and skills in the following ways:

- To reinforce positive efforts;
- To stimulate thinking about future intervention issues;
- To teach others to monitor the student's behavior for subtle positive or negative changes in performance;
- To provide information about preparing or structuring the home environment to promote good communication;
- To obtain information about the family's goals for the student and home routines that might be valuable for planning future treatment or services;
- To suggest ways to incorporate specific treatment techniques and strategies into the home and classroom environments;
- To explain mystifying terminology and confusing procedures;
- To better understand the others' concerns and needs;
- To answer questions that arise; or
- To provide encouragement and motivation when progress seems slow or limited.

Role Modeling

Perhaps one of the most valuable and effective mentoring techniques is role modeling. Much can be learned from observing the mentor in action. Other than rare events like "Open House" when family are invited to visit the school, opportunities are generally limited for getting an "up close and personal" look at a professional in action. Teachers don't often take time to go to the therapy room to observe the SLP. However, there are opportunities for role modeling when the SLP goes into the classroom.

Mentors can use role modeling during the following activities:

- Team planning meetings;
- Classroom and treatment sessions; and
- Phone calls (for example, to establish contact with another service provider or agency; transmit or exchange information about the person's program or needs; inquire about available services; seek assistance; or look for answers to difficult questions).

Demonstration

Similar to role modeling, demonstration also provides opportunities to "see how it's done." It goes a step further, however, and enables the proteges to practice techniques under the guidance and supervision of the mentor. Demonstration is a more purposeful activity than role modeling.

Demonstration is particularly useful for teaching significant others to execute treatment strategies in the home and school environment. One of the primary goals of involving other people directly in the treatment process is to help them develop skills needed to encourage and teach the student more effectively. It also enables them to develop confidence about their efforts and skills. To implement this approach, plan functional therapy activities based on expectations and demands of the school situation. This approach makes it easier to involve other people and it makes treatment more relevant. Discuss the purpose and design of specific tasks planned for the day. Demonstrate the clinical techniques the teacher or parent watching, including ways to praise or reinforce the student's positive behaviors and make changes to elicit improved responses and behaviors. After demonstrating the activity, ask the person to conduct the same activity with the student. If the technique is not demonstrated in the proper way, the mentor again demonstrates, adding suggestions. The family should also be asked to critique their own performance of the task and ideas for making changes. For some, just a little guidance and encouragement is enough, for others more reinforcement is needed. The extent of reinforcement needed is as diverse as the personalities and cultures represented. Mentors have to evaluate each mentee to determine individual needs for instruction, explanation, and reinforcement. The suggestions made should be matched to the mentee's ability, tools, and technology available.

Demonstration can be particularly effective in many of the same situations as presented for role modeling. Mentors should cue mentees to listen for the way the mentor elicits a response or identifies the steps followed while performing a specific therapy task.

Observation and Feedback

A key factor in the mentorship process is providing meaningful feedback to the mentee as quickly as possible after the completion of a task or activity. In this way, the performance will still be fresh in each person's mind and the mentee will still be enthusiastic and receptive to suggestions. This conference time should be viewed as a time to recall the experience with the mentee and exchange information as well as provide guidance.

Allow time to express fears, frustrations, and feelings of success. Provide feedback. It enhances learning. Therefore, positive interaction is a must. Positive relationships do not just happen; they need to be cultivated. This is not always an easy task. The mentor must be very sensitive to the other person's level of understanding, communication style, feelings, hopes, and attitudes. Awareness of these factors will help the mentor formulate and deliver comments.

For example, after observing a teacher interact with the student, the mentor can comment on his or her perception of how the conversation went. Reinforcement can be given for positive interactions. Suggestions for rewording or rephrasing comments can be made if misunderstandings occurred.

As the mentor-mentee relationship is refined, it will be easier for the mentor to deliver feedback and for the mentee to receive it. With the goals in mind of transferring responsibility for case management, it is essential for the others to learn to recognize when they are doing well and when their efforts are not as successful as they could be. Observing the teacher in action and providing feedback during times such as those listed below will provide opportunity for them to refine their skills and build their confidence.

Mentors can observe and provide feedback when they observe others in the following situations:

- Conducting therapy activities;
- Talking about the student's disability and discussing the impact on learning and treatment strategies;
- Making recommendations during an IEP meeting;
- Conveying their thoughts, concerns, and recommendations during a team planning meeting;
- Interacting with staff personnel to ask questions, relate experiences, or express concerns;
- Conversing with the individual with student or giving instructions;
- Inquiring about desired services or procedures; and
- Interpreting reports about the student's skills and capabilities.

Plan for the Future

Mentees should be given guidance as they plan for the student's future. Issues of concern should be addressed and either brought to solution or recommendations made for seeking additional assistance. Many families ask service providers to clarify the "next step" they will need to take. Planning together will help alleviate future shocks. Here are some steps that can be taken:

- Provide referral lists and information about community services;
- Help establish networks with families with similar needs and concerns;
- Determine roles all family members can play (immediate as well as extended family) in caretaking, transportation, implementing treatment, and providing respite for primary caregivers.

Selecting Mentors and Mentees

It is unrealistic to think that all service providers can serve as mentors or all families can be mentored. Disposition, willingness, personality, knowledge, and experience are important factors for consideration. A high level of energy is generally devoted to mentoring relationships. Therefore, mentors as well as mentees have to be committed to effectively working together. Professionals who have a proven record of commitment to working with students with disabilities make excellent mentors. They demonstrate an attitude of willingness to help as well as learn from others. As the protégé shows progress, the mentor will need to modify his or her role, thus building independence and confidence.

Mentor Responsibilities

One does not implement this model without advance preparation. Here are some helpful hints for success:

- Remain available to talk and meet when needed;
- Develop and maintain a resource library with materials about communication disorders;

- Prepare instructional materials explaining how family can be active in developing the IEP or transition plan;
- Conduct workshops and training sessions about topics such as understanding the evaluation process, how language relates to reading, and inclusion;
- Promote networking among people with similar needs and interests;
- Prepare and distribute a calendar illustrating the focus of treatment sessions and inviting others to visit;
- Establish a Hotline or Web address for quick responses to questions that arise;
- Prepare a listing of opportunities such as camps, schools, and classes;
- Prepare a directory of agencies and services available in a community; or
- Prepare a calendar of upcoming workshops, meetings, classes that would be of interest.

The schedules and demands of all that are involved will dictate the amount of effort and time that can be devoted to mentoring relationship. Mentoring means assisting not assessing. The mentor facilitates the mentee's learning rather than controls it. The mentor functions as a teacher and role model and promotes growth through encouraging self-reliance. The most important aspect of mentoring is establishing a cooperative spirit between the family member and service providers. The speech-language pathologist engaged in a mentoring approach is able to help establish the spirit needed. How does one go about mentoring? There are a number of mentoring techniques depending on the circumstances, time frame, expertise, goals, unique personalities, and relationships that evolve. Try these techniques as you interact with other professionals and family members.

Intervention Assistance Teams

To promote collaborative planning, many school systems have organized teams of educators who represent different disciplines and perspectives. They are charged them with collaborating to find ways to help students who are struggling or experiencing challenges in the classroom. The composition, goals and names of these teams vary from district to district. Some call them the Student Support Team. Others refer to them as the Intervention Assistance Team. Some districts refer to them as the Problem-Solving Team.

In recent years, schools have adopted a service practice referred to as Response-to-Intervention (RtI). The educators may be called the Response-to-Intervention Team. Regardless of the label, the teams are generally comprised of the child's teacher/s, a school administrator such as the principal, the school psychologist, a special education teacher, and other instructional support professionals who have knowledge of the child's skills and needs. This includes the speech-language pathologist, the occupational therapist, the physical therapist, and others.

The focus and practices of the team models vary from school to school and state to state. In some schools, the team serves as a resource or advisory committee. Educator colleagues can provide help insights and recommendations to teachers who are puzzled by a child's behavior. In the team framework, teachers bring problems to the committee and receive recommendations of teaching or intervention strategies that may work. Meeting time is often spent asking probing questions or reviewing classroom work. These activities give insights into the child's problems and needs. In another version of the team model, the team members and the child's parents make decisions regarding assessment procedures needed and intervention strategies to be used. In the RtI model, the team assigns specific responsibilities and tasks, recommends specific intervention strategies, and designates a specified time period and context for implementation. Checkpoints are also established to determine progress. This step often occurs prior to a formal referral for a multifactored assessment and may result in resolution of the problem without enrollment in special education services. It may be referred to as a prereferral process.

To implement a team-oriented process for dealing with children who present learning challenges, the following questions must be addressed: Which children will be served by the team? Who will participate on the team? What philosophy, procedures and rules will guide the team process? How will the team's effectiveness be evaluated? To be most effective, team members must be prepared for the job they are to do. Goals and expectations of what can be accomplished must be realistic. It is wise to keep minutes of team meetings. These can then be used to document assistance as well as to serve as a guide for implementing recommendations in the months following the meeting.

The Principal

The building principal is a key person for the success of the special education programs, including the speech-language pathology program. This individual's attitude regarding the importance of communication in the learning process can make or break a program. Without the understanding and cooperation of the principal it would be extremely difficult to carry out an effective program. The principal is the chief administrator of the building, and in a sense, the school SLP is responsible to that person while in that building. The school SLP is a member of staff of that particular building in the same way that other teachers are staff members.

What can the school clinician expect from the principal? First, the principal is legally and educationally responsible for each child enrolled in the school. Therefore, it is important for the principal and speech-language clinician to work closely together to ensure the delivery of quality services. Principals can be instrumental in creating an educational environment that promotes collaboration among members of the teaching staff, including the SLP. This can be accomplished by providing the staff with time to work together on projects, attend professional development seminars, or form peer-mentoring relationships. In addition, collaboration can be promoted by providing the technological supports for communication such as Internet access, E-mail, and teleconferencing opportunities.

The principal is often the representative of the local education agency in the development of Individualized Education Programs (IEPs) for children and may serve as the coordinator of the placement team.

The principal is responsible for arranging for adequate working space and facilitating the procurement of equipment and supplies. The principal or a representative from the principal's office may acquaint the clinician with the policies, rules, regulations, and all procedures in that school. In some situations, the principal may facilitate the scheduling of screening and testing programs and setting up the caseload and schedule for children to be seen in therapy.

The principal can be expected to visit the therapy sessions and observe. Indeed, a wise clinician will invite the principal to observe therapy sessions and will encourage questions.

The interpretation of the program to other members of the school staff, the parents, and the community is ongoing. The principal may arrange opportunities for the clinician to explain the program to staff and parents as well as professional and lay groups in the community. The principal is the liaison between the school and the community and between the school clinician and the school staff. When a parent, a classroom teacher, or a member of the community has a question regarding the speech, language, and hearing program, that person will ask the principal, who may answer the query or refer it to the school SLP.

On the other hand, the school clinician has some important responsibilities to the principal. Providing information about the program to the principal is one of the most important factors in maintaining a good relationship. The clinician will want to confer with the principal regarding major aspects of the screening, assessment, and intervention program. For example, the clinician should provide information to the principal on screening policies and procedures, grades and numbers of children to be screened, plans and time scheduled for follow-up testing, criteria for case selection, scheduling policies and procedures, and plans for developing intervention goals jointly with parents and teachers. The principal needs to know the children on the active caseload, the children dismissed from therapy, and the children being monitored indirectly. It is helpful to identify children by name, age, grade, communication problems, room number, and teacher and to provide a brief statement of progress on a periodic basis.

It is advisable to furnish the principal with written reports both periodically and systematically. Some information is valuable if submitted on a monthly basis; other information can be submitted semiannually or annually. Any plans for inservice programs for teachers and group meetings with parents and local professionals should be discussed with the principal prior to inception. Written reports or correspondence pertaining to a child in that school should be shown to and approved by the principal prior to sending them to parents or other professional personnel. Reporting information to the principal in this manner will help keep your program activities visible and it will keep the principal aware of the important role you play in the school.

If the clinician is itinerant, more than one building and more than one principal will be involved, therefore, the clinician needs to know the policies and procedures in each assigned school. Because clinicians often work in several buildings and with several principals at one time, it is good practice to keep all the principals informed in a general way about the programs in the other schools. This practice serves to keep the principals well informed about the total program in the school system, facilitates cooperation and coordination among schools, and helps keep the clinician's workload well balanced. Care should be taken not to share private information from one building to the next and never gossip about colleagues.

The Classroom Teacher

In the speech-language pathologist's role as a collaborator and consultant to the classroom teacher, several areas should be considered:

- the strengths and needs of the student with the communication impairment;
- the academic and social demands placed upon him or her in the classroom;
- the student's interaction with peers; and
- the teacher's interest in and capability for collaborating and providing assistance.

This means that the SLP must understand the education process in addition to having competency in the communication disorders profession. It also means that the SLP must know what is going on in the classroom as well as making sure that the classroom teacher understands the speech-language intervention program and the role of the speech-language pathologist.

In most school systems there is an administrator for curriculum development. With assistance from teachers, principals, directors of special services, or other administrators, this person is responsible for the selection of textbooks and instructional supplies and materials. The business of educators is the selection of what will be taught, at what level, and in what sequence. The content and sequence of what is taught to students is the curriculum. Teachers organize the curriculum into instructional units, each made up of lesson plans.

One of the ways in which the speech and language program can be integrated into the curriculum is for the SLP to participate on the school's curriculum committee, either as a member or in an advisory capacity. In this way the speech-language pathologist can be perceived by the rest of the staff as someone who contributes to students' learning program. As a communication specialist the SLP can provide information on pragmatics, communication in the classroom, how to help the children follow directions, how to encourage children to ask questions, and how teachers can become better communicators in the classroom. The SLP can offer suggestions on how the teaching of improved communication skills can be integrated into language arts, social studies, science, art, physical education, math, reading, spelling, and writing.

The speech-language program should be fully integrated into the school's curriculum. It is essential that the classroom teachers understand the program, but it is equally important that the speech clinician understand what is going on in the classroom. It is not enough to give lip service to the idea of integrating the program into the educational framework; it must be put into practice. How can this be accomplished? The answer is not a simple one. Let us first consider some of the things the school pathologist can expect of the class room teacher; then let us look at some of the expectations of the classroom teacher in regard to the clinician.

The school SLP can expect the teacher to provide a classroom environment that will encourage communication and will not exclude the child with the stuttering or articulation problem or the child who is hearing impaired. A teacher who shows kindness and understanding toward the child with a disability is not only assisting that child but also is showing other children in the classroom how to treat individuals who are disabled. Sometimes, it takes more time and patience to deal with children who are disabled, but the rewards in terms of the child's performance are many. The teacher in the classroom takes the lead by establishing the emotional climate, and the children learn by example.

The classroom teacher is also a teacher of speech and language by example. If you doubt this, watch a group of children "playing school" sometime. Teachers provide the models for communication and children imitate the teachers. Teachers must have an awareness of their use of language, the quality of speech, the rate and volume of speech, and the use of slang or dialect.

The SLP can expect the teacher to help identify children in the classroom with speech, language, or hearing problems. Some children with communication problems are not spotted during a routine screening, and teachers who see children on a day-to-day basis will have more opportunity to identify the children and refer them to the SLP.

The clinician can expect the classroom teacher to send the children to and therapy at the time scheduled. The SLP will need to supply the teacher with a schedule, and both teacher and clinician should stick to it. The SLP can also expect the teacher to inform him or her of any changes in schedules that would necessitate absence from therapy.

A very important goal of collaboration between the SLP and the classroom teacher is the effective integration of speech and language intervention into the classroom setting so the student can access the curriculum and succeed. This means that the teacher becomes a meaningful partner in the process of improving speech and language skills. For this to be accomplished is necessary for the SLP to keep the teacher well informed about the child's goals in therapy, progress in therapy, steps in development of new patterns, and intervention strategies. This must be done, not in general terms, but in very specific ones. The teacher needs precise information on the child's problem and what is being done in therapy before there can be a carryover into classroom activities. The teacher can provide the SLP with information concerning how well the child is able to utilize the new speech or language patterns in the classroom.

When confronted with the idea of helping the child with communication problems in the classroom, the teacher's reaction is apt to be, "I don't have time to work with Megan on her speech when I have 25 other children in the room." The SLP's role in this situation is to give the teacher specific suggestions on how this can be accomplished as a part of the curriculum. Of course, this means that the clinician will have to be well acquainted with classroom procedures, practices, and activities. It also means the SLP will have to know what can be expected of children of that age and on that grade level. This will happen if there is a continuous pattern of sharing ideas and information between the SLP and the classroom teacher. Knowledge of the core curriculum, especially in subjects such as language arts, will create context for mutually establishing goals and plans.

We have considered what the SLP can expect of the classroom teacher. Now let us look at the other side of the coin: what the teacher can expect of the clinician.

If you are new in the school, starting off on the right foot is important. Being friendly and open with teachers, showing an interest in what they are doing in their classrooms, and showing a willingness to give them information are all steps that can be taken to help build trust and understanding. There are many ways in which this can be accomplished. One way is to plan to get to know what the teachers are like on a personal basis. For example, eat lunch with the teachers or join them in school social activities. Because clinicians deal with many teachers in different schools care should be taken to avoid becoming identified with cliques or those with negative attitudes. Outside the school you will have your own circle of friends, but inside the school be friendly with everyone.

Adhere to your schedule and if you make changes in it, as you surely will, be sure to tell the classroom teachers who are affected. If you send a child back to the classroom late, you will have no basis for complaint if the teacher fails to send a child to you on time. Share information with teachers through informal conferences, arranged conferences held periodically, invitations to observe therapy sessions, and observation in classrooms. Always make arrangements in advance for conferences and observations. The principal can often help make arrangements for any of these activities.

Information can also be transmitted in written form. Short descriptions or definitions of the various speech, language, or hearing problems or any aspects of the program will help teachers understand the program better. *Short* is emphasized because realistically teachers are not going to take the time to read long treatises.

In working with classroom teachers, the school SLP is a partner in effecting the best possible services for the child who has a communication disability. The more help that is given to the teacher, the more opportunity there will be for integrating the speech, language, and hearing program into the schools.

As schools strive to improve their inclusive practices, teachers are increasingly faced with the task of integrating children with special needs into regular classrooms. Providing in-service programs or arranging university courses for credit are excellent ways of supplying teachers with information about children with communication disorders.

What are some of the things that classroom teachers will need to know about communication and communication disorders? Following is a list of topics that can be included in an in-service program:

- The mission and goals of the speech and language program in the school, including the preventive, diagnostic, and remedial aspects. Describe policies and procedures for case identification, selection, eligibility, and dismissal.
- Normal patterns and milestones for speech, language, and hearing development.
- A brief description of the major types of communication impairments to be expected in the school-age population (i.e., articulation, delayed language development and language/learning disorders, fluency, voice disorders) and impairments associated with specific disability conditions including autism, developmental disabilities, emotional disturbances, traumatic brain injury, organic disorders, and the like. Briefly describe the characteristics, range of severity, possible causes and related factors, diagnosis and assessment procedures, criteria for selection, intervention strategies, impact on school performance, and the role of the classroom teacher for each disorder category.
- The importance of hearing for learning and information related to hearing problems including the anatomy of the ear, nature of sound, types of hearing loss, causes of hearing loss, identification and measurement of hearing loss, role of the classroom teacher, rehabilitation and habilitation of hearing deficiencies, hearing aids, and assistive listening devices.
- The relationship of speech, language, and hearing to the educational/learning process.
- Medical and dental intervention where applicable for specific disorders.
- The roles of other professionals in treatment such as physicians, physical therapists, occupational therapist, psychologists, and counselors.
- Treatment techniques and intervention strategies that can be successfully implemented in the classroom.
- Aspects of the curriculum where focus can be placed on improving students' communication skills and where communication goals can be integrated.
- Assistive devices and augmentative communication systems used to facilitate communication in students with severe impairments.

Figure 10–2 shows an observation form developed to facilitate teachers' awareness and understanding of their own instructional communication style. It can be shared with teachers (or others) for self-evaluation or used as an observation tool. Analyzing the responses jointly with the teacher can lead to meaningful discussion about how to modify communication

COMMUNICATION MANNER AND STYLE OBSERVATION FORM

During communication with (____________________), pay close attention to your own communication manner and style. As completely as possible, describe the characteristics of your communication manner and style in the categories listed below. In consultation with a Speech-Language Pathologist, determine those characteristics which can potentially pose difficulty for the student. Place a minus sign (–) next to them. Place a plus sign (+) beside those behaviors which can be used to promote the use of good communication skills.

1. ______ Average rate of speech
2. ______ Typical length and complexity of sentences
3. ______ Use of sarcasm, humor, and puns
4. ______ Word choice (simple, difficult, technical)
5. ______ Attentiveness to students during conversation
6. ______ Organization of conversations
7. ______ Use of hand and body gestures
8. ______ Use of objects to help make explanations
9. ______ Manner of responding to students' questions
10. ______ Manner of giving directions and instructions
11. ______ Patience while waiting for someone else to talk or answer
12. ______ Ability to understand students with communication impairments

Figure 10–2. Communication style observation form.

style in order to meet a particular child's needs. For example, if Renick cannot process language at a fast rate and the math teacher, Mr. Butler, speaks very quickly, Renick will be at a disadvantage for learning math. Therefore, a reasonable and doable modification for Mr. Butler would be to slow his rate of speech when presenting important information or new concepts to his class. Figure 10–3 outlines numerous communication strategies which can be recommended to teachers to encourage them to modify their instructional communication styles in order to accommodate children in their classroom who demonstrate communication impairments.

Special Education Teachers

Speech-language pathologists relate to all the providers of special instructional services in the schools. This includes teachers of children who present autism, emotional disturbances, specific learning disabilities,

Recommended Communication Strategies for Communication Partners
Based on the results of formal and informal assessment procedures, indicate those strategies which will facilitate development of communication skills or correct speech and language productions. For example, when **Giving Instructions and Directions**, it is recommended that the communication partner make attempts to modify his or her communication style by reducing the length of complexity of the utterance, reducing the rate of utterance, repeating the instructions, altering the mode of instruction delivery, or giving prompts and assistance.
Giving Instructions and Directions
_____ Reduce length of instructions _____ Reduce complexity of instructions _____ Reduce rate of delivery _____ Repeat instructions more than once _____ Alter mode of instruction delivery _____ Give prompts and assistance _____ Vary voice and intonation patterns to emphasize key words
Explaining New Concepts and Vocabulary
_____ Give definitions for terms _____ Show visual representations of concepts and vocabulary _____ Present only a limited number of new concepts at a given time _____ Ask questions to verify comprehension
Reading to the Student
_____ Reduce rate _____ Reduce complexity _____ Reduce length _____ Determine comprehension through questioning _____ Redirect student's attention to important details and facts
Practicing Memory Skills
_____ Encourage the student to categorize information and make associations _____ Provide opportunities for rehearsing information _____ Encourage the student to visualize information

Figure 10–3. Recommended strategies for modifying communication style to accommodate the needs of children with communication impairments. *continues*

Practicing Higher-Level Thinking and Communicating

_____ Provide opportunities for problem solving

_____ Provide opportunities for decision making

_____ Provide opportunities for making judgments

_____ Ask questions to elicit solutions, judgment, decisions

Announcing and Clarifying the Topic of Discussion

_____ Introduce the topic to be discussed

_____ Restate the topic frequently throughout the conversation

Attending to the Student's Behaviors, Queries, Comments

_____ Reinforce queries and comments

_____ Inform the student if the message is not understandable

_____ Request repetition of utterances not understood

Relaying Important Information to Students

_____ Avoid sarcasm, idiomatic expressions, puns, humor

_____ Reduce rate, complexity, length of utterance

_____ Use or reduce gestures dependent on student's responses and needs

_____ Incorporate visual cues and imagery for clarification

_____ Permit ample time for student response

_____ Introduce alternative and/or augmentative communication systems if necessary

_____ Arrange the physical environment to reduce distractions, eliminate barriers, and invite communication

_____ Invite questions

_____ Present information in clusters and groups

_____ Introduce information with attention-getting words

_____ Select materials appropriate for skills, age, interest levels

Figure 10–3. *continued*

cultural and linguistic diversity, developmental disabilities, physical impairments, visual impairments, and hearing impairments. Instructional services are available to children in all of these groups and more as mandated by public laws. The collaborative team should be comprised of those educators who have the greatest expertise in the areas of need defined for each particular student.

Because the laws do not clearly define the areas of professional specialization which must be involved in the delivery of services to particular groups of children, confusion sometimes arises concerning the professional scopes of practices. This is especially evident between SLPs and learning disabilities specialists because many children with learning disabilities demonstrate problems processing and producing spoken or written language. Their deficits negatively effect learning and result in academic problems in subject areas such as reading, spelling, writing, mathematics, and other academic and social areas that require adequate language abilities.

The working relationship between the SLP and other special educators is dependent on the local school and the individual professional persons involved, including the principal and the classroom teacher. The SLP has the academic background, interest, and competence in language development and communication disorders.

Using the continuum of service delivery options, cooperation between special educators may be provided under different plans. The service delivery options are not mutually exclusive. The SLP may function as a member of the diagnostic team during the initial evaluation procedures or on an ongoing service delivery basis. Specific remediation may be provided to children placed in full-time special classes or in regular education classes. The SLP may function as the resource room professional or as a consultant to the other specialists in relation to general or specific problems. Obviously, different service delivery models would depend on each local school system's situation. The possibilities have not been fully exploited, and the creativity of the SLP may be utilized in determining innovative approaches to helping pupils with language-learning disabilities.

In some school districts, SLPs function as resource specialists for children with language-learning disabilities. To function successfully, communication specialists must have a theoretical background in language and literacy development. They must be able to identify and develop prescriptive techniques for problems related to phonology, syntax, and semantics; and should be able to relate these aspects of linguistics to all levels of oral and written language. In addition, the speech pathologist must be a generalist as well as a specialist. In other words, the speech-language pathologist must know much about the learning process.

The Educational Audiologist

The most evident interrelationship between specialists in education to children with hearing impairments and members of the speech-language profession is in audiology. Educational audiology, a comparatively new specialization in the field of communication disorders, was born out of a need for improved services for the children with hearing impairments in the school.

The adverse effects of hearing loss on school children has been well documented (Flexer, 1999). Hearing loss causes delay in the development of receptive and expressive communication skills (speech and language). As a result, youngsters experience learning problems and experience poor academic achievement. Children's ability to understand the speech of others and to speak clearly often results in social isolation and poor self-concept.

The educational audiologist plays a primary role in identifying children who are have impaired hearing through mass screening programs and/or teacher or parent referrals. The children who fail screening tests are given a comprehensive audiological assessment. Air and bone conduction pure-tone tests are administered as well as speech-reception and speech-discrimination tests. Immittance or impedance testing evaluates the function of the middle ear and can provide valuable information about the presence or absence of middle-ear pathology (for example, otitis media).

Additional evaluative and/or therapeutic recommendations may be made by the audiologist if indicated by the tests. If audiological and medical evaluations reveal that amplification is necessary, the educational audiologist helps the parents to obtain the aid or assistive device. Parents are taught to monitor the child's behavior and hearing ability to ensure their acceptance and proper use.

In addition to advising parents, it is necessary to provide classroom teachers with information to help them deal with students who are hearing impaired. The educational audiologist participates in multidisciplinary team meetings. The audiologist also monitors classroom acoustics, measures noise levels, makes recommendations for sound treatment, and calibrates audiological equipment. Ideally, all these functions are performed by the educational audiologist. Unfortunately, they are in short supply and often must spread themselves very thin.

The quality of educational services provided for youngsters who are hearing impaired creates some concern. Case management must be comprehensive to ensure optimum coordination of services. The educational audiologist appears to be in the best position to be a case manager if the optimization of residual hearing is the starting point for learning. Moreover, the classroom teacher typically monitors hearing aids even though the educational audiologist is the best-equipped person for this function.

Direct services provided for the child with a hearing impairment in the classroom are often termed aural habilitation and are essential if the child is to develop skills that will enhance learning opportunities. Other areas of concern include the availability of counseling for parents and for the child as well as consultative services for teachers, administrators, and other resource personnel. All services provided for the child should be coordinated.

There are many possible areas for cooperation between the SLP and the educational audiologist. The SLP is specifically prepared to provide a program of language and speech intervention and is the person best qualified to do so. As information is obtained from the audiologist concerning the child's need for auditory development, it can be incorporated into the speech and language program. Because most audiologists service a wide geographical area, they are not in a specific building with the same regularity as the SLP. Thus, the clinician is considered to be the critical link between the student in the classroom and comprehensive audiological services.

The SLP may work with the educational audiologist in the evaluation of the child with a hearing disability. Consultation with classroom teachers and visits to the classroom may be scheduled by both the SLP and the educational audiologist in an effort to better assess the needs of the student.

To summarize, it may be said that to provide the child with a hearing impairment with the best possible services, the SLP and the educational audiologist must work together in the evaluation, habilitation, and psychosocial adjustment of the child.

School SLPs would do well to encourage the employment of educational audiologists who are either by training or by experience familiar with schools and the process of education. Educational audiologists must utilize their clinical knowledge and awareness of the educational and communicative needs of the child with a hearing impairment in the classroom.

Although the number of educational audiologists employed in the schools is increasing, there are still many schools with partial or limited audiological services. The school SLP may be playing a larger role in the delivery of services in these situations. Without an educational audiologist in the school system the task of caring for the child with a hearing impairment falls to the SLP.

The school clinician's role is to provide appropriate components of supplemental services directly to hearing-impaired children. The SLP serves as a hearing consultant to teachers, administrators, and resource specialists, helping them make reasonable accommodations to meet the special needs of the child in the integrated class setting. He or she is a member of the interdisciplinary team and develops new components of comprehensive hearing services within the school district.

Speech-Language Pathology Assistants

The involvement of Speech-Language Pathology Assistants is becoming a more common component in service delivery in schools as well as health care settings. The use of assistants has increased in recent years as professionals have sought mechanisms for expanding service delivery options and containing costs. As caseloads grow in size and diversity, there is a need to broaden the services that are offered. SLP Assistants perform tasks that are prescribed, directed, and supervised by ASHA-certified speech-language pathologists. Thus, assistants support clinical services provided by the SLP. By incorporating an assistant into the intervention services, many SLPs have been able to focus their attention on more complex treatment issues rather than the day-to-day operational activities such as filing, preparing clinical materials, recording data, etc. Although the SLP's relationship with the assistant is usually in a supervisory capacity, it is clear that by working as a team the value of services can be expanded to better serve the needs of youngsters. The Code of Ethics of the American Speech-Language-Hearing Association (2010) clearly deals with the issue of supportive personnel and the supervision of same in Principle of Ethics 11: "Individuals shall honor their responsibility to achieve and maintain the highest level of professional competence."

In the school setting, support personnel have been referred to by different titles (e.g., speech-language pathology assistants, communication aides, paraprofessionals, speech aides, teacher's aides, classroom aides, educational associates, and volunteer aides). Sometimes, they are paid employees or they may be volunteers. In some states, they are licensed. The background and educational levels and amount of training may vary, depending on the requirements of the state and local school district. Speech-language pathology assistants may receive training provided through on-the-job training, formal course work, workshops, observation, supervised field experiences, or any combination of these activities. Some universities and community colleges have training programs leading to state certification of assistants. Appropriate areas of training may include:

- Normal processes in speech, language, and hearing;
- Disorders of speech, language, and hearing;
- Behavior management skills
- Discrimination skills including, but not limited to, the discrimination of correct and incorrect verbal responses along with the dimensions of speech sound production, voice parameters, fluency, syntax, and semantics
- Instructions for presenting stimuli to students, collecting data, reporting observations, and utilizing instructional materials;
- Management of equipment and materials used in speech-language pathology programs; and
- Overview of professional ethics and their application to the assistant's activities

The American Speech-Language-Hearing Association has promoted greater understanding of the potential scope of responsibility of speech-language pathology assistants and issues surrounding the use of this group of support personnel. Some state licensure boards have also developed a set of criteria for the use of aides and assistants.

The use of assistants has spurred great debate in the profession over the years. Those who support the use of assistants believe it to be a good mechanism for expanding the delivery of services to an increasingly diverse client base. Administrators often see it as a way to be more cost efficient. Some SLPs fear that the use of speech-language pathology assistants will eventually lead to the replacement of qualified, licensed, and/or certified practitioners. This will not happen as long as professionals continue to maintain responsibility for the types of work assistants are permitted to do. The public expects speech-language pathology services to be delivered by the highest qualified practitioner. That is the speech-language pathologist who holds the appropriate credentials. ASHA guidelines and state licensure laws mandate what those credentials are. Assistants can only function in supportive roles and must be supervised by qualified professionals. If properly integrated into the speech-language pathology program, assistants can be very beneficial. The use of assistants permits the SLP to do those professional level tasks that require expertise and clinical judgment while still enabling the completion of day-to-day tasks that may be necessary but time-consuming.

ASHA published a document, "Guidelines for the Training, Credentialing, Use, and Supervision of Speech-Language Pathology Assistants" (ASHA, 1995, 2004). These guidelines included the definition of supportive personnel, qualifications, training, roles, and supervision.

The legal, ethical, and moral responsibility to the client for all services provided cannot be delegated; that is, they remain the responsibility of the professional personnel. Supportive personnel can be permitted to implement a variety of clinical tasks given that the speech-language pathologist responsible for those tasks provides sufficient training, direction, and supervision. Examples of tasks that assistants may perform under the supervision of a qualified speech-language pathologist are listed in the ASHA Guidelines:

- Conduct speech-language and hearing screenings;
- Follow documented treatment plans or protocols including implementing reinforcement activities to strengthen skills previously introduced by the SLP;
- Document patient/client progress; this may include observing the student in settings around the school including classrooms, cafeteria, and playground;
- Assist during assessment;
- Assist with informal documentation and other clerical duties;
- Prepare, fabricate, and maintain clinical materials, equipment, and tools;
- Program augmentative communication devices as prescribed by the clinician;
- Add information to students' records as dictated by the SLP, including attendance and filing data;
- Schedule activities, prepare charts, records, graphs, or otherwise display data;
- Perform checks and maintenance of equipment;
- Participate in research projects, in-service training, and public relations programs; and
- Escort children to and from the classroom and therapy room.

The SLP must maintain the primary responsibility for the speech and language services for students with communication disorders. By specifying those tasks that assistants are permitted to do, the SLP clarifies the expectations of the job assignment for the assistant as well as for other personnel in the school system such as the principal. Instructions should be communicated to the assistant verbally and in writing. The clinician must establish a plan for observing how these activities are executed to confirm that the assistant is not over stepping his or her boundaries.

The ASHA guidelines document also provides an extensive list of what assistants cannot do, including:

- Performing standardized or nonstandardized diagnostic tests or evaluations;
- Interpreting test results;
- Provide counseling to the student or family;
- Write, develop, or modify a student's individualized education plan;
- Implement any aspects of the treatment plan without being supervised;
- Select or discharge students from the speech-language program;
- Share clinical or confidential information orally or in writing to anyone;
- Make referrals;
- Communicate with the student, family or educators regarding any aspect of the student's status or service without being directed to do so by the supervisor; or
- Represent himself or herself as a speech-language pathologist.

Supervision of a speech-language pathology assistant is an important responsibility and should not be entered into lightly. The use of assistants will be much more effective if you take this responsibility seriously and learn how to provide the guidance and supervision that is needed to ensure they execute their role appropriately. Supervision of support personnel must be regular, comprehensive, and documented to ensure that the student working with the assistant receives the highest quality services he or she needs. The amount of supervision should be based on the assignments and skills of the assistant. The ASHA 1995, 2004 speech-language pathology assistant guidelines recommend supervising 30% of the assistants' weekly work for the first 90 workdays and 20% after the initial work period. Supervision includes onsite, in-view observation and guidance while an assigned activity is being performed. Care should be taken to follow stated guidelines since funding is often linked to the qualifications of the person providing services.

Once a speech-language pathology assistant is employed, it becomes the SLP's responsibility to assure others that the assistant is doing the job appropriately. Evaluation protocols serve two purposes. They serve as a mechanism for clarifying expectations, and they enable supervisors to identify performance that is good as well as that which is problematic. A sample evaluation form is provided in Figure 10–4.

Paraprofessionals have been used effectively in the health, education, and human service fields for many years.

Assistant's Name					
Data of Evaluation					
School					
Reviewer					
Check Items E = Excels S = Satisfactory NI = Needs Improvement U = Unsatisfactory NA = Not Applicable					
	E	S	NI	U	NA
A. General: Record Keeping					
1. Knowledge of program goals.					
2. Ability to update standardized pupil information records.					
3. Knowledge of school organization and operation.					
4. Performs routine clerical duties.					
B. Work With Students					
1. Ability to work with individual students.					
2. Ability to work with small groups of students.					
3. Ability to assist student with SLP-planned activities.					
4. Knowledge and ability to use instructional materials and teaching aides.					
5. Knowledge and ability to use instructional materials and teaching aids.					
6. Ability to maintain control and discipline.					
7. Ability to manage behavior of students when SLP is not present.					
8. Awareness of students' therapy goals.					
9. Ability to describe students' performance.					
C. Work Habits and Personal Relations					
1. Performs adequate amount of work.					
2. Work is accurate.					
3. Maintenance, storage, and clean-up of materials.					
4. Initiative and resourcefulness.					
5. Neatness of work product.					
6. Attendance.					
7. Observation of work schedule.					
8. Compliance with rules, policies, and directives.					
9. Communication with students and school staff.					
10. Cooperative and flexible.					
11. Exhibits positive attitude.					
12. Shows tact and good judgment.					
13. Accepts constructive criticism.					
14. Implemented appropriate suggestions for improvement.					
15. Understands assigned responsibilities.					
16. Performs effectively under stress and opposition.					
D. Overall Performance					
E. Summary of Recommendations					

Figure 10–4. Speech-language pathology assistant evaluation form.

The need for supportive personnel in our fields undoubtedly will increase in the coming years. As a profession it is incumbent upon us to determine the competencies and preparation needed to perform the duties of a speech-language pathology assistant. We must then monitor and supervise them closely in order to ensure that our services continue to be effectively and efficiently delivered with their involvement.

The Psychologist

The school psychologist is a member of the team of professional persons helping the child with communication impairments. The National Association of School Psychologists defines four major areas of practice including psychological and psychoeducational assessment, consultation, direct service, and planning/evaluation (Levinson & Murphy, 1999). The psychologist can provide valuable information regarding the student's cognitive and academic abilities. The psychologist assesses a student's eligibility for special education services as well as identifies and tests the effectiveness of interventions designed to solve academic, social or behavioral difficulties. Psychologists' knowledge of learning and behavior theory is valuable in determining the optimal conditions for learning. Educators and the school clinician may make referrals to the psychologist to obtain additional information about educational diagnosis, school adjustment, personality, learning ability, or achievement. The child's speech, language, or hearing problem may be closely related to any of these factors, either as a result, a cause, or an accompanying factor.

The school SLP and the psychologist will find that a close working relationship is mutually beneficial. The school clinician will want to know the kinds of testing and diagnostic materials the psychologist uses. On the other hand, the clinician may be helpful to the psychologist in interpreting the child's communication problem so that the best possible tests may be used. In making a referral to the psychologist the clinician should ask specific questions in regard to the kind of information being sought. The school clinician can also furnish the psychologist with helpful information that would facilitate working with the child.

The school psychologist's role differs from one school system to another, so the clinician should make a note of that role and find out what additional kinds of psychological help are available in the community.

The Social Worker

Social workers can contribute much to programming and transition planning for students with disabilities. The Council on Social Work Education (CSWE) describes the social work profession as "committed to the enhancement of human well-being and to the alleviation of poverty and oppression" (Hepworth et al., 1997, p. 4). The major role of the social worker is to help students and their families access support services. They facilitate interagency linkage among tax-supported and voluntary agencies. They may assist in gathering data needed to determine eligibility for special education services. The social worker pays particular attention to self-advocacy.

This professional's thorough knowledge of social agencies in an area can be of considerable aid to the school clinician. The social worker is a key person in helping families find places where they may receive needed help. The social worker may provide counseling, make home visits, and serve as the liaison between the school and the family. They can be particularly helpful in advocating for your students with disabilities as they transition from school to work or postsecondary education (Markward & Kurtz, 1999). When financial assistance is required for supplemental services, the social worker is the one who can be of assistance to the family in locating that aid. Not all school systems are fortunate enough to have a social worker on the staff, but if there is one, the school clinician should explore ways in which they may work cooperatively.

The Bilingual Educator and/or English-as-a-Second Language (ESL) Teacher

America is truly a multicultural nation. Across the country there are children in our schools who do not speak the same language as their teachers and classmates. They may speak a language other than English or a nonstandard dialect. They may be from families who have recently moved to the United States, have parents who do not speak English, or live in communities where a unique dialect is spoken. These children are classified as presenting cultural and linguistic diversity. Their traditions, values, attitudes, and beliefs may be different from their teachers and classmates. They often struggle in the school setting while trying to learn to communicate and participate in school activities. Schools refer to this group of children who are learning English as a second (or third) language as English Language Learners (ELL).

Class placement and service to children in these groups varies widely. In communities where there are large numbers of children from different cultures, programs and protocols for meeting their needs may be established. The speech-language pathologist is often called upon to assist these children in developing communication skills that will permit them to learn and benefit from the education setting. In these cases, SLPs should work cooperatively with the bilingual educators or English-as-a-Second Language (ESL) teachers in the district to determine how to best assess and establish a plan for intervention.

IDEA mandates that assessment materials and procedures should not be racially or culturally discriminatory and must be provided in the child's native language. Similar to assessment of children with disabilities, determination of eligibility and services cannot be based on one procedure alone. The SLP's role is to help the education team determine if the child is demonstrating a communication impairment that impacts on learning or if the learning difficulty is a result of being an English Language Learner. Children are only eligible for speech-language services if there are clinical implications.

When working with multicultural populations it is important to select individuals who can act as informants or interpreters during interviewing, testing, planning, and intervention procedures. Inclusion of a person who speaks the child's native language and understands the child's culture will help ensure that the program developed is appropriate and relevant for the student's needs. If a bi-lingual SLP is not available, federal law mandates that we must collaborate with an interpreter. ASHA and other organizations, such as the National Association of School Psychologists have provided guidelines for working with interpreters. The ASHA Code of Ethics support the involvement of an interpreter and recommends that they should be trained to administer activities and transcribe the student's responses. Furthermore, the Code indicates that it is critical to prepare interpreters for this role.

Chamberlain and Landurand (1990) and Bader (2011) indicated several competencies that are preferred when selecting informants. These include proficiency in both English and the child's language, an ability to navigate between both languages, good auditory memory skills, sensitivity to dialects and cultural differences, and other cognitive, personality, and experience factors that would facilitate cooperation during the time that the person is acting as an interpreter or informant. School districts often identify individuals within the community to serve as interpreters. If using informants or interpreters to assist with a speech-language assessment or intervention, it will be important to provide training for them so they clearly understand their role and duties.

Bader (2011) prepared a comprehensive overview of recommendations and guidelines for working with interpreters in the assessment process, including desired qualifications and skills, the SLP's roles and responsibilities, and training recommendations (Figure 10–5).

The Guidance Counselor and Vocational Rehabilitation Counselor

The guidance counselor works with students with adjustment or academic problems, helps students plan for future roles, and makes available to them information pertinent to their situation. This individual may also do individual counseling.

The guidance counselor is especially helpful in dealing with students in middle and high school. Students with communication problems are often known by the guidance counselor, so the school clinician may depend on this person for referrals, supplementary information, and cooperative intervention.

The vocational rehabilitation counselor is usually employed by a district or state agency. This individual assists students 16 years of age and older in overcoming handicaps that would prevent them from being employable at their highest potential. The vocational rehabilitation counselor, although not a member of the school staff, may work in conjunction with the school system.

Why Use Interpreters?	• Assessment materials and procedures should not be racially or culturally discriminatory. • Assessment materials and procedures should be provided in the child's native language. • Demographics—high numbers of non-English speakers in the community. • Clinical implications of not using an interpreter or testing in the native language. • Most SLPs are not bilingual.
SLP's Role	• Select and interpreter who can be trained to meet the qualifications, skills, and knowledge required for effective interpretation. • Prepare the interpreter. • Establish a working relationship with the interpreter.
Desired Interpreter's Skills	• High degree of proficiency in English and the child's native language. • Ability to navigate between both languages. • Understand cultural differences. • Sensitive to regional dialects. • Good auditory memory skills. • Ability to follow instructions.
SLP's Responsibilities	• Train the interpreter to administer activities and transcribe the student's responses. • Implement a 3 pronged process: – Briefing – Interaction – Debriefing • Teach the interpreter vocabulary unique to special education. • Watch for verbal and non-verbal cues from the interpreter and student to ensure validity of the assessment process.
Interpreter's Role	• Act as a bridge to facilitate interaction between the SLP and student. • Ask for clarification. • Provide accurate interpretations. • Remain neutral. • Respect confidentiality.

Figure 10–5. Recommendations and guidelines for working with interpreters. Adapted from Bader, S. (2011). *Bilingual Assessment: Speech-Language Pathologists Working Effectively With Interpreters*. Baltimore, MD: Progressus Therapy. *continues*

Three-Pronged BID Process When Working with Interpreters
Briefing
Discuss meeting logistics and planned agenda.
Provide overview of assessment plan — purpose and activities
Review pertinent student behaviors.
Discuss importance of confidentiality.
Provide assessment materials.
Discuss technical terms and vocabulary.
Explain importance of translating precisely.
Specify the importance of limiting non-verbal cues, gestures, hints.
Audio record the session.
Verify the accuracy of the student's responses and interpreter instructions.
Interaction
Welcome student (and family if present).
Inform the student of the interpreter's role and the SLP's role.
Speak directly to the student.
Speak in short, concise sentences.
Allow time for the interpreter to translate information.
Avoid using idioms and slang.
Observe and take notes on the interaction between the student and interpreter.
Observe and take notes on the relevant interpreter's behaviors.
Debriefing
Review the student's responses.
Discuss difficulties that may have arisen.
Example the language sample and ask questions to clarify.

Figure 10–5. *continued*

The School Nurse

Depending on the size of the system, there may be a number of school nurses, only one, or one working part time. In some regions the school nurse may be part of the staff of the city, county, or district health department and work either part time or full time with the school. The role of the school nurse has expanded in recent years to provide several very valuable services to schools and their students.

The National Association of School Nurses describes seven roles including: providing direct health care to students and staff; providing screening and referral for health conditions; promoting a healthy school environment; promoting health education; serving in a leadership role for health policies and programs; providing leadership for the provision of health services; and serving as a liaison between school personnel, family, community, and health care providers.

In situations where students present health care issues that may impact their educational performance, the school nurse may serve as a manager of medical and health information. He or she may monitor the health-related components of medically ill or fragile students. The nurse maintains the health and medical records of the children in the school. Children with hearing loss, brain injury, cleft palate, cerebral palsy, and other physical problems should be known by the school nurse. The nurse is often the one who arranges for medical intervention when it is needed, makes home visits, and knows the families. It goes without saying that the school nurse and the speech-language pathologist work closely together and need to share information on a continuing basis.

In some states, the school nurse is legally responsible for conducting hearing screenings. The nurse, the school clinician, and the educational audiologist may work together to organize and administer the hearing-conservation program for detection, referral, and follow-up. Medical referrals and follow-ups involving family doctors, otolaryngologists, and other medical specialists may be carried out by the school nurse. Medical problems in addition to those connected with hearing loss would be included. The school nurse is one of the best sources of information for the school clinician and should be one of the clinician's closest working allies.

The Occupational Therapist

The profession of occupational therapy is concerned with human lives that have been disrupted by physical injury, accident, birth defects, aging, emotional, or developmental problems. Occupational therapy services are designed to enhance a person's development, establish independence, and prevent disabilities. Occupational Therapists work to help individuals improve their function in their "daily occupations." The word occupation does not necessarily refer to the individual's employment but rather to being occupied in meaningful day-today activities, including work, leisure, and play. In the school setting, occupational therapy is considered a related service to support a student in accessing his or her educational curriculum. OTs address sensory-motor, cognitive, and psychosocial skills and habits. Their intervention helps students learn to perform tasks related to self-care, work and play tasks in multiple contexts such as the classroom, gym, cafeteria, playground, work setting, and community (AOTA, 2002; Bullock, Delli-Fraine, & Torrez, 2010). A student's daily occupation within the school setting may include skills such as coloring, cutting, writing, dressing, throwing balls in gym class, using utensils, and other tasks that occur during the school day.

Occupational therapists work in a variety of settings, and today an increasing number are employed in public school systems. The occupational therapist and the SLP will find many areas for collaboration and cooperation that will enhance students' potential. These same areas, however, may also give rise to conflicts regarding professional responsibility as well as differences in therapeutic approaches. The answer to this problem seems to be the establishment of a truly cooperative working relationship. Each profession has unique skills, and the recognition and respect for each other's expertise will only serve to help the handicapped individual.

Working within classrooms enables occupational therapists to identify important routines and to modify the learning environment so it is more conducive to student success. In educational environments OTs may engage in activities such as adapting the environment, introducing adaptive equipment, using assistive technology, coaching teachers about how to help students with writing difficulties, and participating on education teams. OTs help students develop basic self care including using transportation systems. They encourage students to develop interests and skills necessary to engage in work or transition from school to work. They identify age appropriate toys and leisure experiences so students can participate in art, music, sports, and after school activities.

OTs may work with children to provide adaptive devices, such as conversation boards and writing tools aid greater independence. They may work with children with visual-spatial perceptual problems or with children who are having trouble adjusting to handicaps. They may work with a child individually or with groups of students in such activities as role playing, games, work adjustment sessions, and discussion groups. Some examples of activities OTs may implement in the classroom setting are helping a student achieve independence while dressing by playing dress-up, putting on a jacket, pants or sweater, and so forth. As with integrating speech-language services, collaboration and planning time are essential.

Several factors are considered by occupational therapists and educational team members when determining eligibility for special education and occupational therapy services. Following are some questions that may be asked to determine if school-based occupational therapy is necessary for the student to access the curriculum. Does the student present motor or sensory goals that cannot be addressed by adaptations or modifications to the classroom environment or curriculum? Will typical educational strategies result in a reasonable expectation of success? Can educators conduct a program of activities designed by an OT specifically for a student, with reasonable expectations of success? Must activities be delivered only by a professional OT?

The Physical Therapist

A certified physical therapist (PT) provides services to children in the general area of motor performance. PTs strive to increase students' independence, engagement, and social play. They focus on correction, development, and/or prevention of gross motor and sensory motor problems. Physical therapists work with children who experience difficulty with functional mobility, balance, stability, posture, coordination, motor control, motor planning, and endurance required for educational performance. PTs often help children develop improved use of the lower extremities for sitting, standing, walking, and movement with and without aids. The school SLP and the physical therapist may work together to serve children with orthopedic and neurologic problems and to provide developmental programs for high-risk infants. Physical therapists may also provide information and assistance to SLPs in achieving good posture for optimal breath support and control and in the stabilization of extraneous movements for cerebral palsied children. In addition, physical therapists may evaluate motor abilities for students who are possible candidates for communication boards or augmentative communicative equipment. Physical therapists can assist in maximizing the students' physical functioning so they can participate in various daily living, leisure, and vocational activities.

More physical therapists can be found working in hospitals or home health care agencies than in public schools. Some school systems contract with external agencies to provide physical therapy services. Children are often referred for physical therapy services by medical professionals. Like other instructional support personnel, physical therapists must develop a written treatment plan for each student. Before a student is referred for PT services, it is recommended that teachers and others first attempt to modify the environment and provide extra assistance or cues.

Physical therapists suggest referring students if the following behaviors are observed: the inability to safely negotiate the school building or grounds; significant difficulty in the child's gross and/or fine motor skills; difficulty maintaining appropriate sitting posture during classroom activities; difficulty participating in school tasks without the use of adaptive equipment or modifications; unusual walking or movement patterns; poor hand use; or difficulty learning new motor tasks (Carothers-Liske, 2010).

SLPs and physical therapists can work together to establish methods of communication for children with severe physical disabilities. Similar to speech-language services, physical therapy services can be integrated right into classroom activities by coordinating physical therapy treatment strategies with classroom routines and by collaborating with teachers. Some examples are PTs helping children with their gross motor skills on the playground, joining children during circle time to facilitate sitting balance or helping a child learn to pull to a standing position during playtime, and adapting materials to optimize participation. When PTs help in this way, they model activities for teachers so that a teacher can implement the strategy when the PT is not present.

The Health and Physical Education Teacher

One staff member who may be in as close of contact with pupils as the classroom teacher is the health and physical education (HPE) teacher. This individual sees students in an environment where movement is stressed, where pupils are engaged in activities in which they may be more relaxed, and where talking may be more spontaneous. School SLPs may be able to work with the HPE teacher in generalized activities for the pupil with an articulation problem. The HPE teacher can also help with the pupil with a voice problem who yells too much. The HPE teacher is competent in teaching relaxation strategies and may help the children who are dysfluent or who present motor disorders. The HPE teacher on the elementary or secondary level can be a valuable resource person for the SLP.

Vocational Counselors and Employers

Schools are becoming more concerned and involved in planning for the student's success after leaving school. From the time a student is around 14 years of age, the planning focuses on transition from school to postsecondary activities, either additional education or work. A variety of professionals can contribute to the vocational assessment and transition planning necessary to assist students.

The vocational evaluation process should be conducted by a qualified vocational evaluator who can help collect, synthesize, and interpret complex information (Leconte, 1999). High school educators are often charged with this responsibility. Vocational assessment and training strategies are a major component of transition planning. The SLP can be a valuable contributor to the discussion. However, oftentimes SLPs are not asked or do not volunteer to participate. Discussions should center on the type of communication that is required and expected for successful performance, strategies employers can use to ensure effective performance, and advance preparation of the students' communication skills including vocabulary, direction following, reading instructions, and conversing with to customers and coworkers.

Nonteaching Support Personnel

In every school building, there are many nonteaching support personnel with whom speech-language pathologists, audiologists, and students interact. This includes the clerical staff, cafeteria workers, bus drivers, gardeners, custodians, and volunteers who make the school function.

These individuals, who often know the students in different ways than the teacher, are important people without whom the school could not run smoothly. The SLP can rely on them for information on where to get things and where to find things as well as information on the school buildings, equipment, and classroom housekeeping. The custodian may be the only one who knows that in the back of a storage closet there are some textbooks, workbooks, chairs, or a portable chalkboard that the clinician could use.

All of these individuals can contribute something to the success of a school therapy program even if it is just a positive comment now and then. Their work and contributions to the operation of the school should be acknowledged. They will provide you with more efficient and effective services if you take the time to share information about your program with them. Often these individuals live in the school district community and will promote your program to their neighbors if they understand what it is that you do. In addition, they interact with children on a daily basis and can provide compliments and reinforcement to children on your caseload.

Working with Physicians in the Community

A good relationship with the physicians in the community enhances the speech, language, and hearing program. School clinicians should take every opportunity to establish such relationships by conducting their programs in a professional manner-following established local protocol in referral procedures, writing letters and reports that are professional in content and style, and giving talks to local medical groups if invited to do so.

A competent school clinician never oversteps professional bounds by giving medical advice or advice that could be construed as medical in nature. For example, the school clinician may think that a child's persistent husky voice may be the result of either vocal abuse or vocal nodules, or possibly a combination of both conditions. After collecting as much information as possible from parents and teachers and the child, the clinician must follow local referral policies established by the school system. These policies will differ from school system to school system. In some places all medical referrals are done through the school nurse, the school social worker, or some designated administrator. The school policy may allow the clinician to discuss the contemplated referral with the parents, who then follow through by taking the child to the family physician. The referral is accompanied by a letter from the clinician and includes results of diagnostic procedures, general impressions, and specific questions, as well as any other helpful information. The clinician should also include a request for the results of the physician's diagnosis and suggestions. It is best to request that the physician's results should be sent to the SLP, with a copy to the parents. When parents ask the clinician to suggest a physician in the event they don't have a family doctor; the acceptable policy is to give the family the names of at least three doctors from which they can choose.

Care should be taken when referring for a medical evaluation or opinion. In some circumstances the school system is required to pay for the evaluation; in others payment is the responsibility of the family. Each school district will have guidelines specifying the circumstances for making referrals to physicians and determining the responsible payer. Be sure to discuss and clarify this important information before recommending a visit to the doctor. Although it is imperative to understand who will serve as the pay source, the decision to refer for a medical opinion should be based on the child's physical condition versus the pay source.

Nothing is more important than good health. The child who is ill or in need of medical attention cannot be expected to perform well in school. School clinicians should be alert to the child's physical condition. If there are any behaviors or symptoms that might be related to a health condition, the school clinician should discuss this with the school nurse and/or the principal. Proper referral steps should be taken to ensure the youngster's health and safety.

Working with the Dentist

There are a number of areas of specialization within the dental profession, among them pedodontists, who are concerned with children's dental care; orthodontists, who are concerned with dental occlusion; and prosthodontists, who are concerned with designing and fitting appliances to compensate for aberrations within the oral structure. SLPs may make referrals to, or may be the recipient of referrals from, these dental specialists as well as the dentist in general practice within a community. The referrals may be children whose articulation problems are related to dental or oral cavity problems, such as cleft palate or other craniofacial anomalies. Children with dysarthrias associated with cerebral palsy, as well as children with developmental disabilities, may require special handling by dentists. Thus, the professional relationship between the dentist and the SLP requires cooperation.

Working with Family

Throughout this book references are made regarding the importance of working with family. State and federal legislation have mandated the inclusion of parents and/or guardians in the planning and intervention process. This is not a new role for the SLP; most have always worked with the parents of children on their caseloads and the parents of children at risk. In this section the term family shall be used to include parents, guardians, and significant other family members who can contribute to the program designed for a child.

Involving families can facilitate development of meaningful intervention goals, better implementation of recommendations, and effective transfer of skills from the therapy room to daily life. Families are the constants in the child's life. Clinicians, teachers, and other service providers enter temporarily. It is for this reason that families should be considered equal partners in the assessment and intervention process. The treatment plan should be designed to foster families' decision-making skills as well as their capabilities for providing their child with assistance. Professionals need to recognize the individuality of clients and families and modify services to meet those needs. This means that services must be delivered in contexts which are considered "normal" for the youngster. All services should be coordinated so that the family and youngster are not stressed by having to go in too many directions at one time.

Although there is not one set of rules on how the school SLP should work with families, the beginning clinician might find it helpful to have some general ideas. Most clinicians develop their own "style" of working with family members as they gain confidence and experience.

The first and most important thing to remember is that parents are people. The basic ingredients for effectively working with people are understanding and respect. The inexperienced clinician sometimes approaches parents with a preconceived idea of how they are going to react and behave and, therefore, expects resistance. At the same time the parents may anticipate the clinician's role as that of the "expert" who has at hand all the information and know-how to "cure" their child's problem. Obviously, then, everyone gets off on the wrong foot. If the clinician approaches the parents in a friendly open way and lets them see her or him as a person whose task is to apply the most appropriate principles of rehabilitation (or habilitation) to the situation, the clinician will set the stage for the next step in the process. It is the clinician's responsibility to establish the ground rules and create the climate for a positive working relationship.

The climate that is established for the parent conference can help formulate the foundation needed for success. Make sure parents are seated comfortably. Avoid leaving spaces between parents and other professionals. This will make them feel isolated and as though they are not a part of the team. Be sure there are no obstructions such as desks between you and the parents. This creates a barrier to open communication. Equip the conference setting with adult-size chairs. There is nothing more uncomfortable than trying to have a serious conversation with your knees up against your chin. Check to be sure that chairs are arranged neatly so that a conversation can be conducted. Ensure that lighting is adequate, not too bright or too dim. Draw the drapes if the sunlight is directly on your face or that of the parents'.

Parent Groups

In schools it is common for clinicians to work with parents in a group as well as individual format. Parent groups may be organized by the school clinician as support groups or by the parents themselves as a result of the need for more information about their child's disability. Many parents are interested in assuming a greater amount of involvement in the treatment program. The professional in this kind of relationship assumes the role of a resource or support person. Parents should be encouraged to express both positive and negative feelings without being judged about what they say or how they say it. Parents of children with disabilities often have feelings of guilt, as if something they did or didn't do caused the child's handicap. Professionals need to understand this response and help parents use the group situation as an opportunity for change, growth, and personal development. The use of the words ought and should are best dropped from the SLP vocabulary when dealing with anxious parents.

Parents can be the most reliable sources of information concerning the child's speech, language, and hearing behavior. For example, if a parent insists that her child cannot follow simple directions or stammers when playing with an older sibling, accept her word for it. Subsequent observation will often prove her correct.

Involving Siblings

Brothers and sisters may experience several emotions related to their sibling's communication problems. They may be embarrassed about the way people react when they cannot understand the child. Some siblings feel the need to defend or translate for their brother or sister. All members of the family can play a positive role in the treatment of a communication problem if they understand the nature of the disorder and the ways they can help. Be sure to make brothers and sisters feel welcome to visit the therapy room. Describe the speech and language problem. Explain simple tricks for increasing their understanding of unintelligible speech. Show them how to model good speech patterns, how to stimulate correct productions, or how to help with homework assignments. Stress the need for patience and understanding. By providing the sibling with positive ways to respond, the likelihood of embarrassment and teasing will be reduced.

Changing Family Patterns

Family patterns are changing in the modern world. There are many single parent families or divorced and remarried parents in families in which children are "his," "hers," and "ours." Many children are cared for on a daily basis by someone other than a parent. Others are "latchkey" children who care for themselves and/or their siblings many hours each day. Some children are negatively affected by family situations such as these; others aren't troubled. The speech-language clinician needs to be sensitive to the child's emotional well-being.

Unique family situations that are new to the school clinician may arise such as abuse, neglect, or poverty. One can never be prepared for all circumstances. However, situations such as these will be easier to handle if you strive to increase your knowledge about them and learn recommended strategies and solutions. The school clinician should keep in mind that children who come to school hungry, malnourished, inadequately clothed, or frightened have difficulty learning and concentrating on tasks such as speech and language production. Make no assumptions about a child's worth or capabilities or a parent's love and interest in her child based on the family income. Many poor families have homes that are rich in love.

Involving the Student

Too often, children with impairments are treated as inanimate objects. People talk about them and decide how to teach them or how to "fix" their communication problems. They are eliminated from the decision-making process. This approach does not enable us to understand if the student feels the communication impairment is important or not. It also prohibits us from gaining insights about the student's interest or motivation for improving communication skills. Some students can even provide their recommendations about how to structure therapy to benefit them most.

Reports in the professional literature have demonstrated that families, educators and others are being included in the decision making process more frequently. We often read recommendations that the patient/client should be included, but anecdotal reports from clinicians appear to indicate that this recommendation is not commonly practiced. Perhaps that limitation results from a lack of clinician awareness of how to involve the client meaningfully in program planning and decision-making.

What kind of information can we obtain from the children we serve? When people participate in planning a treatment program, they are likely to be more actively engaged in the success of the program. The student has expectations and opinions about what their treatment should be. Intervention will be much more effective if the treatment meets the client's expectations and if motivation is high. The plan that is developed should reflect the client's goals and special needs regardless of age. Students' comments should lead to specific recommendations to be incorporated into the treatment plan.

According to IDEA, students are supposed to be a part of the team, especially when transition services are discussed. The regulations state that the coordinated set of activities developed for the transition plan must be based on the student's needs, taking into account the "student's preferences and interests. This directive has sound implications for servicing all clients regardless of age. There is nothing "magical" about the age of 14 (the time period when transition plans are developed for children). Children of other ages and adult clients have opinions and expectations that will impact on their commitment and performance in treatment.

Individuals who have a sense of control over their own destiny generally are more successful at the tasks they attempt. It is vital that service providers do everything possible to encourage the development of the client's ability to understand his or her communication disability and participate in meaningful ways in the treatment process.

The IEP meeting is one opportunity for soliciting youngster's opinions about strengths, needs, preferences, and interests. If that opportunity is not possible due to barriers such as time constraints, cost, conflicting schedules, and so on, the clinician can take other opportunities to obtain relevant information. In the initial weeks of enrollment in a therapy program, the youngster's opinion can be sought through dialogue and questioning to obtain information that would contribute to determining treatment priorities and procedures to be used for the coming year. Ideally, these questions would be asked during a team planning conference attended by the child, parents, key teachers, speech-language pathologist, other specialists, and administrators. If that is not possible, the SLP can ask the questions during a therapy session. The student's responses can then be considered and incorporated into future treatment plans, thus increasing the quality of the treatment plan and the student's motivation to perform.

Some youngsters may find it difficult to participate in the team process. They may be reluctant to be in a meeting with several adults. They may be too shy to say what is on their minds. They may not be able to find the words to clearly express their thoughts, feelings, and opinions. In addition, they may not feel doing so in such a forum. Youngsters can be prepared for making contributions ahead of time through coaching. Or, their opinions can be sought during one to one discussions with the parent or speech-language pathologist. Ultimately the goal is for students to have control and manage their own intervention program including selecting goals and identifying treatment procedures.

Efforts should be made to provide the student with a clear understanding of the communication impairment and how it affects the performance academically and socially. The student should be asked to contribute ideas for developing a treatment plan that can effectively meet his or her personal needs. Of course, the quality and quantity of a student's involvement as a member of the collaborative team will depend on how the involvement is sought and on the student's capability for understanding the problems and for providing information. The level of involvement should be commensurate with the student's cognitive and social maturity.

Satisfaction with Services

It is reasonable to believe that children, like adults, have opinions and expectations about the situations in which they participate. Manufacturers of children's products such as toys and food often seek children's opinions via simple questionnaires and surveys. Clinical experiences and anecdotal evidence show that clinicians have been less likely to sample children's likes and dislikes or satisfaction with the services they receive. Perhaps we assume that we already know what's good for the children we serve. The consumer satisfaction tools that have been devised to sample satisfaction with speech-language pathology services have not been geared to our young consumers. However, the principles that apply to meeting the needs of our adult consumers apply equally to meeting the needs of the young children and adolescents we serve. Blosser and Park (1996) developed a "Kids Are Consumers Too" satisfaction survey to sample children's opinions about speech and language services. The survey questions can be found in Figure 10–6. Responses to questions such as these could be used to guide the improvement of services.

Maintaining Ongoing Communication with Collaborative Partners

How do SLPs bridge gaps in understanding? First, it must be emphasized that understanding is a two-sided coin and that, although clinicians seek to be understood, they must also understand the roles and responsibilities of school administrators and personnel. Second, this is a continuous, ongoing process requiring a vigorous and assertive stance on the part of the SLP. Third, the responsibility for communicating with others about the profession should be shared with others including members or the state and national professional organizations.

Administrators and teachers may not invite us to tell them who we are or what we can do. The SLP must be take the initiative and invite others to learn more about our profession. An assertive, proactive approach is needed to gain administrative support. To accomplish this, administrators must first be educated about the profession and be encouraged to work with the SLP to facilitate effective service delivery. The SLP needs to establish a more visible position in the school so that administrative attention, understanding, and cooperation can be attained. The following School Personnel Education Program can be initiated in school buildings throughout the school district:

- Conduct a quality program. No program change or growth can occur unless quality is already in operation.

STUDENT SATISFACTION SURVEY

Name ______________________________ Age __________

School ______________________________ Grade __________

Teacher ______________________________

SLP ______________________________

Communication Needs

❑ Articulation ❑ Language ❑ Voice ❑ Fluency ❑ Hearing ❑ Other

Directions

Read each question. Place an X on the face that describes how you feel. (If the child cannot read, the SLP should read the sentence.)

---

1. Do you know what you are learning in your speech-language therapy class?

Yes Sometimes No Don't know

2. Do you sound as good as other children in your class when you talk?

Yes Sometimes No Don't know

3. Do you think the speech-language therapy room is an interesting place to learn?

Yes Sometimes No Don't know

4. Do you think you should come to speech-language therapy more often?

Yes Sometimes No Don't know

5. Do you like the learning activities you do when you come to speech-language therapy class?

Yes Sometimes No Don't know

6. Do you think that what you are learning in speech-language therapy is helping you to talk and listen better in class?

Yes Sometimes No Don't know

Figure 10–6. Kids are consumers too! *continues*

7. Do you think you can talk better with your family and friends because you come to speech-language therapy class?

8. Do you tell your friends about what you do and learn in speech-language therapy class?

9. Would you tell one of your friends to come for speech-language therapy if he or she had a problem talking or listening?

What are 2 of your favorite speech-language therapy activities?

____

____

What are 2 activities you did not like?

____

____

What is the best thing about speech-language therapy class?

____

____

What is something you'd like to change about speech-language therapy class?

____

____

Figure 10–6. *continued*

- Identify the key decision-makers within the school district. Determine who needs to be "educated." This may include principals, teachers, curriculum directors, central office administration, school board members and parents.
- Continually supply key administrators at the building, central administration and top administration levels with facts and information that will challenge them to act on behalf of the speech-language therapy program when decisions are being made.
- Increase the visibility of the speech-language therapy program district wide:
  - ☐ Join school committees and attend building activities.
  - ☐ Participate in prevention services and in-service activities.
  - ☐ Host invitational days ("Board of Education Day"; "Principal's Day"; "Administrator's Day"; "Teacher's Day"). Invite important people to observe therapy sessions.
  - ☐ Establish an ongoing mechanism for communication such as a newsletter.
  - ☐ Offer to speak at Board of Education meetings, parent groups, church groups, and so forth.
  - ☐ Serve as a source of information to other educators regarding communication skills.
  - ☐ Forward informative clippings and articles about communication disorders and the relationship to learning. An "FYI" ("For Your Information") approach could be effective.
- Inform administrators of your aspirations and goals for your program. Arrange for a meeting with district leaders to share your ideas about the program's strengths, weaknesses, and potentials.

Seize every opportunity possible to form working relationships with parents, students, and fellow professionals. Because there may be conflicting schedules and time is a precious commodity for all, it is essential for clinicians to be creative and use a wide range of mechanisms for exchanging information with others about communication disorders, program goals, and intervention strategies. These mechanisms can include face to face conferences, written communication (letters, reports, newsletters), audio and videotape recordings, discussion groups, in service meetings, news articles, and observations.

Figure 10–7 shows a variety of mechanisms that can be used to form effective working relationships with specific constituency groups.

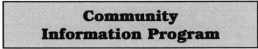

Community Information Program

There are a number of advantages that will result from keeping the community informed about the speech-language pathology program in the schools. Begin by

Listed below are several communication and engagement methods that can be used to form effective working relationships with others in order to develop awareness of the SLP program and cooperation for effective intervention.

Students
Visits to classrooms
Observations during learning activities
Interactions throughout the building
Visual displays inside and outside the therapy room
Attendance at school events

Students' Parents
Discussion groups and training programs
Written communication (newsletters, progress reports, homework notes, E-mails)
Conferences (face to face and telephone)
Observation days and school visits

Teachers and Other Education Professionals
Meetings and conferences to develop educational plans
Written communication (notes, letters, reports, newsletters, summarizing relevant articles)
In-service meetings and training
Audio and videotapes
Discussion groups
Informal interactions (lunch, school events, after school activities)
Curriculum team meetings
Building level meetings
Social activities

Administrators
In-service trainings
Meetings and conferences
Written communication (budget requests, annual reports, summaries of relevant professional literature, service statistics, thank you notes, state association newsletters, reports describing conferences attended)

Community
Participation in school events
Speaking and/or membership in community organizations
Grant and sponsorship requests
Free testing days
Articles for newsletters

Local Professionals
Networking through professional organizations
In-service meetings
Written communication (newsletters, letters, reports, articles)
Committees and offices

Figure 10–7. Methods for communicating with others.

describing the services that are designed for prevention, assessment, and intervention. This will help remove any possible stigma attached to having a child enrolled in the program. It will also build a feeling of trust and confidence in the program and toward the school system in the community.

A community information program should not be a haphazard affair; it should be well planned and executed. It should not be a "one-shot" deal but rather continuous, consistent, and persistent. It should also be varied, informative, and interesting.

The school clinician may want to survey the types of media available within the community. The most commonly utilized are newspapers, radio, television, Web sites, service clubs, lectures, presentations, E-blasts, and poster displays. Consider making arrangements with the local newspaper to run a series of articles. Topics of interest include: characteristics of communication problems, how parents can help children learn to talk, helpful suggestions for families of children with fluency problems or hearing impairments, and the importance of early referral. Many other topics will be of interest to parents and community members.

In preparing articles for release in the local newspapers, it is best to inquire of the editor how long the article should be and then stick to the length suggested. If an article submitted is too long the editor is likely to trim it and may inadvertently cut out an important part. Most editors like to have articles submitted, but they should be well written and interesting. The school clinician can usually obtain from a member of the newspaper staff the pertinent facts on style and length. If pictures are used and they contain any children, it is an absolute must first to obtain written consent of the parents.

Some school systems have community information or public relations offices. The person responsible for internal and external communication for the district can often assist the clinician in preparing articles for publication or contacting the appropriate person at the news office.

Radio interviews or other types of programs are a good way of getting information across to the public. Local radio stations often welcome suggestions on programs of special interest. Clinicians can utilize such timely events as Better Speech and Hearing Month to focus attention on the needs of persons with speech, language, and hearing disorders. The same can be said of television programs. Often, local television stations have programs during which various personalities are interviewed. Or the television station may cooperate in preparing a program on a particular type of disability or various aspects of the speech, language, and hearing program.

Talks to community service clubs, professional organizations, and other groups can yield innumerable benefits. Many of these groups sponsor special projects or programs as part of their community service activities. Another effe ctive way of informing the community about the program is through displays at health fairs and similar events. Public libraries are often willing to add to their shelf books of interest to parents of handicapped children. The school clinician can make suggestions for specific books, which then could be made available to the public.

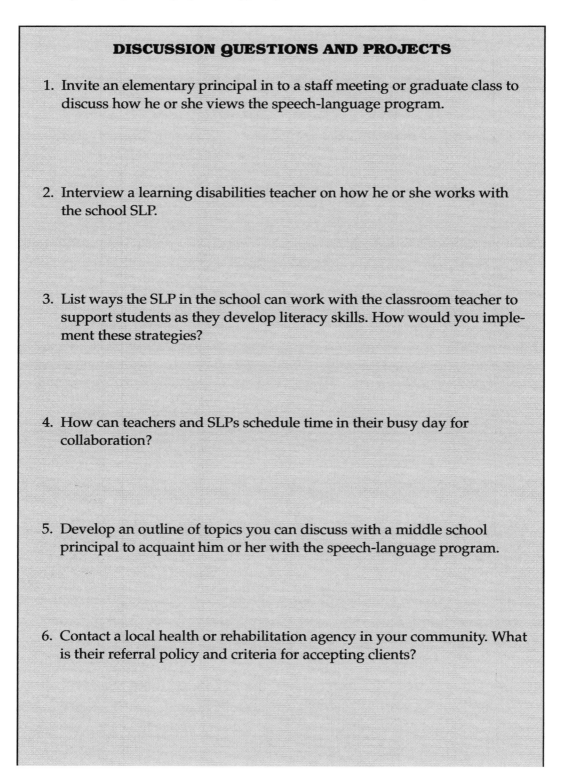

DISCUSSION QUESTIONS AND PROJECTS

1. Invite an elementary principal in to a staff meeting or graduate class to discuss how he or she views the speech-language program.

2. Interview a learning disabilities teacher on how he or she works with the school SLP.

3. List ways the SLP in the school can work with the classroom teacher to support students as they develop literacy skills. How would you implement these strategies?

4. How can teachers and SLPs schedule time in their busy day for collaboration?

5. Develop an outline of topics you can discuss with a middle school principal to acquaint him or her with the speech-language program.

6. Contact a local health or rehabilitation agency in your community. What is their referral policy and criteria for accepting clients?

7. Ask a practicing school SLP to explain the policies for making a medical referral in that school system.

8. Write a brief article about a speech-language topic that could be submitted to a local newspaper or organization for their website.

9. Role-play the following situations with your colleagues or teammates. What would you say? How would you respond?

   - Parents ask whether having their child's tonsils removed will help his speech problem.

   - Parents ask how long Jennifer will be enrolled in therapy in order to cure her fluency problem.

   - Parents ask how they can stop the neighborhood children from teasing their child because she "can't talk right."

   - A parent asks if her smoking during her pregnancy caused her child to be learning disabled.

11

Experience Schools

A step along the academic and clinical pathway to becoming a professional in the field of speech-language pathology involves experiencing first-hand practice in a variety of settings and with a broad range of individuals across the age and disability continuum. Schools are one of the best settings to acquire experience with pediatric populations. Completing a school-based clinical externship experience prepares you to take advantage of the joys and benefits of working in that setting.

The school-based externship experience is sometimes regarded with trepidation by the graduate student speech-language pathology major. This is probably because, like all new experiences, there is an element of the unknown. The experience is usually anticipated with a mixture of fear, curiosity, and excitement. Students enter their clinical and externship experiences at differing levels. Some may have limited experience with children and others may have had a wider exposure. The actual experience may bear out what was anticipated, and it may also contain some wonderful surprises. The following comments made by graduate students during their externship provide insights for contemplation by students and their supervisors.

> "The thought that occupied my mind as I drove home after the first day of my externship was, 'How will I ever make it? How am I going to remember everything I need to know about all of the disorders? How will I write so many reports?' I foresaw the weeks ahead as consumed with writing lesson plans and thinking up activities. And now, here I am twelve weeks later. I can look back to that first day and laugh when I think of how my ideas have changed. It doesn't seem possible that I could have experienced all that I did. All aspects of my school externship made it a great learning situation."

> "My externship has been a great experience and has been more of a benefit than I ever imagined it would be; from both a personal as well as professional point of view. There has been a lot of hard work and a lot of time invested, but the satisfaction, rewards,

and learning that this experience has created has made it all worthwhile."

"I suddenly realized that I didn't need to be unsure, for I could handle the situations that I feared, adequately and surprisingly well."

"I feel much more confident being out in the schools since I am no longer regarded as a *student*. When the teachers ask my opinion about various children, their confidence in me boosts my confidence in myself."

"I feel the most important lessons that I learned from my school placement were learned through my own mistakes. I had a very excellent extern supervisor who allowed me to experiment and try new things on my own. When I failed, I learned a great deal. Instead of telling me my ideas were inappropriate, she allowed me to find out for myself through my own mistakes."

"As a student extern I have grown to understand the daily routine, unexpected problems and hassles a school clinician must go through and accept. I have also experienced the rewards an SLP gains when a child achieves progress and success. Being able to take over many of the responsibilities has opened my eyes and allowed me to see how fulfilling it is to be able to help children improve their communication skills."

"One mistake I feel that I made at the beginning of my externship was a failure to ask questions about everything that was going on around me. I don't know if I was afraid to ask them or if I didn't know which questions to ask but either way it was a mistake. I think I went in with the attitude that I was *supposed* to know everything. This is, of course, the wrong attitude to have. The whole purpose of off campus practicum and externships is to learn. What better way to learn than by asking questions?"

"My supervising clinician was very helpful when I asked questions. She gave me her professional opinions and/or referred me to other professional sources. Although she informed me of reasons why some therapy sessions were less successful, she did not fail to commend the progress she saw and my success in therapy."

"My externship has shown me how a school can function, how to deal with faculty, staff and parents, and possible procedures to follow in making referrals and recommendations."

The Externship Program

The ultimate goal of the school-based experience is for student clinicians to actively apply knowledge that is learned in the classroom and prior clinical experiences, to the school setting, Independence is the mark of success. Universities have many ways of providing graduate students with opportunities to broaden their skills and perspectives. In order to obtain the Certificate of Clinical Competence, all students must gain experience in different settings and with different age groups and disabilities. Obviously, there are many different placement options depending on the location, relationships, university philosophy, and availability of sites and supervisors. There are, however, some commonalities that we consider.

Universities generally establish a formal agreement, often referred to as an affiliation agreement, with schools or other facilities in order to clearly outline requirements of the experience and expectations for all who are involved in the externship placement. This is also a requirement of the organizational entity that oversees academic accreditation. Reviewing the agreement document helps set the foundation for the experience and clarifies roles and responsibilities of all parties.

It is common practice to conduct courses or seminars for the students participating in an extern experience during a given time period. Seminars may be held weekly or less often, depending on the organization if the university curriculum. The seminar time may be used to discuss best practices, exchange information and seek solutions to challenges. Guest speakers and panels are often invited to discuss pertinent issues and familiarize externs with current information or controversial issues. Demonstration therapy or diagnosis may be carried out, visits may be made to agencies or centers, and some seminar time may be devoted to an explanation of school policies and practices.

In addition to fulfilling the university's requirements for consistent attendance, the student clinician must also consider the importance of verifying their experience for certification by the American Speech-Language-Hearing Association, licensing in various states, and certification by state departments of education. Universities establish reporting systems and specific forms for documenting the acquisition of pertinent knowledge, attitudes, skills, and experiences. The knowledge and skills, acquisition is delineated in the standards for the Certificate of Communication Competence. Besides the identifying information, the forms should include a system for documenting that the student is able to develop and implement setting specific appropriate evaluations and interventions with measurable and achievable goals. In addition, there is documentation that the student clinician can select appropriate materials and instruments and measure performance and progress. Of course, it is imperative that the student also gain understanding and experience with the administrative and reporting functions. The SLP who supervises the experience verifies that the student has gained the experiences and demonstrated the skills.

The externship provides an excellent forum for learning to develop and execute on therapy plans, including IEPs and IFSPs. Teachers prepare lesson plans and must make them available for review by administrators. The counterpart to this for therapists is the daily therapy or treatment plan. The plan should indicate each child scheduled for a given day, their goals, procedures, materials to be used. As a follow-up, the child's progress should be noted. It is helpful to receive feedback from the supervising clinician and to compare notes on observation of the effectiveness of the procedures and the materials. There is no one universally accepted form for a treatment or lesson plan, but most forms include the same basic elements.

Goals of the School-Based Extern Experience

Although each school placement differs, there are several common goals that can be accomplished through the placement. Keeping these goals in mind will ensure a rich experience:

1. Explore a variety of disorders or disabilities, service delivery models, workload and case management procedures that are unique to the school setting and may not be available in the university program.
2. Consider the demands and responsibilities unique to the school setting and school speech-language pathologists.
3. Concentrate on gaining confidence and qualifications for future employment.
4. Gain the specific clinical experiences and exposure needed to meet the requirements for national certification and/or state licensure.

The School Externship Team

Three key individuals are directly involved in execution of the externship experience. The first is the **student** who is doing his or her practicum in an off-campus school system. The second is the **master SLP** clinician who is directly responsible for the day-to-day guidance, mentoring, and supervision of the student clinician. Third is the **university supervisor** or program coordinator.

Clearly defining the roles and responsibilities of these three participants in the externship process ensures that participants know what is expected of them, what to do, when to do it, and how to do it.

Following is an explanation of the roles, qualifications, and responsibilities of the persons involved in the school externship program. Although this description is not exhaustive, it can serve as a foundation for understanding.

The Graduate Student Clinician

Prior to beginning the school-based experience, it is advisable to complete enough graduate coursework and clinical practicum experiences to be considered ready for an off-campus experience in a complex setting that serves a wide range of communication disabilities. Many school districts and other types of organizations consider the student's previous academic coursework and clinical experiences as essential components when deciding whether or not to accept a student for a placement. As an example, many settings expect students to have gained the theoretical base necessary to understand the disorders/disabilities they will encounter; observed and directly worked with a number of clients of various ages with different disability types and levels of severity; participated in practical experiences commensurate with their academic level and clinical training and prepared to select and implement appropriate diagnostic, intervention, data collection, and report-writing procedures; and learned about the resources that can be accessed for clinical decision-making and problem-solving. Students who are ready for a school-based experience should demonstrate the physical, mental, and emotional stability, and possess acceptable communication patterns.

Responsibilities

- Recognize status as a learner and the opportunity as a learning situation from which much can be gained.
- Adhere to the Code of Ethics of the American Speech-Language-Hearing Association.
- Carry out the university's requirements for the externship experience.
- Adhere to the policies and practices of the school and district.
- Comply with the directives of the SLP supervisor regarding delivery of speech-language services and execution of all aspects of the program.
- Demonstrate professional behavior at all times.
- Demonstrate dependability and assume responsibility while realizing that the supervisor is legally responsible for the children being treated.
- Establish and maintain appropriate interpersonal relationships and rapport with children, families, and educational colleagues.
- Self evaluate performance and willingly accept and utilize constructive criticism.
- Demonstrate interest in continued professional growth by making use of resource centers and attending in-service meetings, workshops, and professional meetings.

University Supervisor or Program Coordinator

The university has the ultimate responsibility for the student's placement and participation in the experience. The person who is assigned to the role generally has knowledge about practice in the school setting, including the unique aspects and comparison to practice in other settings. They should guide students through discussions of current issues and trends including how schools are organized, relationships with educators and administrators, general and special education policies and laws, and the processes for identifying, evaluating, and treating children with disabilities. Universities must establish an official relationship with the school setting or sponsoring agency through an affiliation agreement.

Responsibilities

- Evaluate the student's readiness for the externship experience.
- Assist with the selection of the placement site.
- Provide information about the student's background and advanced preparation for the experience.
- Inform the student and school-based supervisor of the university's requirements for experiences and evaluation.

- Provide guidance and training for the school-based SLP who will be supervising the experience.
- Supply pertinent procedural guidelines and materials.
- Provide students with feedback regarding their performance and recommendations for continued professional development.
- Respond to queries from the SLP supervisor and discuss any problems that may arise.
- Provide a wide variety of resource materials, approaches, and techniques that are based on sound theory, successful therapy, or documented research.
- Keep everyone informed of the university's polices and requirements.
- Observe the student during the experience (if geographically possible).
- Solicit the student's feedback on their experience both during and after the externship.
- Promote communication between the university, school district personnel, supervisor, and student.
- Act as mediator between the student and supervisor when questions or concerns arise.
- Evaluate students' performance.
- Submit appropriate paperwork to document the student's completion of the experience.

SLP School-Based Supervisor

The person who provides the supervision for the student plays a pivotal role in shaping the future of another professional. By agreeing to serve as an externship supervisor, he or she acknowledges the important responsibility of being in a position to influence the career path that the student may follow. Based on the quality of that experience, the student may decide whether working as an SLP in the schools is for them or not. They make judgments about the place of speech-language services within the educational setting, how services should be delivered, relationships with other educators, and the link between learning and communication. The supervisor imparts philosophy as well as strategies, techniques. and attitudes. If they are positive, passionate, and enthusiastic, it is likely that the student will also become that way. If they are negative and do not provide evidence-bases services, the student's desire to practice in the schools may wane. The supervisor guides all day-to-day aspects of the experience. They share their knowledge and expertise as well as their caseload, schedule, resources, and relationships.

Responsibilities

- Encourage the student to develop measurable goals and objectives for the experience.
- Share information about each child, their diagnosis, intervention plan, and records.
- Acquaint the student with available materials and equipment for screening, diagnosis, and treatment.

- Provide the student with information regarding the school system in reference to school policy, location of schools, the community, dismissal, check-in/ check-out procedures, fire drill procedures, and other appropriate information.
- Supplement the student's previous academic and clinical information with additional references and resources.
- Provide the student with opportunities to:
  - ☐ Observe the supervising therapist doing therapy.
  - ☐ Assist in screening and diagnostic programs.
  - ☐ Understand how to make clinical decisions and establish a caseload and workload.
  - ☐ Plan for and evaluate therapy sessions.
  - ☐ Visit classrooms where children with disabilities are enrolled.
  - ☐ Meet other school personnel informally and also confer with them about specific children.
  - ☐ Write progress reports, case history reports, letters, therapy logs, and individual educational programs.
  - ☐ Prepare for meetings with parents and teachers.
  - ☐ Become familiar with the reporting, recording, filing, and retrieval systems used by the supervising therapist.
  - ☐ Learn about varying treatment approaches and service delivery models.
- Provide feedback to the student regarding strengths and weaknesses using predetermined evaluation guidelines and multiple mode of communication.
- Encourage the student to become increasingly independent in self-analysis, self-evaluation, and problem-solving.

Laying the Groundwork for Success

The role of extern supervisor is one of leadership. There is opportunity to influence the direction a student takes in their profession. Experiences that are well planned and executed will lead to much greater knowledge and understanding of the school SLP's role. Table 11–1 illustrates suggested experiences that will ensure a broad exposure to school-based practices. This will help students get off to a great start and gain more from their placement.

Recommendations for Making the Most of Your Experience

Take the time to get to know the community in which you are getting the experience. Knowing the region's demographics and socioeconomic backgrounds of the families in the school district provides a base for understanding the school's goals and the children to be served. This may be especially important for student clinicians whose own backgrounds are different from those of their prospective clients.

Table 11–1. Recommended Experiences for the School-Based Externship

Prior to Initiation of the Externship Experience

- Review the procedural guidelines provided by your university and/or department.
- Review the school district's guidelines for university students if available.
- Contact the clinician who will be supervising you to learn about the school district, program and caseload.
- Visit the clinician and school in advance of your start date if possible.
- Obtain a background check
- Obtain a physical exam and inoculations (if required by your university or school district).
- Review procedures, test protocols and policies required by the supervisor or school.

Week One

- Confirm the work schedule and school calendar.
- Get oriented to the school system and meet key administrators and staff.
- Obtain school I.D. (if required).
- Observe the supervisor and various classrooms (if permitted).
- Tour school to learn about important facilities and resources.
- Attend school staff meeting (if one is being held).
- Become familiar with school procedures, code of conduct, emergency procedures, etc.
- Discuss expectations and goals of therapy program and school-based experience program.
- Discuss lesson plan and IEP procedures and forms.
- Review student records making sure to maintain confidentiality.
- Schedule a time for a weekly meeting with your supervising therapist to discuss progress, issues, concerns, and strategies.
- Discuss and orient to assessment and intervention materials.
- Obtain information about risk management and infection control procedures to be followed.
- Assist the supervisor in preparing your assignment and daily schedule.
- Start a personal journal to document your observations, perceptions, feelings, and goals.

Week Two

- Observe and jointly participate in assessment and intervention sessions with your supervisor.
- Continue with orientation to paperwork, IEPs, student records, assessment, and intervention materials.

Week Three

- Plan and independently implement intervention and/or evaluation for 2 to 10 students.
- Collect and document data on student performance and maintain daily attendance records, parent/teacher communication logs, etc.
- Complete appropriate paperwork regarding treatment and evaluations conducted.
- Observe students in classrooms.

Table 11–1. *continued*

Week Four
• Demonstrate greater independence.
• Continue to collect and document data on student performance and maintain daily attendance records, parent/teacher communication logs, observations, etc.
• Plan and implement intervention and/or evaluation for more students.
• Complete appropriate forms, records and reports for students.
• Attend child study or IEP planning meetings.
Week Five Through the End of the Externship Experience
• Increase independence at planning and implementing intervention and/or evaluation.
• Assume entire caseload with about 4–5 weeks left in the experience.
• Draft IEPs/ISFPs and other reports and participate in team meetings when appropriate.
• Continue to collect and document data on student performance and maintain daily attendance records, student progress reports, parent/teacher communication logs, etc.
• Consult with teachers regarding communication skills and intervention strategies in the classroom of students on caseload. Follow recommendations of the supervisor. Pre-plan the purpose and content of the conversation.
• Communicate with parents regarding student progress. Follow recommendations of your supervisor. Pre-plan the purpose and content of the conversation.

Source: Adapted from Blosser, J. (2009). *Progressus Therapy's Explore Schools Program: Recommended Experiences for the School-based Externship or Fieldwork Experience.* http://www.ProgressusTherapy.com

Many university training centers have found it productive and valuable to assist students in making the most of the experience. An example is providing the student and the extern site with a checklist of prerequisite experiences the prospective SLP should have before starting their experience. It might include information on any experience in child care such as baby-sitting or teaching church school; observational experience; clinical practicum experience; diagnostic experience; academic experience; and experience with recorders, audiometers, assistive listening devices, computers, video equipment, copying and scanning machines, computers, and augmentative devices.

Each university program has developed its own requirements and often includes policies regarding the behavior of student externs. There are numerous school activities the student clinician can take part in during the weeks of student teaching. It is important for the cooperating clinician to have a list of priorities or activities that seem most valuable for the student. The list can be compiled from various sources: university information, other clinicians, published articles, and discussions with the therapists in the district or other students. The student should have the opportunity to take part in as many phases as possible of the school therapy program. Besides learning to organize and carry out a therapy program, the student clinician will want to become familiar with related activities. For instance, it is helpful for the student to attend meetings of the clinicians as well as those meetings held in the individual schools.

The cooperating clinician should discuss with the student clinician how to begin and how to wrap up the school year. The clinician will want to include the student in obtaining referrals for therapy and in conferences with teachers and parents. Furthermore, the cooperating clinician can discuss with the student clinician bulletin board ideas, newsletters for parents, parent conferences, and special therapy ideas that have proven successful. The student should learn to use technology and equipment that is applicable to the therapy program. Also, the student clinician will want to have information about the many sources of therapy materials.

Competency-Based Evaluation of Student Externs

Self-evaluation and evaluation by supervisors is a critical aspect of any clinical practicum or externship experience. This provides opportunity for two-way feedback and exploration of ideas for improvement. Generally, there is a midpoint and final evaluation at the conclusion of the experience. The forms used for these evaluative procedures vary from university to university. Obtain a copy of the form prior to beginning the experience so that expectations are clear from the beginning. This enables the experience to be shaped to accommodate the need for particular types of experiences or disabilities. The midpoint evaluation provides an opportunity to discuss strengths, areas in need of improvement, and how to shape the experience to yield the best results. As a learner, the graduate student should then assume the responsibility of acting on the suggestions. The final evaluation generally provides an overview and summary of performance during the entire experience. It can serve as a reflection of the potential for the student's success in the school setting and provide the groundwork for further professional growth and development.

Performance and competency evaluation is an ongoing process. The evaluation process should be based on observations and data that measure a student's performance using predetermined criteria. Generally, time is spent discussing the student's performance in a conference that is designed to promote self-reflection and feedback. The supervisor has the responsibility of letting students know where they stand and their level of competency at a given time. If their performance is not adequate, then goals can be set to foster improvement.

Although universities vary in the process and forms they use to evaluate student's performance and provide feedback, there are several common skills areas and criteria that the extern supervisor generally uses. Skill areas that are evaluated typically include:

- Caseload and workload management

- Knowledge of disorders and how they impact on children's performance in the classroom
- Evaluation and recommendations
- Intervention plans and techniques
- Recordkeeping, reporting, and documentation
- Professional manner
- Communication, interaction and collaboration with supervisors and educational colleagues
- Managing behavior
- Personal qualities such as responsibility and professional attitude.

ASHA Certification and State Licensure Requirements

The American Speech-Language-Hearing Association has set standards for the supervision of student clinicians. They have specified that in states where credential requirements and/or state licensure requirements differ from ASHA certification standards, the supervised clinical experiences must be supervised by ASHA certified personnel (CCC) to ensure that the student satisfies ASHA requirements. Students seeking ASHA certification should take responsibility for understanding differences between ASHA requirements, state education certification requirements, and licensure requirements.

A Word of Advice to Student Externs

Are you ready to start your school externship experience? Here are 10 suggestions that might be helpful:

1. Work in harmony with your supervising SLP and university supervisor. Their job is to help you become a better speech-language pathologist.
2. Be enthusiastic about your work and sincerely interested in the children with whom you will be working.
3. Stay healthy. Get plenty of rest and eat the right foods.
4. Take advantage of every opportunity to become involved in the unique experiences a school has to offer.
5. Ask questions when you aren't sure, and even when you are sure. Find out why things work the way they do.
6. Know what you can expect of children at various ages and ability levels.
7. Be firm, fair, consistent, and compassionate in all your dealings with children. Every human being deserves respect.
8. Know the ground rules of your assigned schools and adhere to them.
9. When making professional decisions always ask yourself, "Is this in the best interests of the child?"
10. Enjoy your externship experience.

DISCUSSION QUESTIONS AND PROJECTS

1. Interview a current graduate student who is involved in an externship assignment in the schools. Ask for suggestions to ensure that your experience is successful.

2. Invite a principal to talk to your university class about what he or she expects of the student seeking an externship experience in the school setting.

3. Make a list of the experiences you'd like to gain during your externship experience.

4. Interview a school SLP about what he or she expects from a student clinician.

5. Ask a first-, second-, or third-grade child what he or she likes best about a favorite teacher. Ask a junior high and high school student the same question. Did you find any differences or similarities in their answers?

12

Life After College

Changes in the field of speech-language pathology are occurring rapidly. Heraclitus once said that one may not step in the same river twice, not only because the river flows and changes, but also because the one who steps into it changes, too, and at any two moments is never identical.

What does this mean to you as a beginning SLP? And, more specifically, what does it mean to those of you who will be employed in education? First, it means that this is an incredibly interesting time to be alive and in the field of communication and education. You will need to be knowledgeable and involved in the world, not only the world of the therapy room and the classroom, but also your local and professional communities and beyond.

In this chapter we consider some of the ways you can stay abreast of current information through professional reading and continuing education programs. Your role as a researcher is also examined. Issues such as the core curriculum, school improvement, evidence-based practice, and collective bargaining will become important issues to you. We also look at ways you may provide interviewers and prospective employers with information about your skills, knowledge, and attitudes to enhance your employment opportunities.

The importance of being familiar with state and federal laws is discussed. Due process procedures in the light of malpractice claims are described, as well as liability insurance.

There *is* life after college. Welcome to a very interesting, challenging, and important profession. Be your best self and do your very best.

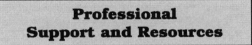

Professional Support and Resources

As the role of the school SLP expands, there is a need to keep abreast of current information. This is particularly crucial for school clinicians working in remote areas or in areas where access to academic institutions, medical centers, or even libraries may be limited. There is no need to worry if these institutions are not near your home. We are thankful that we can connect with the top resources in the world through the Internet.

Many states have established a statewide or regional network system with resource centers that provide a broad range of services to support educators and families of children with disabilities. They provide continuing education as well as information about products and materials. They may also help school personnel create new materials when commercially produced products are not available. Announcements are generally made through mail and online newsletters and other media forms.

National and state associations publish professional journals that discuss state-of-the-art research and intervention. Each of the special interest divisions of ASHA maintains an E-mail listserv, offers continuing education opportunities, and publishes newsletters. It is difficult to keep up with all the written communication that crosses our desk. One possible way of accomplishing this daunting task is to schedule a reserved time for reading professional materials each week.

The Internet provides access from your home or office to information from throughout the world 24 hours a day. Surfing the "net" can connect you to leading experts who specialize in diagnosis and treatment of communication disorders. Through digests, listservs, chat rooms, and discussion groups you can pose complex questions and obtain answers from fellow SLPs and special educators. You can obtain research findings, intervention protocols, and clinical resources. Technology continues to change the way we learn and do business. Take care, however, that you do not become so absorbed in communicating via technology that you forget to develop relationships on a person-to-person basis. Create good habits regarding use of your time at the computer, including how you file materials for later retrieval.

Continuing Education

Another way in which the SLP keeps current on professional matters is through continuing education, in the form of workshops, short courses, seminars, mini-seminars, in-service training courses, professional meetings, university courses, teleconferences, Web-based or televised courses, and video presentations. Continuing education can be in the form of a structured program or on a more informal basis. Learning must be a lifelong process for an individual expecting to remain accountable and qualified. It is a process by which one keeps one's skills and knowledge up to date.

Continuing education is valuable to practitioners and to clinicians who have stopped out of their professional lives and wish to reenter at a later date. Continuing education is not the responsibility of any one institution or agency but should represent the coordinated efforts of a number of groups. Universities cannot offer courses in a geographic area unless there is an expressed need concerning the content area of such a course. For the university to plan for such courses, the need should be expressed to the university staff by the school clinicians. By the same token, universities should be willing to offer courses at a time that would be convenient to the school clinicians and in a location that would be accessible to them. Advances in technology have enabled universities and school systems to form partnerships to deliver advanced education via the Web, television, videotapes, or other forms of distribution. Many states have formed collaborative projects to enable school practitioners to get specialty certificates or advanced degrees while still working full-time. The education "anywhere, anytime" concept is very beneficial.

Members and nonmembers of the American Speech-Language-Hearing Association who are holders of the Certificate of Clinical Competence may apply for an award called the ACE (Award for Continuing Education). Credits are earned through continuing education activities under ASHA-approved sponsors. A specific number of CE units are awarded to the participant for each instructional activity, and a national CE registry is maintained. Upon completion of the required number of units, the ACE is awarded. Some state licensure boards have similar requirements and maintain registries. Each SLP is responsible for knowing the required number of continuing education units required to maintain their certification and licensure.

Research

It is doubtful that anyone would argue against the need for research about pediatric communication disabilities and appropriate services. There is widespread agreement that public school is a fertile field for research to identify solutions to the challenges of providing services in the school setting. To add further emphasis, federal legislation has created pressure to find answers to questions about prevalence of speech-language disorders, impact on learning, treatment outcomes, comparison of delivery systems, efficacy of treatment methods, qualifications for service delivery, and other important issues.

Due to our responsibility to the children we serve, it is imperative that we must seek the highest quality of evidence to support our clinical decisions. Perhaps one of the most impressive recent professional movements is the systematic review of evidence from multiple sources. Those reviews lead to the development of clinical practice guidelines that practitioners can use to make clinical decisions. IDEA requires implementation of evidence-based assessment and intervention approaches.

Unfortunately, many school-based clinicians don't engage in research activities. There are a number of possible reasons given by school clinicians. Among the most frequently cited reasons are lack of time, funding, support by school administrators, and limited interest by journal publishers. The fear of performing statistical analyses, the lack of training in research methods, and the lack of rewards have also been suggested as reasons for limited research in the schools. Another reason may be that SLPs may simply be more interested in being clinicians than researchers. This is understandable in light of their employment setting. On the other hand, school clinicians eagerly read journals and attend professional meetings in the hope of finding answers to questions.

A profession must be based on a body of knowledge, and this body of knowledge is accumulated by research. There must be thoughtful individuals to pose questions as well as interested individuals to seek answers and solutions. Collaboration by researchers in universities, specialists in departments of education and special education on both the state and federal levels, and school SLPs is one of the best methods for generating research on the public school level. Public schools provide a good base for research projects, and university personnel are a good source of information for consultation on research design.

Research projects that employ a single-subject design are especially appropriate for school SLPs. So is research on treatment outcomes, program management, and the relationship of communication disorders to learning. The clinician can carry out most types of research without disruption of schedule and without ethical constraints on using school-age clients for research. School administrators should be advised and parents should be informed and must give their consent of the student is to be considered a "human subject" in the research project.

Longitudinal studies in which a single subject or a group of subjects are followed for months or even years are ideally suited for public school researchers in speech-language pathology. Examples of this type of study can be readily found in journals such as *Language, Speech and Hearing Services in the Schools* and the journal published by the National Students in Speech, Language, Hearing Association (NSSHLA).

The school clinician of the future will undoubtedly be involved in research on the local level, the state level, or as part of a national research project. The questions are everywhere, and the need to find answers is urgent. The questions of the school clinician in Mississippi may be the same ones asked by the clinician in Montana. Not only is the search for answers important, but equally important is the need to exchange professional information. There are many venues for sharing professional findings including state and national conferences and association publications.

Influencing Decision-Makers

Often we believe that our hands are tied and that it is impossible to obtain the support or special changes that we seek. In reality, we can make great gains if we learn advocacy strategies for influencing decision makers, especially school administrators and leaders. For example, Estomin (2010) discussed the steps she followed to convince her colleagues in the Pittsburg School System to provide the SLPs with the funds generated through their Medicaid related service delivery to purchase assessment and therapy instruments. Here are the key steps she and others recommend:

1. Decide what goal you want to achieve. What is most important to you?
2. Share your ideas and thoughts with your colleagues. See if others share your goal and agree with you. Most importantly, find out if they will be willing to work with you achieve the goal or bring about the desired change.
3. Choose a person to lead the group's effort. They will be responsible for calling meetings, facilitating the group's development of an action plan, and making sure that everyone stays focused and on track.
4. Create a logical plan of action that outlines all of the steps to be followed.

5. Research all aspects of the issue, asking questions about whether the topic has been explored before, similar actions in other districts, support needed to be successful, and impact of making the change versus not making it.
6. Determine who needs to hear your message or your request.
7. Prepare your proposal, including statement of the problem, impact on the program or district, and your recommended solutions.
8. Gather data and facts to support your case.
9. Develop talking points so you can present your case in an organized fashion. Talking points should be clear and succinct: defining the problem, highlighting the desired change, and supporting with facts.
10. Be ready to answer tough questions about funding, rationale, and priorities.

Collective Bargaining and the School SLP

In school districts where there is a teachers union and collective bargaining, speech-language pathologists must determine in advance their role and response during negotiations or strikes. Collective bargaining has a long history in the private sector and since 1962 when New York City teachers negotiated a collective bargaining agreement it has become a significant factor in American education. Collective bargaining is an outgrowth of the desire to have a fair discussion in such issues as salary, fringe benefits, and working conditions. Teachers unions are organized and powerful voices in education politics.

Whether the American Federation of Teachers (AFT) and the National Education Association (NEA) call themselves labor unions or professional organizations is a moot point. If they bargain collectively with management they are functionally labor unions. The American Speech-Language-Hearing Association and the various state speech, language, and hearing associations are professional organizations because they do not negotiate salaries, contracts, and fringe benefits.

Many, but not all, states have collective bargaining laws and the laws differ from state to state. Your state labor relations board can give you information on your state's collective bargaining law. Whether you, as a speech-language pathologist, are considered management or labor will depend on your state's collective bargaining law. If your state classifies you as management, during a strike you may be called upon to staff a classroom. If you are classified as labor, it is important to become involved in and work with the union or unit at the local level to make sure the issues and concerns important to you are brought to the bargaining table.

The decision of whether or not to affiliate with a local collective bargaining unit depends on the local situation. If you belong to the local unit of either AFT or NEA you also must belong to the state and national organization. Even if you choose not to join the locally designated unit, the law requires the unit to bargain for you regardless.

School speech-language pathologists may be at a disadvantage primarily because they comprise a very small percentage of persons covered by the bargaining unit. During negotiations when concessions are made it would be easier for a unit to give up a demand affecting the few speech-language pathologists in favor of a demand affecting all the classroom teachers.

Some SLPs have undertaken leadership roles in their teachers union. As a result, they have been able to bring key issues to the discussion table such as caseload size, workload, school assignments, and compensation. Being a leader in any organization enables individuals to gain a better understanding of how the organization works and how to bring about change.

If speech-language pathologists and audiologists are going to be able to use the collective bargaining process to improve their working conditions it is important to become knowledgeable about their state's collective bargaining law and how negotiations are handled locally.

The bargaining unit can also be a good vehicle for informing colleagues about speech-language and hearing services that members should consider in the health care plans that are offered to employees. For example, you can be a good advocate for your profession by advocating for coverage for hearing aids, therapy services after stroke, and services for children with developmental disabilities.

You and the Law

Free Appropriate Public Education (FAPE) for all children with disabilities has been mandated by federal legislation since 1976. The laws also describe procedures for parents and other parties to appeal when they believe it is not being provided. The laws ever provide for the recovery of attorney's fees when the parents prevail in disagreements with school district decisions. Over the years this legislation has opened the door for an increase in the number of appeals generated. Due process hearings are the administrative legal proceedings between the school and the family, presided over by a presumably impartial hearing officer. Due process hearings occur when there is disagreement between the parents and the Local Education Agency (LEA) regarding the services that are to be provided to a child. Often, prior to the due process hearing, the school district attempts to amicably resolve the misunderstandings.

Corbin (2008) outlines several strategies schools and professionals can take to avoid a due process hearing. Unfortunately, many clinicians find themselves in a situation of having to participate in a hearing. Here are Corbin's recommendations for preparing for a hearing if you are called to testify as a witness. These activities include the following:

1. *Case Background.* Review student school files; review speech/language file, note the reason for referral; consult with pertinent staff (teachers, therapist, etc.); compile a chronology of significant dates and events.
2. *Individual Education Program (IEP).* Check inclusion of and be familiar with: disability codes; model of service recommended and intensity of program; evaluative instruments, including validity and norms; data reported; strengths and needs; goals and objectives related to needs; mastery criteria; committee members, parent's presence; and other special education services.

3. *Program Implementation.* Review therapy logs and note attendance, group composition, techniques, and materials, and progress; review observations of the student in the educational program; and note parent contacts, frequency, and content.
4. *Testimony.* Be prepared to summarize your credentials, educational background and experience; discuss your knowledge of the case; discuss evaluative finds and the basis for recommendations; describe test characteristics, validity and normative data; discuss the program in relation to student needs; describe progress and how measured.

Some behavioral do's and don'ts were also recommended. They suggested maintaining professionalism and formality at all times, taking notes on any points you hear that may help your case presenter, and stop testifying and wait until the question is resolved if there is an objection from either side. They also advise not to panic if you are placed under oath and not to talk except when testifying. Conversing with the hearing officer and discussing hearing issues with the opposing side during breaks should not occur.

Malpractice claims are a continuing risk for speech-language professionals. There are preventive measures such as maintaining good client relationships, careful documentation of therapy procedures, and knowledge of current state and federal regulations. But the best guide to avoiding malpractice claims is strict adherence to the American Speech-Language-Hearing Association's Code of Ethics. The Code of Ethics not only serves as a model of behavior for you, as a professional person, but also protects the consumer (in this case, the student) against dangerous practices of inexpert and injudicious individuals.

As a school speech-language pathologist, you may be the subject of a claim in a malpractice suit but you are much more likely to be called as an "expert witness" in a trial. An expert witness does not have direct knowledge of the case at hand but by virtue of education, research, or experience is qualified to testify.

Your Role as a Grassroots Advocate

As frequently noted, state and federal legislation greatly impacts the delivery of services to individuals who have communication impairments. This cannot be taken lightly. The laws affect the qualifications you need to do your job, the environment in which you work, the salary you earn, the students you see, and the service delivery options you can offer. This translates to a very important need to get involved in the political process through grassroots political advocacy. You can make an important contribution by talking with your legislative representatives about your profession and the people you serve.

Meeting with state or national legislators can seem like a very frightening experience; but only for the first time. Once you have done it you will soon realize that they want to hear from you. They are interested in what you have to say. And they will listen to your message. After all, you have the power to vote them into or out of office.

ASHA and many state professional organizations have developed simple procedures to help you understand the process and feel comfortable in your role as an advocate for the communication sciences and disorders profession and for individuals with communication disabilities. Following is a summary of recommended steps for advocating with your legislators.

Lay the Groundwork

First identify who your local, state, and national legislators are. You can obtain this information by reading the newspaper, contacting your Board of Elections, or checking the government Web sites. ASHA's website links to the congressional Directory which lists the representatives for all states. Once you have identified the elected officials you want to contact, learn as much about them as possible including their political party, voting record on key issues, legislative committees, personal facts, and profession. Many state and national associations have done the legwork for you.

Contact Your Representative or Senator

Decide if you can visit or if you simply want to write to your lawmaker. If you want to visit, make arrangements to do so. You can call for an appointment by contacting the U.S. Capitol Switchboard. Be ready to state the intended purpose of your visit in one or two brief statements. Select only one or two priority issues. ASHA, CEC, or your state association will be able to suggest timely issues.

Most likely you will be visiting with the legislator's congressional aide who is assigned to health or education issues. That individual will in turn communicate your message and opinion for the representative or senator. He or she is most likely working in the office as an intern trying to learn the political process. If the legislator or aide cannot see you, ask the receptionist if you may stop by the office to drop off materials. This is generally acceptable.

Prepare for Your Meeting

If your organization offers the opportunity, attend a briefing session to learn the key issues that legislators are dealing with at the time. Learn to discuss the issue and be familiar with how it affects the students you serve or you. Take a few well-chosen written materials with you when visit. It you are visiting with a group of colleagues, decide in advance who will act at the spokesperson. When it is time for the visit, be punctual and to the point.

Present Your Issues

Make your issue clear. What is it you want the lawmaker to do? Do you want them to vote on a particular bill or sponsor a specific law? Then let them know that is what you are asking. Concentrate only on one or two issues. Be sure to listen to the lawmaker's opinion even if you disagree. Some examples of issues that professionals have brought to their legislators lately include: inclusion of SLPs in education funding, infant hearing screening, funding cutbacks, capping services to Medicare patients, and the like. If you are asked a question you can't answer, don't be embarrassed. Find the answer and phone or mail it to the person who asked it.

Follow Your Visit with a Thank You

Be sure to let the lawmaker and his or her aide know that you appreciate the time they allotted for your visit. Re-emphasize your key points. Offer to provide additional information upon request.

Go Political

If you really enjoy the political arena, consider expanding your activities to contact more legislators or serve on a grassroots committee. If you really like the environment, consider running for office. Local, state, and national governments need individuals who are committed to important causes.

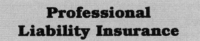

Professional Liability Insurance

As the school speech-language clinician's caseload and role expands to include a wide variety of communication disorders and intervention tasks, the possibility of situations occurring for which the clinician may be held liable is increased. Although this may be a sad commentary on the state of our world today, it is nevertheless a reality. The school-based SLP and other educators are treating youngsters with complex disabilities such as autism, dysphagia, traumatic brain injury, and severe emotional disorders. The increased complexity leads to increased risk because the intervention treatment may be more invasive or involve physical contact. Thus, it is important to maintain professional liability insurance in case such an event should occur. Many districts and employment settings require liability insurance coverage. Others provide the coverage for educators and practitioners. Check with your local school system to see if there is coverage through an educational agency. Another source of information is ASHA or your state speech-language-hearing association. Liability insurance for speech-language pathologists and audiologists would cover all professional activities but may not cover corporal punishment, transportation by private auto, and travel by aircraft or watercraft. Your personal insurance agent is also a source of information; you may already be covered under your own insurance plan.

Insurance for students is usually offered by universities at a nominal sum and is often treated the same as a course fee. It is incumbent on the student to find out what is specifically covered. Students may also be covered under their parent's insurance plans.

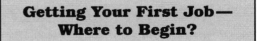

Getting Your First Job—Where to Begin?

The job search for you, as a beginning SLP, may start any time during your master's program. Your university's placement office can provide guidance and recommendations. The service is available at most universities and is usually free to students and alumni. Contact them or visit their Web site to find out the specific services available to you. You can also research the Web for tips of how do conduct an effective employment search. Generally speaking, these are the services career placement centers and Web sites provide:

- Individual counseling
- Vacancy listings
- Credential services
- Career fairs
- Seminars and guest speakers
- Mock interview training and critique sessions
- Resource centers with information concerning employment strategies, career opportunities, alumni placement services, videotapes, and slide presentations.

After you find out what services are available, which ones are applicable to you, and those you want to utilize, it is time to plan your strategy. Timing is important here. You will want to visit the placement office after you have completed most of your academic work and clinical practicum.

Your Credential File and Portfolio

Employers expect to see well-organized and up-to-date credential files on prospective SLPs. The credential file you accumulate should document your past achievements and support your candidacy for a position. It is important to begin early to collate representative samples of your work and appropriate letters of recommendation from faculty members and past employers.

A complete credential file should include the following information.

Letters of Recommendation

Most university placement services and school districts use a standard reference form on which reference writers make statements regarding your professional or personal relationship and how long the writer has known you. There should be a description of your academic or career growth and potential, a review of your major achievements, an estimate of future promise at this point, a paragraph on your personal qualities, and a final summary paragraph. If you intend to use someone's name as a reference it is always necessary to request that person's permission in advance. The reference letter may be sent directly to the potential employer or you. You may want to request a copy for your records. Always enclose self-addressed stamped envelopes. Some persons who provide references may prefer not to send a copy. If this is what your reference indicates, you may want to probe the reason to be sure that it is not because they won't be providing a positive reference.

Professors are often asked to provide references for many students just prior to graduation. When asking for a reference, allow ample time for the person to fit the writing into their schedule. Otherwise, the reference may not be compelling enough to help you get the job. Select your references carefully. Think of people who know you in different ways and can provide different perspectives about your skills and experiences. A good combination would be your academic advisor, a supervisor from your student teaching or extern site, and your summer employer.

Externship Evaluation

An evaluation is made by the person who supervised you during the experience. You want them to highlight your experiences and summarize your performance and strengths. They may also include their perception of your professional potential.

Transcript of Grades

This is obtained from the registrar of the university. Be sure you check to see if the employer wants an "official" transcript. If so, it you must request to have it sent out from the registrar's office.

Examples of Work

One of the most successful "marketing tools" is the use of the pre-professional portfolio. Your resume, samples of treatment plans, photographs of displays or bulletin boards, and statements verifying your participation in educational projects both before and during the externship should be placed in the portfolio. Your extern supervisor can offer excellent recommendations concerning the content and layout of your portfolio.

Regardless of immediate or long-range plans, establishing a credential file that you can use during your job search is strongly advised. Be sure you keep it up to date by adding new addresses and positions and by periodically including letters of reference from employers.

The Interview

One of the keys to successful interviewing is advance preparation. It is also one of the best ways to combat nervousness during the interview. The beginning point of your preparation is to know yourself. Review your personal inventory and background thoroughly and always in light of the position you are seeking. Be prepared to answer questions regarding your education, grades, courses, jobs, extracurricular activities, goals, strengths, weaknesses, and other information. Keep in mind that the interviewer is wondering, "Why should I hire you?" In answering this question be prepared to give examples and illustrations of your abilities, skills, leadership, effectiveness, and potential.

Successful preparation for the interview also entails knowing the school system. Your placement office may be able to assist you. Other sources for general information include newspaper articles, the school district's Web site, school board minutes, parent-teacher organizations, or your university education department. However, you should also be interested in learning about the speech-language pathology programs. You may obtain this information by contacting colleagues in the profession and by asking the interviewer questions. Pertinent questions would include the following: How many SLPs are presently on the school staff? How long has the program been in existence? What is the school population? How many buildings and grade levels do the speech-language pathologists in the district service? Will you be assigned to a particular age or disability group of children? To whom is the speech-language clinician directly responsible?

Another important way to prepare for the interview is to practice. Role-play a mock interview with a friend, instructor, relative, fellow student, or a placement staff counselor. Pay especially close attention to questions that may deal with some weaknesses or problem areas in your background. Don't wait until you reach the interview to think about responding to a question concerning a weakness.

Another facet of interview preparation is appropriate dress. First impressions are often lasting impressions, and you must look as if you fit the role before an employer will let you act the role. How you dress is a statement about how you feel about the significance of the interview and whom you will be meeting. Careful attention to dress and grooming is a way of putting your best foot forward. When in doubt it is best to be conservative in your dress.

What can you expect the interviewer to be like? Because you really don't know in advance you will need to take your cues from the content of the interview. If the interviewer wants you to do most of the talking and wants to assess your ability to communicate and reason, this individual's style will be nondirective. If the interviewer is concerned with eliciting specific and precise responses, the style will be more formal and structured. Sometimes interviewers will create some stress to ascertain how the candidate will react. How you handle the interview is important. Avoid short responses, as they tell the interviewer little or nothing or perhaps the wrong things, about you. Use this opportunity to capitalize on your assets. Use anecdotal information to demonstrate your strong points, for example, "During my spring vacation I helped the school clinician in my hometown with the preschool screening program. We screened over 500 children for speech, language, and hearing problems. She was pleased with my work and wrote a letter describing my contribution. The letter is in my portfolio and I would like to have you read it." This tells the interviewer not only that you were able to function well in a professional situation and that you have gained some experience but that you were also interested in improving your skills by spending your spring vacation doing so.

Be prepared for questions like these: What is your philosophy of education? How would you plan to work with the learning disabilities teacher? What do you think a speech, language, and hearing program can add to a school system? What special preparation do you have for working with children with autism spectrum disorders? How would you manage a referral of a student who does not speak English? Have you completed PECS training?

Inappropriate behaviors elicit negative impressions during an interview. They include candidates who show up late, chew gum, smoke without permission, bring uninvited guests, have poor hygiene, are braggarts and liars, are overly aggressive or too shy, lack confidence and poise, fail to look the interviewer in the eye, show lack of interest and enthusiasm, and ask no questions or poor questions.

Follow-up on the interview is important. Write a thank-you letter, noting anything that was said that you want to reemphasize. Thank the interviewer for the opportunity to discuss your mutual interests and clarify any questions or ambiguities from the meeting. If you are interested in this position restate your desire to work for this particular school system. If you are undecided, write a thank-you letter anyway.

Your Resume

Another important tool is the resume, a written document that introduces your education, background, skills, and experience to the prospective employer. It is a document that is used not only for the first job but also for subsequent employment searches throughout your professional life. The resume is a cornerstone of the job-hunting process. Its worth is seldom questioned; its necessity is simply assumed. However, despite its importance as a marketing tool, many people express anxiety and frustration about preparing it.

A resume is neither an autobiography nor merely a listing of your employment history. When properly done, it is an advertisement that excites an employer's interest in a particular product, *namely, you*. Because there are no absolutes in resume writing, you will ultimately decide how it looks and what it says. Its style, format, and length should be determined by your employment interests or target markets and your background and qualifications.

An effective resume can be prepared in different styles or formats and contain widely diverse information. Making the strongest presentation of your unique and individual qualifications will contribute to the kind of distinction that will set your resume apart from others. So although there are no absolute rules on what "all" resumes should contain, except who you are and how you can be contacted, the following general rules address issues of honesty, accuracy, neatness, grammar, layout, and content that should be carefully observed:

- Do not exaggerate your accomplishments to give the impression that you did more than you did. Employers know the difference between a restaurant hostess and an executive vice president for customer relations.
- Be reasonably brief. You are writing a resume, not an autobiography. Tailor your information to fit the employer's needs.
- Be careful with your grammar and the design and layout of your resume. There is no excuse for sloppy writing and poor grammar.
- Be sure the font size and style are legible, not too small or too fancy.
- Do not include information that will work to your disadvantage. Negative or harmful information is best handled in a personal interview.
- Use strong action verbs to make your resume as impressive as possible. This is essential as employers will most often see your resume before they see you.
- Always present accurate information. Honesty really is the best policy.
- Use an E-mail address that is professional. Avoid cute or unusual names.
- Make sure that your personal social network Web sites do not contain information that would create a

negative perception of you as a person.

A sample resume is provided for your review (Figure 12–1). It is designed to help you produce a document that strongly reflects your interests, qualifications, and potential. By itself, a resume cannot get you the job you want; yet without it, you most likely will not even get started.

Although there is a critical shortage of speech-language pathologists interested in working in the school setting, not all interviews result in a job offer. School administrators may be looking for an individual with a specific set of qualifications and credentials. In a few regions of the country the supply of SLPs may even exceed the demand. The individual who is willing to be flexible about location and types of disabilities on the caseload has a much better chance of finding a job.

There are many avenues for searching job openings including school district websites, national staffing organizations, career boards, state and national newsletters, and alumni publications. And don't neglect the classified pages of the newspapers although these are unlikely to yield a great amount of information about positions in school systems. The newsletters of state speech, language, and hearing associations often list job openings in schools, and the state consultants in speech-language pathology know of job openings within that state. The names and addresses of the state consultants can be obtained by writing to the state department of public instruction, division of special education. They are located in or near the state capital cities. Information can be found in educational directories or on the state government Web pages.

Begin now to build a network of persons who may be able to provide you with information concerning job possibilities. This will be valuable not only for your first job but also for subsequent job searches. When you meet professionals on your campus or at conferences, introduce yourself to them and exchange contact information. Retain their information in an organized way so that you can access it when needed. Don't hesitate to send them a letter or E-mail to let them know that you are searching for a position.

Discussing Salary and Benefits

Realizing that you will finally be earning a salary is perhaps one of the most exciting aspects of getting your first job. The salary discussion is a very difficult one for most individuals. Make sure that the position meets your career goals and needs prior to entering a discussion about salary. Take time to create a list of features you desire in a job. Ask questions that will ensure that you understand everything there is to know about the job. When evaluating your offer, consider the following:

- Nature of the work (caseload demographics and composition, workload expectations, match to your skills and qualifications)
- Support, mentoring, and supervision
- Organizational structure—key administrators
- Work hours and expectations for productivity

Name
Address
City, State, Zip
E-mail Address
Phone / Fax

PROFESSIONAL OBJECTIVE

This is really the most difficult section to write. Listing a particular job objective on a resume may be limiting. However, if you have a clear objective that applies to many organizations, it is to your advantage to include it. You may also state your professional objective in your cover letter rather than resume. Include the job function desired and the type of organization.

EDUCATION

List the highest or most recent degree first. Include name of college(s), major(s), minor(s), graduation dates. Add any special emphasis in your studies, such as relevant courses, practica, externships, populations served, and so forth.

EXPERIENCE AND WORK HISTORY

This section provides a summary of your work experience, highlighting your most recent or most relevant employment first. Include descriptions of your responsibilities, titles of positions held, names of companies or organizations, and dates employed. Summer employment and volunteer work may be included. Stress the level of responsibility, achievement, and motivation you demonstrated in previous positions. This section is an active statement of what you can do. The way you describe the experience is key.

ACTIVITIES / INTERESTS

Extracurricular involvement highlights your leadership skills, sociability, and energy level. Choose activities that support your professional objective by demonstrating your leadership or organizational skills. If you have many activities, select the ones in which you were most involved and describe your degree of responsibility.

REFERENCES

It is not necessary to include names and addresses of references. If references are requested, they can be provided separately or included on an application form. State "Available upon request."

OPTIONAL INFORMATION

In this section you can include information about honors and awards, publications, professional associations, research projects, scholarships, study abroad, recognitions, and personal information. It is illegal for an employer to solicit personal data (age, weight, height, marital status, number of children, or disability) unless a genuine occupational requirement exists. Include this information only if pertinent to the position you are seeking.

Figure 12–1. Sample resume.

- Travel and school locations
- Salary
- Benefits including insurance and professional development opportunities
- Advancement opportunities
- Training/development and continuing education opportunities and financial support
- Therapy materials and resources
- Culture of the school organization
- Employee satisfaction and attitudes
- Technology
- Student information and data tracking/reporting systems.

Often, candidates are perplexed about when and if the question of salary should be raised. Most employment consultants suggest waiting until the job is offered to you and you have discussed the expectations and responsibilities fully. It is at that time that the interviewer will generally "make the offer" and discuss the compensation. The salary in most school districts is linked to the degree or educational level and years of experience. Many districts have salary scales. Some offer SLPs a slightly higher salary than teachers. In public education the information is available for review through public sources.

Be cautious; there is more to consider than money. Compensation includes salary, reimbursement for travel (mileage), and medical coverage. In some districts professional membership and licensure fees might be covered. Be sure to inquire about excused time off and reimbursement for professional materials and continuing education. And, of course, sick days and vacation days are also considered a part of the full compensation package. Here are some tips you might find helpful in preparing for salary discussions with perspective employers:

- Maintain an enthusiastic, polite, and professional attitude throughout the job interview and salary negotiation process.
- Strive to demonstrate your value during the interview process.
- Research the standard salaries that are generally offered to a person with your education, credentials, and in the geographic location. Make sure your requests are reasonable and within the ongoing salary range for the position and your experience. You can find great information about salary trends in the profession in the ASHA literature and on the Web.
- When asked for a salary range by an interviewer, it is appropriate to let him or her know that you are seeking a "competitive salary" or that "salary is negotiable." If asked to provide a salary request on an application form, you can feel comfortable writing statements such as, "open," "willing to discuss following our interview." You can also consider providing salary ranges.
- Take notes about the offer and request that it be put in writing.
- Ask for time to make your decision so that you can think about the

position and the offer to make sure they both meet your career goals and needs.

- Be willing to walk away. Obviously, the less you want the job the easier it is to negotiate.
- Be careful not to jump from job to job in search of more money. There are many factors that lead to job satisfaction and money is not always at the top of the list.

Your Clinical Fellowship Experience

The first year of employment in any profession often sets the tone for a person's career. Some new professionals find the first year experience exciting and a dream come true, whereas others find it overwhelming and may even make a decision that the field or work setting is not for them. Thus, getting off on the right foot is essential to future success and career happiness.

In the speech-language pathology profession, the first year of employment is the Clinical Fellowship experience. It is the final requirement for obtaining the Certificate of Clinical Competence. As it is such a critical experience, it is important consider the quality of guidance and mentoring that you will receive. Many employers and work settings promise to provide a high quality Clinical Fellowship experience. Not all end up fulfilling that promise. Seek to understand the nature of the experience you will have prior to accepting a new position.

A significant number of Clinical Fellows and SLPs select the school-based setting as their first preference for employment or as an alternative setting after completing an externship in a medical, rehabilitation, or private practice setting. This is exciting because the need, challenges, and rewards that come with employment in the school-based setting are so great. Often, Clinical Fellows feel unprepared to meet the challenges and demands of school-based practice. Although every student majoring in speech-language pathology participates in courses and clinical experiences, there is great variation in the content and quality of academic and clinical preparation for practice in school settings. Adding complexity to this situation, there are also great variations in SLP's roles, responsibilities, expectations, and procedures in school districts across the country. These scenarios sometimes combine to create fear, lack of preparation, and low confidence for new practitioners. They may be unsure of their roles and have difficulty translating the professional knowledge and skills they have learned to effective service delivery. It is preferable for SLPs who choose to practice in the school setting to have experiences that enable them develop a passion for school-based service delivery and realize the joys of treating children in that setting.

Being mentored by a professional who has passion and expertise in school-based services can provide the foundation for a wonderful career. Take an active role in shaping your Clinical Fellowship Experience. Learn from your mentor. Engage in lively conversations about the profession. Ask for advice and recommendations of solutions to the challenges you face.

Some school districts and employers offer structured, formalized mentoring programs for new professionals. Blosser and Silverman (2010) described two programs that were designed differently but focused on similar goals of preparing new professionals to succeed as school-based SLPs. Both programs parallel the school year so that Clinical Fellows are provided with support and resources as challenges arise. Mentors can provide an "insider's perspective" on how to navigate the school system. They enhance understanding of key policies and practices. In addition, they can help identify knowledge gaps and ways to acquire new skills and expertise.

Silverman's (Blosser and Silverman, 2010) program in Maryland's Anne Arundel Public Schools, Speech-Language Induction Program (SLIP) designates a seasoned SLP to serve as mentor to all new clinicians. The program is designed to accelerate learning of the district's policies and procedures.

Blosser explained that the Progressus Therapy Career Launch Program (2010) matches newly graduated Clinical Fellows (Mentees) with experienced therapists from within the Progressus organization (Mentors). SLPs who serve as Mentors are those who have demonstrated professional expertise and leadership and who are seeking opportunities to pursue leadership roles and expanded experiences within their careers (Mentors). Through planned interactions and experiences, the Career Launch Program facilitates professional development and growth. The Career Launch Program strives to prepare professionals to be knowledgeable and to deliver efficient and effective services. Mentees are guided to do the following:

- Map out their first year of services delivery;
- Meet IDEA compliance requirements;
- Access support systems, professional expertise and resources;
- Implement evidence-based practices;
- Offer varied models of service delivery;
- Solve problems and address challenges;
- Acquire new skills; and
- Identify future career directions and professional development opportunities.

Alternative Career Paths

Preparation for the profession of speech-language pathology is complex, yet rewarding. The coursework is difficult; there are multiple points along the way where you must demonstrate your capabilities such as on the national examination or comprehensive exams at the university. You must work long hours alone or on teams to prepare for clinic and student teaching. You should be very proud of your efforts on the journey.

Some students reach the end of the trail and can't wait to begin practicing. Others decide that the profession is not for them. They may feel frustrated and afraid to tell anyone, especially family members, professors, and student peers who have been supportive all along the way. Some clinicians join the workforce and then decide their interests and talents lie elsewhere or they are not happy doing therapy on a day-to-day basis. All these circumstances are normal. Life is too short to spend years dissatisfied with your work and where you are doing it.

Prior to accepting a job, have a talk with yourself. Decide if the position, responsibilities, caseload, workload, location, people, duties, and culture are right for you. If the answer is no, feel comfortable exploring other opportunities. Your education and experiences have provided you with the tools and qualifications to do many things. Following is a list of representative options illustrating the careers that speech-language pathologists are qualified to pursue:

- Develop, promote, copy edit, or sell products for use in the clinical, education, health care, or rehabilitation fields such as:
    - Clinical materials and equipment
    - Educational materials and resources
    - Assessment instruments and diagnostic tests
    - Augmentative communication devices
    - Voice recognition and production systems
    - Textbooks and reference books
    - Assistive listening devices
    - Intervention software
    - Accommodations for individuals with severe physical disabilities
- Contribute to the "Edutainment Industry":
    - Develop educational programming
    - Review or write scripts
    - Coach actors in dialogue, accents, mannerisms
- Work in related fields:
    - Rehabilitation counseling
    - Job coaching
    - Academic advising
    - Clinical assistants and support staff
    - Clinical intake specialists
    - Technology support staff
    - Group home staff
    - Mentoring youth
    - Assisting families of individuals with disabilities
    - Scouting for individuals with disabilities
    - Community outreach programs
    - Employment search firms
- Consider a degree in a related field such as:
    - Special education
    - General education
    - Early intervention
    - Vocational rehabilitation
    - Mental health
    - Public health
    - Medical fields
    - Education or health law
- Be creative—use your imagination!
    - Scan the want ads.
    - Make suggestions to perspective employers.

Set Time Aside for Yourself

It is easy to get so absorbed in work and forget your own needs once you are no longer a student and begin to take on work, family, and financial responsibilities. Sometimes, we forget to set aside time for ourselves. We don't appreciate the contributions we make. Reward yourself for your success and set aside time to reflect on the positive aspects of life or just have fun. Following are some ideas to get you started:

- Take a class for fun.
- Learn a new hobby.
- Get together with a group of friends and go running or to a play.
- Buy fresh flowers for several rooms in your home.
- Pack a lunch and go with a friend to a park in a different city.
- See a matinee performance of a musical or movie at your local theater.
- When you are visiting a new city for a conference, schedule a vacation day for sight seeing.
- Rent a limousine with six friends for an evening of fine dining and entertainment.
- Go out with co-workers and don't let anyone talk about work.
- Keep a running list of funny things that have happened to you lately.
- Visit the pet store.
- See where $100.00 will take you.
- Enjoy a spa day with a friend—get a massage and facial.
- Learn a new sport. Join a neighborhood team.
- Sit by the fire and read a good book.
- Volunteer for an organization of your choice.
- Host a theme party.
- Add 10 ideas to this list.

Best of Luck

Best of luck as you pursue your career path whether it be as a speech-language pathologist in the schools or another setting, as an administration, as a professional in a related field, or as a parent. Continue to grow and learn and enjoy helping people with communication disorders reach their full potential.

DISCUSSION QUESTIONS AND PROJECTS

1. Look on ASHA's Web site. Note the range of information available and the wide variety of topics listed. Read two Position Statements.

2. Find out which universities, organizations, or other facilities in your state are ASHA approved sponsors of continuing education programs leading toward the ACE? Do you think continuing education should be mandatory?

3. Do you think it is feasible for school SLPs to conduct research studies? What is the rationale for your answer?

4. Using the resume format in this chapter, prepare your resume.

5. Discuss the benefits list with an educator in a local school district. Determine the benefits offered in that district.

6. Start assembling your credential portfolio. What will you include?

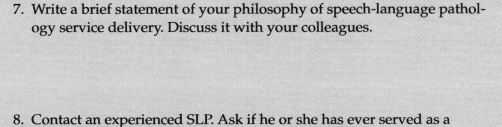

7. Write a brief statement of your philosophy of speech-language pathology service delivery. Discuss it with your colleagues.

8. Contact an experienced SLP. Ask if he or she has ever served as a Mentor. Find out how the Mentee and Mentor worked together.

APPENDIX

A

ASHA Roles and Responsibilities of Speech-Language Pathologists in Schools

Source: Reprinted with permission from Roles and responsibilities of speech-language pathologists in schools [overview]. Copyright 2010 by American Speech-Language-Hearing Association.

Roles and Responsibilities of Speech-Language Pathologists in Schools

American Speech-Language-Hearing Association

NEW!

Policy Documents

- Position Statement
- Professional Issues Statement

Available from **www.asha.org/policy**

School-based speech-language pathology is at a crossroads where SLPs seek to contribute significantly to the well-being and success of children and adolescents in schools as ever-increasing demands are placed on them with an expanded scope of practice.

\+

It is essential that SLPs' roles and responsibilities be redefined in light of substantive changes that have taken place in schools, as well as in the discipline of speech-language pathology.

Critical Roles

Working Across All Levels
Serving a Range of Disorders
Ensuring Educational Relevance
Providing Unique Contributions to Curriculum
Highlighting Language/Literacy
Providing Culturally Competent Services

Collaboration

With Other School Professionals
With Universities
With the Community
With Families
With Students

Position Statement:

Driven by educational reform, legal mandates, and evolving professional practices, it is the position of the American Speech-Language-Hearing Association (ASHA) that based on their unique skill set, speech-language pathologists (SLPs) in schools (1) have integral roles in education and are essential members of school faculties, (2) help students meet the performance standards of a particular school district and state by assuming a range of responsibilities, (3) work in partnership with others to meet students' needs, and (4) provide direction in defining their roles and responsibilities and in ensuring appropriate services to students, as described more fully in the 2010 professional issues statement, Roles and Responsibilities of Speech-Language Pathologists in Schools. Further, it is anticipated that this position may require a realignment of existing roles and responsibilities in the context of a reasonable workload with appropriate professional preparation and lifelong learning.

Range of Responsibilities

Prevention
Assessment
Intervention
Program Design
Data Collection and Analysis
Compliance

Leadership

Advocacy
Supervision and Mentorship
Professional Development
Parent Training
Research

WHAT IS NEEDED

Role and Responsibility Realignment
Reasonable Workloads
Professional Preparation
Lifelong Learning

Not one more thing!

Who should know about these documents?

- Other SLPs in your school district
- The special education director in your district
- Your supervisor
- Your principal(s)
- Reading specialists, school psychologists, and other support personnel with whom you work
- RTI leaders in your district and building
- Leaders of local professional organizations or unions
- Teachers
- Parents

What can you do to spread the word?

- Provide a hard copy or link to the documents for key stakeholders.
- Excerpt relevant sections for specific people.
- Provide an overview at a district professional development activity.
- Provide an overview at a faculty meeting.
- Post a blurb with a link on your school website.
- Engage in (or design) professional development to enhance implementation of these roles.
- Talk with your local university about how they prepare SLPs for these roles.

Replaces Guidelines for the Roles and Responsibilities of the School-Based Speech-Language Pathologist (2000)

Ad Hoc Committee on the Roles and Responsibilities of the School-Based Speech-Language Pathologist: Barbara Ehren (chair), Frances Block, Catherine Crowley, Ellen Estomin, Sue Ann Goldman, and Susan Karr (ex officio). Vice President for Professional Practices in Speech-Language Pathology Brian Shulman (2006–2008) and Vice President for Speech-Language Pathology Practice Julie Noel (2009–2011) served as the ASHA monitoring vice presidents, with contributions from ASHA staff member Deborah Adamczyk.

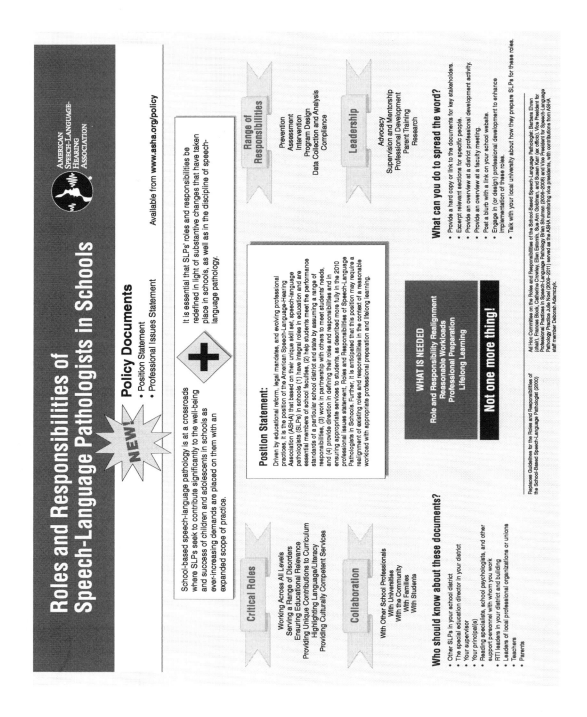

APPENDIX

B

ASHA Code of Ethics

Source: Reprinted with permission from American Speech-Language-Hearing Association. (2010). *Code of Ethics* [Ethics]. Available from www.asha.org/policy .

AMERICAN
SPEECH-LANGUAGE-
HEARING
ASSOCIATION

Code of Ethics

Reference this material as: American Speech-Language-Hearing Association. (2010)*Code of Ethics* [Ethics]. Available from www.asha.org/policy.

Index terms: ethics

doi:10.1044/policy.ET2010-00309

Preamble

The preservation of the highest standards of integrity and ethical principles is vital to the responsible discharge of obligations by speech-language pathologists, audiologists, and speech, language, and hearing scientists. This Code of Ethics sets forth the fundamental principles and rules considered essential to this purpose.

Every individual who is (a) a member of the American Speech-Language-Hearing Association, whether certified or not, (b) a nonmember holding the Certificate of Clinical Competence from the Association, (c) an applicant for membership or certification, or (d) a Clinical Fellow seeking to fulfill standards for certification shall abide by this Code of Ethics.

Any violation of the spirit and purpose of this Code shall be considered unethical. Failure to specify any particular responsibility or practice in this Code of Ethics shall not be construed as denial of the existence of such responsibilities or practices.

The fundamentals of ethical conduct are described by Principles of Ethics and by Rules of Ethics as they relate to the responsibility to persons served, the public, speech-language pathologists, audiologists, and speech, language, and hearing scientists, and to the conduct of research and scholarly activities.

Principles of Ethics, aspirational and inspirational in nature, form the underlying moral basis for the Code of Ethics. Individuals shall observe these principles as affirmative obligations under all conditions of professional activity.

Rules of Ethics are specific statements of minimally acceptable professional conduct or of prohibitions and are applicable to all individuals.

Principle of Ethics I

Individuals shall honor their responsibility to hold paramount the welfare of persons they serve professionally or who are participants in research and scholarly activities, and they shall treat animals involved in research in a humane manner.

Rules of Ethics

A. Individuals shall provide all services competently.
B. Individuals shall use every resource, including referral when appropriate, to ensure that high-quality service is provided.
C. Individuals shall not discriminate in the delivery of professional services or the conduct of research and scholarly activities on the basis of race or ethnicity, gender, gender identity/gender expression, age, religion, national origin, sexual orientation, or disability.
D. Individuals shall not misrepresent the credentials of assistants, technicians, support personnel, students, Clinical Fellows, or any others under their supervision, and they shall inform those they serve professionally of the name and professional credentials of persons providing services.
E. Individuals who hold the Certificate of Clinical Competence shall not delegate tasks that require the unique skills, knowledge, and judgment that are within the scope of their profession to assistants, technicians, support personnel, or any nonprofessionals over whom they have supervisory responsibility.

F. Individuals who hold the Certificate of Clinical Competence may delegate tasks related to provision of clinical services to assistants, technicians, support personnel, or any other persons only if those services are appropriately supervised, realizing that the responsibility for client welfare remains with the certified individual.
G. Individuals who hold the Certificate of Clinical Competence may delegate tasks related to provision of clinical services that require the unique skills, knowledge, and judgment that are within the scope of practice of their profession to students only if those services are appropriately supervised. The responsibility for client welfare remains with the certified individual.
H. Individuals shall fully inform the persons they serve of the nature and possible effects of services rendered and products dispensed, and they shall inform participants in research about the possible effects of their participation in research conducted.
I. Individuals shall evaluate the effectiveness of services rendered and of products dispensed, and they shall provide services or dispense products only when benefit can reasonably be expected.
J. Individuals shall not guarantee the results of any treatment or procedure, directly or by implication; however, they may make a reasonable statement of prognosis.
K. Individuals shall not provide clinical services solely by correspondence.
L. Individuals may practice by telecommunication (e.g., telehealth/e-health), where not prohibited by law.
M. Individuals shall adequately maintain and appropriately secure records of professional services rendered, research and scholarly activities conducted, and products dispensed, and they shall allow access to these records only when authorized or when required by law.
N. Individuals shall not reveal, without authorization, any professional or personal information about identified persons served professionally or identified participants involved in research and scholarly activities unless doing so is necessary to protect the welfare of the person or of the community or is otherwise required by law.
O. Individuals shall not charge for services not rendered, nor shall they misrepresent services rendered, products dispensed, or research and scholarly activities conducted.
P. Individuals shall enroll and include persons as participants in research or teaching demonstrations only if their participation is voluntary, without coercion, and with their informed consent.
Q. Individuals whose professional services are adversely affected by substance abuse or other health-related conditions shall seek professional assistance and, where appropriate, withdraw from the affected areas of practice.
R. Individuals shall not discontinue service to those they are serving without providing reasonable notice.

Principle of Ethics II

Individuals shall honor their responsibility to achieve and maintain the highest level of professional competence and performance.

Rules of Ethics

A. Individuals shall engage in the provision of clinical services only when they hold the appropriate Certificate of Clinical Competence or when they are in the certification process and are supervised by an individual who holds the appropriate Certificate of Clinical Competence.
B. Individuals shall engage in only those aspects of the professions that are within the scope of their professional practice and competence, considering their level of education, training, and experience.
C. Individuals shall engage in lifelong learning to maintain and enhance professional competence and performance.
D. Individuals shall not require or permit their professional staff to provide services or conduct research activities that exceed the staff member's competence, level of education, training, and experience.
E. Individuals shall ensure that all equipment used to provide services or to conduct research and scholarly activities is in proper working order and is properly calibrated.

Principle of Ethics III

Individuals shall honor their responsibility to the public by promoting public understanding of the professions, by supporting the development of services designed to fulfill the unmet needs of the public, and by providing accurate information in all communications involving any aspect of the professions, including the dissemination of research findings and scholarly activities, and the promotion, marketing, and advertising of products and services.

Rules of Ethics

A. Individuals shall not misrepresent their credentials, competence, education, training, experience, or scholarly or research contributions.
B. Individuals shall not participate in professional activities that constitute a conflict of interest.
C. Individuals shall refer those served professionally solely on the basis of the interest of those being referred and not on any personal interest, financial or otherwise.
D. Individuals shall not misrepresent research, diagnostic information, services rendered, results of services rendered, products dispensed, or the effects of products dispensed.
E. Individuals shall not defraud or engage in any scheme to defraud in connection with obtaining payment, reimbursement, or grants for services rendered, research conducted, or products dispensed.
F. Individuals' statements to the public shall provide accurate information about the nature and management of communication disorders, about the professions, about professional services, about products for sale, and about research and scholarly activities.
G. Individuals' statements to the public when advertising, announcing, and marketing their professional services; reporting research results; and promoting products shall adhere to professional standards and shall not contain misrepresentations.

Principle of Ethics IV

Individuals shall honor their responsibilities to the professions and their relationships with colleagues, students, and members of other professions and disciplines.

Rules of Ethics

A. Individuals shall uphold the dignity and autonomy of the professions, maintain harmonious interprofessional and intraprofessional relationships, and accept the professions' self-imposed standards.
B. Individuals shall prohibit anyone under their supervision from engaging in any practice that violates the Code of Ethics.
C. Individuals shall not engage in dishonesty, fraud, deceit, or misrepresentation.
D. Individuals shall not engage in any form of unlawful harassment, including sexual harassment or power abuse.
E. Individuals shall not engage in any other form of conduct that adversely reflects on the professions or on the individual's fitness to serve persons professionally.
F. Individuals shall not engage in sexual activities with clients, students, or research participants over whom they exercise professional authority or power.
G. Individuals shall assign credit only to those who have contributed to a publication, presentation, or product. Credit shall be assigned in proportion to the contribution and only with the contributor's consent.
H. Individuals shall reference the source when using other persons' ideas, research, presentations, or products in written, oral, or any other media presentation or summary.
I. Individuals' statements to colleagues about professional services, research results, and products shall adhere to prevailing professional standards and shall contain no misrepresentations.
J. Individuals shall not provide professional services without exercising independent professional judgment, regardless of referral source or prescription.
K. Individuals shall not discriminate in their relationships with colleagues, students, and members of other professions and disciplines on the basis of race or ethnicity, gender, gender identity/gender expression, age, religion, national origin, sexual orientation, or disability.
L. Individuals shall not file or encourage others to file complaints that disregard or ignore facts that would disprove the allegation, nor should the Code of Ethics be used for personal reprisal, as a means of addressing personal animosity, or as a vehicle for retaliation.
M. Individuals who have reason to believe that the Code of Ethics has been violated shall inform the Board of Ethics.
N. Individuals shall comply fully with the policies of the Board of Ethics in its consideration and adjudication of complaints of violations of the Code of Ethics.

APPENDIX

C

Individualized Education Program (IEP) Forms

Source: The Ohio Department of Education.

IEP Individualized Education Program

SST #13

THIS IEP WILL BE IMPLEMENTED DURING THE REGULAR SCHOOL TERM UNLESS NOTED IN GENERAL FACTORS

CHILD'S INFORMATION

NAME: Suzie Speech ID NUMBER:

STREET: GENDER: GRADE:

CITY: STATE: OH ZIP:

DATE OF BIRTH:

DISTRICT OF RESIDENCE: COUNTY OF RESIDENCE:

DISTRICT OF SERVICE:

Will the child be 14 years old before the end of this IEP? YES ☑ NO ☐
(Changes content of Sections 4 and 5)

Is the child a ward of the state? YES ☑ NO ☐

If yes, provide the name of the surrogate parent:

Foster care, care of Ohio Depart. Job and Family Services. If "yes" and parental rights removed- surrogate parent must be appointed

PARENTS' / GUARDIAN INFORMATION

NAME:

STREET:

CITY: STATE: OH ZIP:

HOME PHONE: WORK PHONE:

CELL PHONE: EMAIL:

OTHER INFORMATION:

- Document the primary language spoken in the home
- Document attempts to get parent to attend the IEP meeting
- Document important information that needs to be "up front" (i.e. medical info)
- Justification for ESY could be recorded here or in Profile (Section 3)
- Information can be put either here or in the Profile (Section 3) but doesn't need to be in both
- Can write N/A

MEETING INFORMATION

MEETING DATE: when team met

MEETING TYPE:

☐ INITIAL IEP
☐ ANNUAL REVIEW
☐ REVIEW OTHER THAN ANNUAL REVIEW

☐ AMENDMENT
☐ OTHER

IEP TIME LINES

ETR COMPLETION DATE:

NEXT ETR DUE DATE: no more than 3 yrs.

IEP EFFECTIVE DATES

START: August 23, 2009

END: August 22, 2010

NEXT IEP REVIEW:

IEP BY 3rd BIRTHDAY ? YES ☐ NO ☐
(If transitioning from EI services)

IEP FORM STATUS

(Check when complete)

☐ 1. FUTURE PLANNING
☑ 2. SPECIAL INSTRUCTIONAL FACTORS
☐ 3. PROFILE
☐ 4. POSTSECONDARY TRANSITION
☐ 5. POSTSECONDARY TRANSITION SERVICES
☐ 6. MEASURABLE ANNUAL GOALS
☐ 7. SPECIALLY DESIGNED SERVICES
☐ 8. TRANSPORTATION AS A RELATED SERVICE
☐ 9. NONACADEMIC AND EXTRA CURRICULAR
☐ 10. GENERAL FACTORS
☐ 11. LEAST RESTRICTIVE ENVIRONMENT
☐ 12. STATEWIDE AND DISTRICT TESTING
☐ 13. MEETING PARTICIPANTS
☐ 14. SIGNATURES

AMENDMENTS: (Complete only if amending the IEP)

IEP SECTION AMENDED	THE SCHOOL DISTRICT AND PARENTS HAVE AGREED TO MAKE THE FOLLOWING CHANGES TO THE IEP	DATE OF AMENDMENT	PARTICIPANT & ROLE
Number/Page	- Specifically describe summary of the changes agreed upon - Actual changes can be made in the body of the current IEP - This can be done without a face to face meeting, - Need written excusals for those not in attendance - If you don't use this part of IEP, attach a page, or rewrite IEP	Date added	Title and name, no signature required May have parent initial and date. If change of placement need section 14 signed

Suzie Speech

IEP Individualized Education Program — CHILD'S NAME: Suzie Speech

1 FUTURE PLANNING

- Based on **discussion with child and family** about child's future (coming year, life after graduation).
- For **younger children** the **emphasis is education** and **older children** on **postsecondary goals.**
- At Age 14+ there needs to be a **specific goal for post high school that is somewhat realistic** (i.e. If they don't become a pro basketball player)
- Summary statement about **student's skills and interests in relation to student's education and employment goals.**
- Can **not go to Due Process** over what is written in this section.
- This could be a **summary of conversations** held on transition

2 SPECIAL INSTRUCTIONAL FACTORS

Items checked "YES" will be addressed in this IEP:

Does the child have behavior which impedes his/her learning or the learning of others?	YES ☐	NO ☐
Does the child have limited English proficiency?	YES ☐	NO ☐
Is the child blind or visually impaired?	YES ☐	NO ☐
Does the child have communication needs (required for deaf or hearing impaired)?	YES ☐	NO ☐
Does the child need assistive technology devices and/or services?	YES ☐	NO ☐
Does the child require specially designed physical education?	YES ☐	NO ☐

3 PROFILE

CHILD'S PROFILE:

- Information which is **NOT tied to a goal.**
- Summarize the **strengths** of the child,
- How the **disability affects progress in the general curriculum** (as compared to typical peers),
- **Background information,**
- **Parent's concerns,**
- Medical/safety concerns
- Results of **state or district wide assessments,**
- Recent **Evaluations** of the child, including growth in any of the 9 assessed ares (preschool)
- Academic, developmental and functional **needs** of the child
- For Preschool: Information about child's **developmental strengths** in adaptive behavior, communication, hearing, vision, sensory and motor functioning, social emotion and behavior and pre-academic skills
- Include information about **Assistive Technology and how it is being used.**
- **Justification for ESY** can be documented here or in the Other Information section on the front page
- Include **needs that were identified on the ETR but are not being addressed on this IEP and tell why** they are not addressed.

4 POSTSECONDARY TRANSITION

FOR 14 YEARS AND OLDER
(or younger if appropriate)

A STATEMENT OF TRANSITION SERVICE NEEDS OF THE CHILD THAT FOCUSES ON THE CHILD'S COURSE OF STUDY

- Child's current courses of study in middle school (i.e. vocational education, prerequisite courses, advanced placement...) Do Not list every course.
- Where the student is going globally (i.e. college prep, vocational).
- Proposed course of study based on the realistic post secondary goal
- Related services needs, that impede the student in getting to their realistic post secondary goal

IEP Individualized Education Program	CHILD'S NAME: Suzie Speech

FOR 16 YEARS AND OLDER
(or younger if appropriate)

AGE APPROPRIATE TRANSITION ASSESSMENTS

Summarize the results of the age-appropriate transition assessment data in the space below, indicating the source of the assessment(s) and the relevant information for transition planning

- i.e. Attendance, work experiences, job shadows, time on task, interest inventories, vocational evaluations, career surveys...
- Courses of study, strengths, what they need to learn to get to the place they want (Section 1 Future Planning vision)

5 POSTSECONDARY TRANSITION SERVICES

POSTSECONDARY EDUCATION AND TRAINING (optional for 15 and younger)

MEASURABLE POSTSECONDARY GOAL:

-Must be based on assessment information.
-If needs will be met through regular ed. curriculum, a measurable goal does not need to be written.
-Write in 3rd person as "Sally will...upon completion of High School".
-District is not responsible for ensuring goals are completed after student leaves IEP coverage - but there should be a good faith effort seen to align all course of study, transition activities/services, and annual goals to post secondary outcome.
- Clarification documents available at www.nsttac.org

COURSES OF STUDY: in which the student receives instruction			NUMBERS OF ANNUAL GOAL(S)
TRANSITION SERVICE/ACTIVITY	PROJECTED BEGINNING DATE	ANTICIPATED DURATION	PERSON/AGENCY RESPONSIBLE
Services or activities needed to support goal. If in section 7 don't repeat	blank if same as front	freq & dura	Name or Title, NOT parent/stud

EMPLOYMENT (optional for 15 and younger)

MEASURABLE POSTSECONDARY GOAL:

COURSES OF STUDY:			NUMBERS OF ANNUAL GOAL(S)
TRANSITION SERVICE/ACTIVITY	PROJECTED BEGINNING DATE	ANTICIPATED DURATION	PERSON/AGENCY RESPONSIBLE
i.e. job shadow, work experience, instruction.. Add boxes if needed			provide services- post sec goal
For each goal there should be 1. Instruction 2. Related service(s)			
3. Community experience(s) 4. Development of employment and other			
post-school adult living objectives 5. if appropriate, acquisition of daily			
living skill(s) 6. if appropriate, provision of a functional vocational			
evaluation listed in association with meeting the postsecondary goal			

EMPLOYMENT (optional for 15 and younger)

IEP Individualized Education Program	CHILD'S NAME: Suzie Speech

MEASURABLE POSTSECONDARY GOAL:			
COURSES OF STUDY:		NUMBERS OF ANNUAL GOAL(S)	
TRANSITION SERVICE/ACTIVITY	PROJECTED BEGINNING DATE	ANTICIPATED DURATION	PERSON/AGENCY RESPONSIBLE

INDEPENDENT LIVING (As appropriate)

MEASURABLE POSTSECONDARY GOAL: Can say " no need for goal as there is no need for specially designed instruction outside the regular ed curriculum" - based on transition assessments			
COURSES OF STUDY: If appropriate there will be information showing the need in this area which would appear either in the Profile or PLOP with a Measurable Goal.		NUMBERS OF ANNUAL GOAL(S)	
TRANSITION SERVICE/ACTIVITY	PROJECTED BEGINNING DATE	ANTICIPATED DURATION	PERSON/AGENCY RESPONSIBLE

INDEPENDENT LIVING (As appropriate)

MEASURABLE POSTSECONDARY GOAL:			
COURSES OF STUDY:		NUMBERS OF ANNUAL GOAL(S)	
TRANSITION SERVICE/ACTIVITY	PROJECTED BEGINNING DATE	ANTICIPATED DURATION	PERSON/AGENCY RESPONSIBLE

Target date for child to Graduate: [ ]

IEP Individualized Education Program	CHILD'S NAME: Suzie Speech

6 MEASURABLE ANNUAL GOALS

NUMBER: 1 AREA: academic content area or area of functioning

PRESENT LEVEL OF ACADEMIC ACHIEVEMENT AND FUNCTIONAL PERFORMANCE

Present levels/Baseline information for this prioritized area. Can be taken from ETR. How disability affects involvement and progress in regular ed. curriculum. Include Academic/Developmental/Functional Needs- Compare to same age peers, Include any Special factors from Section 2, strengths, parental concerns, current assessment data

MEASURABLE ANNUAL GOAL	METHOD(S)
- Accomplished in 12 months - Aligned to content standards - Contains 1. condition (situation, setting or given material) behavior is performed, 2. clearly defined behavior (action) and 3. criteria of mastery, and 4. how frequent the teacher will assess the mastery of skills - Direct relationship between goals and PLOP	a,b or type in your own

METHOD FOR MEASURING THE CHILD'S PROGRESS TOWARDS ANNUAL GOAL

a. Curriculum Based Assessment	e. Short-Cycle Assessments	i. Work Samples
b. Portfolios	f. Performance Assessments	j. Inventories
c. Observation	g. Checklists	k. Rubrics
d. Anecdotal Records	h. Running Records	

MEASURABLE OBJECTIVES

NUM	OBJECTIVE
1.1	Plan for reaching annual goal and means of measuring progress towards those goals - to determine if progressing, or need to revise - Choose Benchmark or Objective from drop down above - Include condition, clearly defined behavior and performance criteria - Goal may be something several disciplines would work on (Intervention specialist, SLP,OT...)
1.2	Reporting Progress: - Objectives provide a mechanism to determine whether the child is progressing to ensure the IEP is consistent with the child's instructional needs and if appropriate to revise the IEP - Progress must be reported on benchmarks/objectives only if the child is taking Alternate Assessment, otherwise just progress on the goals is required - Must be at least as often as report cards and interims are issued to all students

METHOD AND FREQUENCY FOR REPORTING THE CHILD'S PROGRESS TO PARENTS

- ☐ Written report
- ☐ Email
- ☐ Phone call
- ☐ Journal entry
- ☐ The child's progress will be reported to the child's parents each time report cards are issued
- ☐ Other If multiple measures/frequency are used- specify here (be clear about what you will do)

Reported every 6 weeks

Note: Progress Reports must be provided to parents of a child with a disability at least as often as report cards are issued to all children. If the district provides interim reports to all children, progress reports must be provided to all parents of a child with a disability.

IEP Individualized Education Program	CHILD'S NAME: Suzie Speech

7 DESCRIPTION(S) OF SPECIALLY DESIGNED SERVICES

TYPE OF SERVICE		GOAL(s) ADDRESSED	PROVIDER TITLE	LOCATION OF SERVICES
SPECIALLY DESIGNED INSTRUCTION:				
Section #7 is a Synthesis of services -Services section puts all goals together that the person is responsible for - i.e. Adapting the content or methodology or delivery of instruction to access the general curriculum		1,3,5	Intervention specialist- in a group setting, or individual - make it clear! -include name and title	i.e. Resource room - If 2 locations make another drop down box - so it is clear
BEGIN:	END:	AMOUNT OF TIME:		FREQUENCY:
RELATED SERVICES:				
- Developmental, corrective and other supportive services to benefit from special education - Each Service gets it's own box (different location, service, time..BE SPECIFIC - Explain what the specialized instruction is - i.e. Speech and Language Therapy - DIRECT SMALL GROUP		1,4	SLP	Regular Ed. Classroom
BEGIN:	END:	AMOUNT OF TIME: 20 minutes/ Mon & Fri		FREQUENCY: 2 times a week
- i.e. Speech and Language Therapy - INDIVIDUAL		1,4	SLP	Intervention Room
BEGIN:	END:	AMOUNT OF TIME: 80 mins (can be range)		FREQUENCY: a month
-i.e. Speech and Language Therapy - CONSULTATIVE- - Explain what will be done. (i.e. to program AAC devices, select vocabulary, maintain device, and consult with teacher about progress and generalization of skills)		1,4		Consultative
BEGIN:	END:	AMOUNT OF TIME: 15 mins		FREQUENCY: once a week
ASSISTIVE TECHNOLOGY:				
- AT Devices: i.e. Dynamic voice output communication device, switch, keyboard with keyguard, joystick, etc.... - AT Services: (evaluation, purchasing/providing for acquisition, selection/customizing AT devices, coordinating with other therapies/services, maintaining, training) -Services i.e. Data collection on trials of various dynamic voice output communication devices, program leveling voice output communication device , select vocabulary and develop/ program overlays/pages, scan books into scan and read program, obtain narrative text for books from online resources and save as a scan and read document, picture schedule and directions using Mayer Johnson symbols/photographs, social stories done in pictured writing software,etc... - Make sure this is marked in Sections #2 Special Factors and #3 Profile - Don't worry about where you put it - (if you put it under Accommodation, or AT) or if SLP is the one doing it can either be AT or under related service		May or may not be tied to a goal	Individual assistant	Intervention Room
BEGIN:	END:	AMOUNT OF TIME: N/A, or during all classes		FREQUENCY: N/A or all day

IEP Individualized Education Program	CHILD'S NAME: Suzie Speech

ACCOMMODATIONS:			
-Providing access to, but not altering the amount or complexity. - Testing Accommodations should be done for ALL tests - Some may be appropriate for instruction but NOT for state tests (See Appendix H for allowable accommodations) -i.e. extra time for written assignments over 1 page, scribe for papers over 2 pages in length),teacher notes, - BE SPECIFIC - Should be linked to PLOP or needs	Can be left blank		
BEGIN:	END:	AMOUNT OF TIME:	FREQUENCY:

MODIFICATIONS:			
- Altering the content (decreasing amount or complexity). - For those with cognitive impairment, brain injury, multiply disabled	May or not be tied to goal		
BEGIN:	END:	AMOUNT OF TIME:	FREQUENCY:

SUPPORT FOR SCHOOL PERSONNEL:			
- could be an aide, training, resource materials, equipment or consultation with other professionals - i.e. Boardmaker training to create visuals (SLP doing could be here or in Related services or AT ...doesn't matter where)	May or not be tied to goal	Indicate - Who is giving, Who is getting, when and where the support will take place	
BEGIN:	END:	AMOUNT OF TIME:	FREQUENCY:

SERVICE(S) TO SUPPORT MEDICAL NEEDS:			
- Medical services the child needs to receive FAPE -Can include medications, or medical services (i.e. catheterization, feedings...) - Epipen would be in Profile Section 3 - Not Here	May or not be tied to goal		
BEGIN:	END:	AMOUNT OF TIME:	FREQUENCY:

KEY: ☐ OPTIONAL ENTRY ☐ NOT REQUIRED

8 TRANSPORTATION AS A RELATED SERVICE

Does the child have needs related to their identified disability that require special transportation? YES ☐ NO ☐

Does the child need accommodations or modifications for transportation? YES ☐ NO ☐

If yes, check any transportation accommodations/modifications that are needed.

☐ The bus driver will be notified of the child's behavioral and/or medical concerns

☐ Specially Adapted Vehicle ☐ Wheelchair lift ☐ Bus Aide

☐ Securement Systems ☐ Car Seat ☐ Harness

☐ Other Specify: ______________________

Does the child need transportation to and from provider services? YES ☐ NO ☐

9 NONACADEMIC AND EXTRACURRICULAR ACTIVITIES

In what ways will the child have the opportunity to participate in nonacademic/extracurricular activities with his/her nondisabled peers?

Describe

-Document opportunities to participate in non academic activities (i.e. recreational activities, special interest groups/clubs sponsored by the district, counseling services, athletics, ...
- If in IEP (i.e. office helper to help with socialization skills) it MUST happen
- If the parent wants to access one of the opportunities offered, the district must provide what ever they need to participate fully (i.e. interpreter...)

If the child will not participate in non-academic/extracurricular activities, explain.

i.e. parent and child do not wish to participate

10 GENERAL FACTORS

HAS THE IEP TEAM CONSIDERED:

The strengths of the child?	YES ☐	NO ☐
The concerns of the parents for the education of the child?	YES ☐	NO ☐
The results of the initial or most recent evaluations of the child?	YES ☐	NO ☐
As appropriate, the results of performance on any state or district-wide assessments?	YES ☐	NO ☐
The academic, developmental, and functional needs of the child?	YES ☐	NO ☐

The need for extended school year (ESY) services

☐ The team has determined that ESY services are not necessary.

☐ The team has determined that ESY services are necessary for the following Goals and Objectives or Benchmarks: List Goals and Objectives Numbers

☐ The team needs to collect further data before making a determination and will meet again by: Specify the date

11 LEAST RESTRICTIVE ENVIRONMENT

Does this child attend the school (or for a preschool-age child, participate in the environment) he/she would attend if not disabled?	YES ☐	NO ☑
Does this child receive all special education services with nondisabled peers?	YES ☐	NO ☑

12 STATEWIDE AND DISTRICT WIDE TESTING

For each subject tested in the child's grade, choose the method of assessment below. If "With Accommodations" is chosen for any subject, provide a description of the Accommodations for each subject in the right column.
Alternate Assessment, if chosen, must apply to all tests taken.

Will the child participate in classroom, district wide and state wide assessments with accommodations? YES ☐ NO ☑

Is the child to be excused from the consequences of not passing the Ohio Graduation Test (OGT)? YES ☑ NO ☐

The child is completing a curriculum that is significantly different than the curriculum completed by other children required to take the test. YES ☑ NO ☐

The child requires accommodations that are beyond the accommodations allowed for children taking state wide assessments. YES ☑ NO ☐

The child is excused from the consequences of not passing the OGT in the following subjects:

- ☐ Reading
- ☐ Mathematics
- ☐ Writing
- ☐ Social Studies
- ☐ Science

Met Testing Participation Requirement? YES ☐ NO ☐

Is the child participating in alternate assessment? YES ☑ NO ☐

Justify the choice of alternate assessment and address why it is appropriate:

If the team excuses the child from the consequences, NCLB requires that each child must attempt to take the test at least once

☐ Check when complete

IEP Individualized Education Program	CHILD'S NAME: Suzie Speech

13 MEETING PARTICIPANTS

THIS IEP MEETING WAS:

- [ ] Face-to-Face Meeting
- [ ] Video Conference
- [ ] Telephone Conference/Conference Call
- [ ] Other

IEP EFFECTIVE DATES

START: August 23, 2009

END: August 22, 2010

DATE OF NEXT IEP REVIEW: ______

IEP MEETING PARTICIPANTS

THE FOLLOWING PEOPLE ATTENDED AND PARTICIPATED IN THE MEETING TO DEVELOP THIS IEP

POSITION	NAME	SIGNATURE
Student*	If they didn't attend the whole meeting	
Parent	indicate how much they attended	
Parent		
District Representative*		
Intervention Specialist*	* persons need written excusal prior	
General Education Teacher*	to meeting	
Other Agency Representative		

PEOPLE NOT IN ATTENDANCE WHO PROVIDED INFORMATION AND RECOMMENDATIONS

POSITION	NAME	SIGNATURE	DATE
			info provided
			or date signed
			after
			IEP meeting

IF THE REGULAR EDUCATION TEACHER, INTERVENTION SPECIALIST, DISTRICT REPRESENTATIVE OR PERSON KNOWLEDGABLE ABOUT THE INSTRUCTIONAL IMPLICATIONS OF THE EVALUATION DATA HAVE SIGNED AS NOT IN ATTENDANCE AT THE IEP MEETING, A WRITTEN EXCUSE MUST BE ON FILE*.

14 SIGNATURES

INITIAL IEP

☐ I give consent to initiate special education and related services specified in this IEP.*

☐ I give consent to initiate special education and related services specified in this IEP except for **

AREA: ____________________

☐ I do not give consent for special education and related services at this time.**

PARENTS' SIGNATURE: ____________________ DATE: __________

ANNUAL REVIEW/REVIEW OTHER THAN ANNUAL REVIEW (Not a Change of Placement)

☐ I agree with the implementation of this IEP.*

☐ I am signing to show my attendance/participation at the IEP team meeting but I do not agree with the following special education and related services specified in this IEP.**

AREA: ____________________

Note: Not a Change of Placement does NOT require a parents' signature to implement the IEP.

PARENTS' SIGNATURE: ____________________ DATE: __________

ANNUAL REVIEW/REVIEW OTHER THAN ANNUAL REVIEW (Change of Placement)

☐ I give consent for the change of placement as identified in this IEP.*

☐ I do not give consent for the change of placement as identified in this IEP.**

☐ I revoke consent for all special education and related services.**

PARENTS' SIGNATURE: ____________________ DATE: __________

* This IEP serves as prior written notice if there is agreement.
**If there is not agreement or consent is revoked, the district must provide prior written notice to the parents.

TRANSFER OF RIGHTS AT MAJORITY

By the child's 17th birthday, the child and the child's parents or surrogate parent received a copy of their procedural safeguards notice and notice of the transfer of procedural safeguard rights under IDEA will take place on the child's 18th birthday. YES ☐ NO ☐

CHILD'S SIGNATURE: ____________________ DATE: __________

PARENTS' SIGNATURE: ____________________ DATE: __________

PROCEDURAL SAFEGUARDS NOTICE

A copy of the Procedural Safeguards Notice was given to the parents at the IEP Meeting. YES ☐ NO ☐

IF NO, DATE SENT TO PARENTS: __________

COPY OF THE IEP

A copy of the IEP was given to the parents at the IEP meeting. YES ☐ NO ☐

IF NO, DATE SENT TO PARENTS: __________

APPENDIX

D

Sample Language Arts Objectives— Kindergarten to Level 5

Listening Skills— (Kindergarten)

Major Focus

- Direction following
- Sound identification
- Stories
- Poems

Sample Objectives

- Follow oral directions for drawing pictures
- Follow directions for playing games
- Follow directions for marking worksheets
- Demonstrate body awareness of spatial words such as over, under, beside, in front, left, right, and so on
- Name a word that rhymes with a dictated word
- Arrange in the proper sequence, four or five pictures related to the story
- Answer questions using facts from the story
- Recognize the main idea in an oral presentation or story
- Name and describe the main characters of the story
- Repeat short nursery rhymes, poems, finger plays, songs

Speaking Skills—(Level 1)

Major Focus

- Story sequencing
- Sharing experiences

- Rhymes
- Poems

Sample Objectives

- Speak thoughts in complete sentences
- Supply names for concrete items and pictures
- Classification of familiar objects or pictures, (fruit—apple, orange; furniture—chair, table; clothing—dress, suit)
- Retell a story in the proper sequence
- Relate a personal experience in front of a group
- Verbally express human needs and emotions
- Describe how two objects are alike or different
- Take part in an informal exchange of ideas with others
- Present facts and ideas in an organized manner
- Recite familiar rhymes and poems

Oral And Dramatic Interpretation—(Level 2)

Major Focus

- Pantomime
- Role-playing
- Story characters
- Human emotions

Sample Objectives

- Take part in pantomiming activities; pretend to be the animal or character
  - ☐ Animals or real people
  - ☐ Nonliving things
  - ☐ Action or series of actions
  - ☐ Emotion or series of emotions
  - ☐ Story characters
- Act out a situation in the classroom
- Participate in role playing of real-life or storybook characters
- Improvise familiar stories
- Memorize written parts
- Participate in a formal play
- Dramatize a chosen role from a famous book or play

Oral Reading—(Level 3)

Major Focus

- Expression
- Comprehension
- Clear and distinct pronunciation
- Punctuation

Sample Objectives

- Read fluently in thought units

- Use clear and distinct pronunciation when reading
- Use expression to show the mood and emotion in the story
- Reread to location information
- Recall the sequence of the story
- Recall details of the story
- Identify the main idea of the story
- Read orally for the enjoyment of others
- Read a part in a play along with other readers

Grammar Skills—(Level 4)

Major Focus

- Punctuation
- Capitalization
- Abbreviations
- Irregular verbs
- Prepositional phrases
- Pronouns
- Usage
- Contractions
- Possessives
- Verb tense

Sample Objectives

- Write and punctuate sentence types correctly
- Use punctuation correctly in sentences
- Use capital letters
- Use correct plurals
- Identify verbs in sentences
- Identify the pronouns in sentences by underlining
- Identify the two parts of a sentence by underlining the subject and the predicate
- Identify the adjectives in sentences
- Recognize that English sentences have definite word-order patterns
- Show how changing the word order of most English sentences will change their meaning
- Make a list of words that show ownership by adding 's to singular nouns
- Develop skill in proofreading

Written Composition—(Level 5)

Major Focus

- Different points of view
- Advertisements
- Magazine articles, news stories
- Poetry; limericks
- Scripts; dialogues
- Stories—surprise endings, interesting beginnings, science fiction

- Letters
- Note taking
- Organization of ideas

Sample Objectives

- Write from the point of view of animals or other people
- Experiment with writing interesting book cards for a file as a means of pooling information about books
- Develop skill in taking notes
- Write an imaginary news story using notes
- Use information from multiple sources when writing travel ads
- Write a story about the future
- Use correct form for a friendly letter
- Combine concepts, principles, and generalizations in written compositions

References

Ainsworth, S. (1948, December). The speech clinician in public schools: Participant or separatist? *Asha, 7*, 495–503.

American Health Insurance Portability and Accountability Act. (1996). United States Government.

American Occupational Therapy Association. (2002). Occupational therapy practice framework: Domains and processes. *American Journal of Occupational Therapy, 56*, 605–683.

American Speech-Language-Hearing Association. (1984). Committee on Language, Speech, and Hearing Services in the Schools. Guidelines for caseload size for speech-language services in the schools. *Asha, 26*(4), 53–58.

American Speech-Language-Hearing Association. (1985). Committee on the Status of Racial Minorities. Rockville: Author.

American Speech-Language-Hearing Association. (1991). *A model for collaborative service delivery for students with language-learning disorders in the public schools* [Relevant paper]. Retrieved from http://www.asha.org/policy

American Speech-Language-Hearing Association. (1991). Council on Professional Standards. Proposed change in scope of ESB accreditation (revised). *Asha, 33*(11), 63.

American Speech-Language-Hearing Association. (1991). Educational Standards Board. Supervision of student clinicians. *Asha, 33*(6/7), 53.

American Speech-Language-Hearing Association. (1993). *Definitions of communication disorders and variations* [Relevant paper]. Retrieved from http://www.asha.org/policy

American Speech-Language-Hearing Association. (1993, 1998, 2010). *National Outcomes Measurement System (NOMS) for speech-language pathology and audiology*. Rockville, MD: Author.

American Speech-Language-Hearing Association. (1995, 2004). *Guidelines for the training, credentialing, use, and supervision of speech-language pathology assistants*. Rockville, MD: Author.

American Speech-Language-Hearing Association. (1996). *Inclusive practices for children and youths with communication disorders* (Position statement). Retrieved from http://www.asha.org/policy

American Speech-Language-Hearing Association. (1997). *Guidelines for audiologic screening*. Rockville, MD: Panel on Audiologic Assessment.

American Speech-Language-Hearing Association. (2000). Ad Hoc Committee on Reading and Writing Language Disorders. *Roles and responsibilities of speech-language pathologists related to reading and writing in children and youth*. Rockville, MD: Author.

American Speech-Language-Hearing Association. (2002). *A workload analysis approach for establishing speech-language caseload standards in schools* (Position statement). Retrieved from http://www.asha.org/slp/schools/resources/schools_resources_caseload.htm

American Speech-Language-Hearing Association. (2004). *Admission/discharge criteria in speech-language pathology* [Guidelines]. Retrieved from http://www.asha.org/policy

American Speech-Language-Hearing Association. (2004a). *Preferred practice patterns for the profession of speech-language pathology* [Preferred practice patterns]. Retrieved from http://www.asha.org/policy

American Speech-Language-Hearing Association. (2004b). *Guidelines for the audiologic assessment of children from birth to 5 years of age.* Retrieved from http://www.asha.org/policy

American Speech-Language-Hearing Association. (2005). *Quality indicators for professional service programs in audiology and speech-language pathology* [Standards/quality indicators]. Retrieved from http://www.asha.org/policy

American Speech-Language-Hearing Association. (2005). *Speech-language pathologists providing clinical services via telepractice position statement* (Position statement). Available from http://www.asha.org/policy

American Speech-Language-Hearing Association. (2007). *Ethics and IDEA.* Rockville, MD: Author.

American Speech-Language-Hearing Association. (2008). *Incidence and prevalence of communication disorders and hearing loss in children* (2008 ed.). Retrieved from http://www.asha.org/research/reports/children.htm

American Speech-Language-Hearing Association. (2008). *Roles and responsibilities of speech-language pathologists in early intervention: Technical report.* Retrieved from http://www.asha.org/policy

American Speech-Language-Hearing Association. (2010). *Code of ethics* [Ethics]. Retrieved from http://www.asha.org/policy

American Speech-Language-Hearing Association. (2010). *Code of ethics.* Rockville, MD: Author.

American Speech-Language-Hearing Association (2010). *Ethics Q & A for school-based speech-language pathology practice.* http://www.asha.org/slp/schools/profconsult/EthicsFAQsForSchools.htm

American Speech-Language-Hearing Association. (2010). *Omnibus survey.* Rockville, MD: Author.

American Speech-Language-Hearing Association. (2010). *Roles and responsibilities of speech-language pathologists in schools* [Professional issues statement]. Retrieved from http://www.asha.org/policy

American Speech-Language-Hearing Association. (2010). *Professional issues in telepractice for speech-language pathologists.* Available from http://www.asha.org/policy

Annett, M. M. (2004, March 02). Service delivery success: SLPs in Oregon schools tackle workload, enhance recruitment. *ASHA Leader.*

Autism Speaks. (2010). http://www.autismspeaks.org/what-autism

Bader, S. (2011). *An alternative approach to bilingual assessment.* Progressus Pathways Learning Center. Baltimore, MD: Progressus Therapy.

Baker-Hawkins, S., & Easterbrooks, S. (Eds.). (1994). *Deaf and hard of hearing students: Educational service guidelines.* Alexandria, VA: National Association of State Directors of Special Education.

Beitchman, J. H., Nair, R., Clegg, M., & Patel, P. G. (1986, May). Prevalence of speech and language disorders in 5-year-old kindergarten children in the Ottawa-Carleton region. *Journal of Speech and Hearing Disorders, 51,* 98–110.

Bender, R. E. (1960). *The conquest of deafness.* Cleveland, OH: The Press of Western Reserve University.

Bess, F. H. (1988). *Hearing impairment in children.* Parkton, MD: York Press.

Blachman, B. (1998). Early intervention and phonological awareness. A cautionary tale. In B. Blachman (Ed.), *Foundations of reading acquisition and dyslexia, implications for early intervention.* Mahwah, NJ: Erlbaum.

Blosser, J. (2009a). *Progressus Therapy's recommended experiences for the school-based externship.* Baltimore, MD: Progressus Therapy.

Blosser, J. (2009b). *Resource guide for working with teachers. Response to intervention.* Baltimore, MD: Progressus Therapy.

Blosser, J. (2010). Progressus therapy. Innovative solutions. Supporting clinicians to achieve success. Progressus Therapy, http://www.Progressustherapy.com

Blosser, J., & DePompei, R. (2002). *Pediatric brain injury: Proactive assessment and intervention.* Philadelphia, PA: Thompson.

Blosser, J., & Kratcoski, A. (1997). PACS: A framework for determining appropriate service delivery options. *Language, Speech, and Hearing Services in Schools, 28,* 99–107.

Blosser, J., & Park, L. (1996). "Kids are consumers too" satisfaction survey (Class project). Akron, OH: The University of Akron.

Blosser, J., & Silverman, F. (2010). *Mentoring instructional support staff: An effective strategy for achieving recruitment, retention, and successful service delivery.* National Association of Elementary School Principals. Webinar.

Blosser, J., Subich, L., Ehren, T., & Ribbler, N. (1999). *Broward County School District project to determine treatment outcomes.* American Speech-Language, Hearing Foundation Grant. Rockville, MD: ASHF.

Bluestone, C. D., & Klein, J. D. (1996). Otitis media, atelectasis, and eustachian tube disfunction. In C. D. Bluestone, S. E. Stool, & M. A. Kenna (Eds.), *Pediatric otolaryngology* (3rd ed., Vol. 1, pp. 338–582). Philadelphia, PA: Saunders.

Boswell, S. (2009, September 22). Leading change with the workload approach. *ASHA Leader.*

Brain Injury Association. (2011). Retrieved from http://www.BIA.org

Brown, J., Juenger, J., & Forducey, P. (2007). *Addressing shortages in schools via telepractice.* American Speech-Language-Hearing Association.

Bryngelson, B., & Glaspey, E. (1941). *Speech improvement cards,* Scott, Foresman & Company.

Bullock, G., Delli-Fraine, J., & Torrez, B. (2010). *Progressus way: Occupational therapists in schools: Roles and responsibilities.* Baltimore, MD: Progressus Therapy.

Carlin, C. (2011). *OMNIE SLP guidelines: Ohio's workload approach and flexible scheduling.* Ohio Masters Network Initiatives in Education.

Carothers-Liske, J. (2010). Roles of the school-based physical therapist. Personal communication.

CaseliteSoftware.com. (2011). http://www.Caselitesoftware.com

CAST (Center for Applied Technology). (2011). *Universal design for learning guidelines version 2.0.* Wakefield, MA: Author.

Catts, H. & Kamhi, A. (Eds.) (1999). *Language and reading disabilities.* Boston, MA: Allyn & Bacon.

Chamberlain, P., & Landurand, P. (1990). Practical considerations in the assessment of bilingual students. In E. V. Hamayan & J. S. Damico (Eds.), *Limiting bias in the assessment of bilingual students.* Austin, TX: Pro-Ed.

Cheng, L. (2011). Communication in the 21st century. Progressus Pathways Learning Center continuing education course. Baltimore, MD: Progressus Therapy.

Cirrin, F. M., & Penner, S. G. (1995). Classroom-based and consultative service delivery models for language intervention. In M. E. Fey, J. Wondsor, & S. F. Warren (Eds.), *Language intervention: Preschool through the elementary years* (pp. 333–362). Baltimore, MD: Brookes.

Cirrin, F. M., Schooling, T. L., Nelson, N. W., Diehl, S. F., Flynn, P. F., Staskowski, M., Zoann Torrey, T., & Adamczyk, D. F. (2010). Evidence-based systematic review: Effects of different service delivery models on communication outcomes for elementary school-age children. *Language, Speech, and Hearing Services in Schools, 41,* 233–264.

Clark, J. G. (1980). Central auditory dysfunction in school children: A compilation of management suggestions. *Language, Speech, and Hearing Services in Schools, 11,* 208–213.

Clark, G. M., Carlson, B. C., Fisher, S., Cook, J. D., & D'Alonzo, B. J. (1991). Career development for students with disabilities in elementary schools. A position statement of the Division on Career Development. *Career Development for Exceptional Individuals, 14*, 109–120.

Conner, T., & Silverman, F. (2003). Mentoring: Great gains at little cost. *ADVANCE for Speech-Language Pathologists and Audiologists, 13*(10), 10–11. http://speech-language-pathology-audiology.advanceweb.com/Article/Mentoring-Great-Gains-at-Little-Cost.aspx

Council of Chief State School Officers (CCSSO) and National Governors Association (NGA). (2010). *Common core state standards initiative: Preparing America's students for college and career.*

Corbin, C. (2008). How to survive a due process hearing. *Perspectives on School-Based Issues, 9*, 5–12.

Costello, M. R., & Curtis, R. (1989). The early years: History of the Michigan Speech, Language and Hearing Association. *MSHA Journal, 23*, 20.

Crais, E. R. (1991). Moving from "parent involvement" to family-centered services. *American Journal of Speech-Language Pathology, 1*(1), 5–8.

Creaghead, N., Estomin, E., Freilinger, J. J., & Peters-Johnson, C. (1992). Focus on school issues: Classroom integration and collaborative consultation as service delivery models. Teleconference. Rockville, MD: American Speech-Language-Hearing Association.

Damico, J., & Nye, C. (1990). Collaborative issues in multicultural populations. In W. A. Secord & E. H. Wiig (Eds.), *Best practices in school speech-language pathology. Collaborative programs in the schools: Concepts, models, and procedures*. San Antonio, TX: Psychological Corporation.

Davis-MacFarland, E. (2010). *Ethics for school speech-language pathologists and audiologists.* ASHA Schools Conference. Las Vegas, NV.

DeFur, S. H., & Patton, J. R. (1999). *Transition and school-based services*. Austin, TX: Pro-Ed.

Delfosse, A., & Hagge, D. (2011). *Volunteerism and leadership: Let's get started!* Presented at the California Speech and Hearing Association 2011 Annual Convention, Los Angeles, CA.

Dodge, E., & Mallard, D. (1992). Social skills training using a collaborative approach. *Language, Speech, and Hearing Services in Schools, 23*, 130–135.

Downs, M., Mencher, G., Dahle, A., Gerber, S., Stein, L., Cherow, E., & Rubin, M. (1982). Joint Committee on Infant Hearing: Position Statement. *ASHA, 24*, 1017–1018.

Dunn, H. M. (1949, June). A speech and hearing program for children in a rural area. *Journal of Speech and Hearing Disorders, 14*, 166–170.

Education Week. (2004). Achievement Gap.

Education World. (2011). Curriculum resources. Retrieved from http://www.education-world.com .

Eger, D. L. (1998). Outcomes measurement in the schools. In C. M. Fratteli (Ed.), *Measuring outcomes in speech-language pathology*. New York, NY: Thieme.

Eger, D. L., Adamczyk, D., Baker, A., Elkin, M. A., Hartman, K., Klein, D., . . . Wood, M. (1990). *Planned courses: Speech and language program*. Exceptional Children's Program, Allegheny Intermediate Unit, Pittsburg, PA.

Ehren, B. J. (2008). Making informed decisions about literacy intervention in schools: An adolescent literacy example. *EBP Briefs, 3*(1), 1–11.

Ehren, B. J., Montgomery, J., Rudebusch, J., & Whitmire, K. (2011). *Responsiveness to intervention: New roles for speech-language pathologists*. Retrieved from http://www.asha.org/uploadedFiles/slp/schools/prof-consult/rtiroledefinitions.pdf

Ehren, B. J., & Murza, K. (2011). *The urgent need to address workforce readiness in adolescent literacy intervention*. American Speech-Language-Hearing Association. Perspectives on Language Learning and Education.

Ehren, T. (1999). *Developing a professional growth plan for speech-language pathologists.* In-service meeting for Broward County School District, Ft. Lauderdale, FL.

Ehren, T. C. (2005). Responsiveness to intervention: Leadership opportunities. *Topics in Language Disorders, 25*(2), 168–179.

Estomin, E. (2010). Success story: Returning SLP-generated Medicaid funds to the SLP budget. Retrieved from http://www.asha.org

Finn, M. S., & Gardner, J. B. (1984). *Teacher interview: A better speech-language screening technique.* Area Education Agency XI, Ankeny, Iowa and Des Moines Public Schools. San Francisco, CA: American Speech-Language-Hearing Convention.

Flexer, C. (1989). Neglected issues in educational audiology. *Journal of the Aural Rehabilitation Association, 22,* 61–66.

Flexer, C. (1991). Access to communication environments through associative listening devices. *Hearsay: Journal of the Ohio Speech and Hearing Association, 6*(1), 9–14.

Flexer, C. (1992). Management of hearing in an educational setting. In J. G. Alpiner & P. A. McCarthy (Eds.), *Rehabilitation audiology: Children and adults* (2nd ed.). Baltimore, MD: Williams & Wilkins.

Flexer, C. (1999). *Facilitating hearing and listening in young children* (2nd ed.). San Diego, CA: Singular.

Flexer, C., Wray, D., & Ireland, J. (1989). Preferential seating is not enough: Issues in classroom management of hearing impaired students. *Language, Speech, and Hearing in Schools, 20,* 11–21.

Flower, R. M. (1984). *Delivery of speech-language and audiology services.* Baltimore, MD: Williams & Wilkins.

Flynn, P. (2010). New service delivery models: Connecting SLPs with teachers and curriculum. *ASHA Leader, 15*(10), 22–23. Rockville, MD: American Speech-Language-Hearing Association.

Frattali, C. M. (1990). From quality assurance to total quality management. *American Journal of Audiology, 1*(1), 41–47.

Frattali, C. M. (1999). *Measuring outcomes in speech-language pathology*. New York, NY: Thieme.

Friend, M. (2010). Collaboration skills for school professionals. *Journal of Educational and Psychological Consultation, 20*(1).

Fuchs, L. S. (2003). Assessing intervention responsiveness: Conceptual and technical issues. *Learning Disabilities Research and Practice, 18,* 172–186.

Gillette, Y. (2011). *Achieving communication competence. Assessment for intervention: Multimodal communication including AAC.* Progressus Therapy Pathways Learning Center.

Gillette, Y., & DePompei, R. (2009). PDA Intervention Plan. Implementing electronic memory and organization aids. Project produced in partnership with the Assistive Technology Collaboration on Cognitive Disabilities (University of Akron, Temple University, Spaulding Rehabilitation Hospital, and the Brain Injury Association of America. Funded by the National Institute on Disabilities and Rehabilitation Research (NIDRR). Project Number H13A030810.

Gillette, Y., & Robinson, N. (1992). *The individualized family service plan: A systematic approach.* From The CATCH guide to planning services with families: Coordinated transition from the hospital to the community and home.

Golper, L. C. (2007, September 04). Panelists share skills for the future. *ASHA Leader*. Rockville, MD: American Speech-Language-Hearing Association.

Golper, L. C. (2009). Leadership: Finding your inner Throgmartin. *Perspectives on Administration and Supervision, 19,* 39–44.

Grogan, S. (2010). ODE/OMNIE Pilot Telepractice Project. Ohio Speech-Language Hearing Association.

Grogan-Johnson, S., Alvares, R., Rowan, L., & Creaghead, N. (2010). A pilot study comparing the effectiveness of speech-language therapy provided by telepractice with conventional onsite therapy. *Journal of Telemedicine and Telecare, 16*(3), 134–139.

Haines, H. H. (1965). Trends in public school therapy. *ASHA, 7*, 166–170.

Hales, R. M., & Carlson, L. B. (1992). *Issues and trends in special education*. Federal Resource Center of Special Education. University of Kentucky.

Hanson, M., Lynch, E. W., & Wayman, K. I. (1990). Honoring the cultural diversity of families when gathering data. *Topics in Early Childhood Special Education, 10*(1), 112–131.

Harris, G. (1985). Considerations in assessing English language performance in Native American children. *Topics in Language Disorders, 5*(4), 42–52.

Haskill, A. M. (2004). Incorporating state standards in language intervention. *Perspectives on School-Based Issues, 5*, 3–7.

Hepworth, D., Rooney, R., & Larson, J. (1997). *Direct social work practice: Theory and skills* (5th ed.). Pacific Grove, CA: Brooks/Cole.

Herrara, L. M. K., & Burrows, J. A. (2007). *3:1 Model from research to implementation*. Presented at the American Speech-Language-Hearing Annual Convention.

Holzhauser-Peters, L., & Husemann, D. A. (1988). *Alternative service delivery models for more efficient and effective treatment programs*. Alexandria, VA: Clinical Connection.

Homer, E. M. (1997). *Making time in the schools: A program for caseload management*. Presented at the American Speech-Language-Hearing Association Annual Convention.

Hull, F. M. (1964). *National Speech and Hearing Survey interim report*. Project No. 50978. Washington, D.C.: Department of Health, Education and Welfare, Office of Education, Bureau of Education for the Handicapped.

Idol, L., Paolucci-Whitcomb, P., & Nevin, A. (1986). *Collaborative consultation*. Rockville, MD: Aspen.

Irwin, R. B. (March 1949). Speech and hearing therapy in the public schools of Ohio. *Journal of Speech and Hearing Disorders, 14*, 63–69.

Johnson, A. (1997). *ASHA Functional communication measures: Reliability and validity in medical speech-language pathology*. A final report submitted to the American Speech-Language-Hearing Foundation.

Johnson, P. R. (2003). Entry level business practices knowledge and skills document. *ASHA Perspectives on Administration and Supervision, 13*(1), 10–11.

Johnson, P. R. (2004). Documentation and coding for improved reimbursement. *ASHA Perspectives on Administration and Supervision, 14*(2), 7–9.

Johnson, S. M. (1996). *Leading to change*. San Francisco, CA: Jossey-Bass.

Karten, T. (2009a). *Inclusion succeeds with effective strategies (K–5)*. Port Chester, NY: Dude Publishing, an imprint of National Professional Resources.

Karten, T. (2009b). *Inclusion succeeds with effective strategies (grades 6–12)*. Port Chester, NY: Dude Publishing, an imprint of National Professional Resources.

Keane, L. (2011). *SLPs and assistants: Partners in practice*. ASHA Schools 2011 Session Anthology. ASHA's Annual Conference on Speech, Language, Hearing Services in Schools. Rockville, MD: ASHA.

Kreb, R. (1991). *Third party payment for funding special education and related services*. Horsham, PA: LRP Publications.

Krueger, B. (April 1985). Computerized reporting in a public school program. *Language, Speech, and Hearing Services in Schools, 16*, 135–139.

Kulpa, J. I., Blackstone, S., Clarke, C. C., Collingnon, M. M., Griffin, E. B., Hutchins, B. F., . . . Seymour, C. M. (1991). Chronic communicable diseases and risk management in the schools. *Language, Speech, and Hearing Services in the Schools, 22*, 345–352.

Kuster, J. (2010). Monthly Internet guides. *ASHA Leader*. Rockville, MD: American Speech-Language-Hearing Association. Retrieved from http://www.mnsu.edu/comdis/kuster4/leader

Larson, V. L. (2011). *Strategies that motivate adolescents with language disorders*. ASHA Schools 2011 Session Anthology. ASHA's Annual Conference on Speech, Language,

Hearing Services in Schools. Rockville, MD: ASHA.

Lastohkein, T., Glay-Moon, C., & Blosser, J. (1992). Improving collaborative efforts through the QI process. *Hearsay: Journal of the Ohio Speech and Hearing Association, 7*(1), 19–22.

Levinson, E. M., & Murphy, J. P. (1999). School psychology. In S. H. deFur & J. R. Patton (Eds.), *Transition and school-based services: Interdisciplinary perspectives for enhancing the transition process*. Austin, TX: Pro-Ed.

Listen Foundation. (2010). *Options for teaching deaf and hearing-impaired children*. Englewood, CO: Listen Foundation.

Markward, M., & Kurtz, P. D. (1999). School social work. In S. H. deFur & J. R. Patton (Eds.), *Transition and school-based services: Interdisciplinary perspectives for enhancing the transition process*. Austin, TX: Pro-Ed.

Marvin, C.A. (1990). Problems in school-based speech-language consultation and collaboration services: Defining the terms and improving the process. In W. A. Secord & E. H. Wiig (Eds.), *Best practices in school speech-language pathology collaborative programs in the schools: Concepts, models and procedures*. San Antonio, TX: Psychological Corporation.

McCauley, R., & Fey, M. (Eds.) (2006). *Treatment of language disorders in children*. Baltimore, MD: Paul H. Brookes.

Montgomery, J. (2000). *The role of the school-based speech-language-pathologist vis-à-vis IDEA '97*. Retrieved from http://www.asha.org/students/professional_issues/montgomery.htm

Montgomery, J. (2009). *Service delivery models: Effective, efficient, intensive*. Kansas City, MO: ASHA Schools Conference, 2009.

Montgomery, J., & Blosser, J. (2010). Service delivery: Weighing the options. http://www.speechpathology.com

Moore-Brown, B.. & Montgomery, J. (2008). Expanded and specialized services. In B. Moore-Brown & J. Montgomery (Eds.), *Making a difference for America's children: Speech-language pathologists in public schools*. Eau Claire, WI: Thinking Publications.

Moore, G. P., & Kester, D. (1953, March). Historical notes on speech correction in the preassociation era. *Journal of Speech and Hearing Disorders, 18*, 48–53.

Mullins, J. M., & McCready, V. (2002). *The SLP assistant supervisor's companion*. East Moline, IL: Linguisystems.

National Association of State Directors of Special Education, Inc. (2011). Retrieved from http://www.nasdse.org/Projects/ResponsetoInterventionRtIProject/tabid/411/Default.aspx

National Center for Health Statistics. (2010). *International classification of diseases*, 10th revision, Clinical Modification (ICD-10-CM).

National Center on Universal Design of Learning. (2011). Retrieved from http://www.CAST.org

National Governors Association and Council of Chief State School Officers. (2010). *The core curriculum*.

National Joint Committee for the Communication Needs of Persons with Severe Disabilities. (2002). *Adults with Learning Disabilities: Access to Communication Services and Supports: Concerns Regarding the Application of Restrictive "Eligibility" Policies* [Technical report]. Retrieved from http://www.asha.org/policy or www.asha.org/njc

National Institute on Deafness and other Communication Disorders. (1995). *Research in human communication* (Annual report). Bethesda, MD.

National Universal Design for Learning (UDL) Center. (2011). Retrieved from http://www.udlcenter.org

Neal, W. R., Jr. (1976, January). Speech pathology services in the secondary schools. *Language, Speech and Hearing Services in Schools, 7*, 6–16.

Nelson, N. W. (1990). Curriculum-based language assessment and instruction. *Language, Speech, and Hearing Services in Schools, 21*, 170–184.

Nelson, N. W. (2008). *Vision, values, and leadership in the context of shifting policies*. American Speech-Language-Hearing Association Annual Convention.

Nelson, N. W. (2009). *Written language intervention: The writing lab approach*. Kansas City, MO: ASHA Schools Conference, 2009.

North Inland SELPA. (2007). *Communication Severity Scales: The "must have" tool to streamline the eligibility process*. Ramona, CA: North Inland SELPA.

O'Toole, T., & Zaslow, E. (November 1969). Public school speech and hearing programs: Things are changing. *ASHA, 11*, 499–501.

Paden, E. P. (1970). *A history of the American Speech and Hearing Association 1925–1958*. Washington, D.C.: American Speech and Hearing Association.

Pershey, M. G. (1998). Collaboration models and projected outcomes for school-based language therapy: Sampling the buffet. *Hearsay: Journal of the Ohio Speech and Hearing Association, 12*(1), 32–38.

Peterson, H. A., & Marquardt, T. P. (1990). *Appraisal and diagnosis of speech and language disorders*. Englewood Cliffs, NJ: Prentice-Hall.

Phillips, P. (1975). *Speech and hearing problems in the classroom*. Lincoln, NE: Cliff Notes.

Power-deFur, L. (1999, October). Medicaid billing in public schools: Is this health care or education? *Special Interest Division 11: Administration and Supervision*. Rockville, MD: American Speech-Language-Hearing Association.

Power-deFur, L. (2010). *Educational relevance of communication disorders*. ASHA Schools Conference. Las Vegas, NV.

Quigley, S. P., & Kretschmer, R. E. (1982). *The education of deaf children*. Baltimore, MD: University Park Press.

Reynolds, M. C., & Rosen, S. W. (1976, May). Special education: Past, present, and future. *Educational Forum, 40*, 551–562.

Robinson, Jr., T. L. (2010). From the President: Taking the lead in school settings. *ASHA Leader*.

Roth, F. P., Dougherty, D. P., Paul, D. R., & Adamczyk, D. (2010). *RTI in Action: Oral language activities for K–2 classrooms*. Rockville, MD: American Speech-Language-Hearing Association.

Rudebusch, J. (2011). *Speech and language supports in an RTI Framework*. Progressus Therapy Pathways Learning Center continuing education course. Baltimore, MD: Progressus Therapy.

Rudebusch, J., & Wiechmann, J. (2010). *RTI and SLP Services: Road map to implementation*. ASHA Schools Conference. Las Vegas, NV.

San Diego City Schools Office of Instructional Support. (2004–2005). *Articulation differences and disorders manual*. San Diego City Schools: Special Education Programs Division Transdiciplinary Services.

Schoolfield, L. (1937). *Better speech and better reading*. Magnolia, MA: Expression Company.

Secord, W. (2007, May). Learning the deep structure: Elements of school-based leadership. *ASHA Leader*.

Secord, W. A. (2007). Vision and values: Learning the deep structure: Elements of school-based leadership. *ASHA Leader, 12*(7), 10–11.

Secord, W. (2010). *Instructional leadership in language and literacy*. ASHA Schools Conference. Las Vegas, NV.

Selk, F., Bartz, C., Birrenkott, J., & Olmos, J. (2008). The Communication Severity Scales: The "MUST HAVE" tool to streamline the eligibility process. California Speech and Hearing Association Annual Conference.

Silverman, F. H. (1989). *Communication for the speechless*. Englewood Cliffs, NJ: Prentice-Hall.

Simon, C. S. (1987). Out of the broom closet and into the classroom: The emerging SLP. *Journal of Childhood Communication Disorders, 2*(1), 41–46.

Skinner, M. W. (1978). The Hearing of Speech During Language Acquisition. *Otolaryngological Clinics of North America, 11*, 631–650.

Snyder, N. (2010). Accountability: A more accurate description of adequate yearly progress. *ASHA Governmental Affairs*. Retrieved from http://www.asha.org

Soliday, S. (2001). *Implementing a 3:1 service delivery model*. Pilot project. Portland Public Schools. Portland, OR.

Soliday, S. (2010). *The 3:1 service delivery model*. American Speech-Language-Hearing Association. Continuing Education Program.

Spady, W. G. (1994). *Outcome-based education: Critical issues and answers*. Arlington, VA: American Association of School Administrators.

Speedyspeechtherapy.com. (2011). A quick artic program. Retrieved from http//www.speedy speechtherapy.com

Steer, M. D. (1961, July). Public school speech and hearing services. A special report prepared with support of the United States Office of Education and Purdue University. *Journal of Speech and Hearing Disorders, Monograph Supplement 8*: Washington, DC: U.S. Office of Education Cooperative Research Project No. 649 (8191).

Strong-VanZandt, B. (2006). *A comparison of service delivery models: What practicing professionals report*. Miami, FL: American Speech-Language-Hearing Association Annual Convention.

Swift, W. B. (1972, April). How to begin speech correction in the public schools. *Language, Speech and Hearing Services in the Schools, 3*, 51–56.

Swigert, N. (2002, February 5). Documenting what you do is as important as doing it. *ASHA Leader, 7*(2), 14–17.

Taps, J. (2008). RTI services for children with mild articulation needs: Four years of data. *Perspectives on School-Based Issues, 9*, 104–110.

Terrell, B. Y., & Hale, J. E. (1992). Serving a multicultural population: Different learning styles. *American Journal of Speech-Language Pathology, 1*(2), 5–8.

Thompson, M., & Thompson, J. (2002). *Leadership, achievement, and accountability*. Boone, NC: Learning Concepts.

Townsend, A. (2011). *Promoting social-emotional competence in children*. Mariposa Student Success Program.

Ukrainetz, T. (2006). The implications of RTI and EBP for SLPs: Commentary on L. M. Justice. *Language, Speech, and Hearing Services in Schools, 37*, 298–202.

U.S. Congress. (1974). Family Educational Rights and Privacy Rights Act (FERPA).

U.S. Congress. (2006). American Health Insurance Portability and Accountability Act (HIPAA).

U.S. Department of Education. (1998). *To assure the free appropriate public education of all Americans: Twentieth annual report to Congress on the implementation of the Individuals with Disabilities Act* (Pub No 1998-716-372/93547). Washington, DC: U.S. Government Printing Office.

U.S. Department of Education. (2005). *To assure the free appropriate public education of all Americans: Twenty-seventh annual report to Congress on the implementation of the Individuals with Disabilities Education Act*. Retrieved January 16, 2008, from http://www.ed.gov/about/reports/annual/osep/2005/index.html

U.S. Department of Education, America Reads Challenge. (1997). *Read "right" now*. Washington, DC: Author.

U.S. Department of Education, Office of Special Education and Rehabilitative Services. (2003). *A new era: Revitalizing special education for children and their families*. Washington, DC: Author.

Vanderheiden, G. C., & Lloyd, L. L. (1986). Communication systems and their components. In S. W. Blackstone & D. M. Bruskin (Eds.), *Augmentative communication: An introduction* (pp. 49–161). Rockville, MD: American Speech-Language-Hearing Association.

Vanderheiden, G. C., & Yoder, D. E. (1986). Overview. In S. W. Blackstone and D. M. Bruskin (Eds.), *Augmentative communication: An introduction* (pp. 1–28). Rockville, MD: American Speech-Language-Hearing Association.

Vermont Department of Special Education. (2010). Retrieved from Vermont Department of Education Website.

Vicker, B. (2010). The 21st century speech-language pathologist and integrated services in classrooms. Retrieved from www.iidc.indiana.edu/irca/communication/21Century.html

Warren, S., Fey, M., & Yoder, P. (2007). Differential treatment intensity research: A missing link to creating optimally effective communication interventions. *Mental Retardation and Developmental Disabilities Research Reviews, 13*, 70–77.

Weathererly, J. (2010). *Current trends in special education law*. ASHA Schools Conference. Las Vegas, NV.

Wehman, P. (1992). *Life beyond the classroom: Transition strategies for young people with disabilities.* Baltimore, MD: Paul H. Brookes.

Westman, M. J., & Broen, P. A. (1989) Preschool screening for pediatric articulation errors. *Language, Speech, and Hearing Services in the Schools, 20*, 139–148.

Wiig, E., & Secord, W. (1990). *Best practices in school speech-language pathology*. San Antonio, TX: Psychological Corporation.

Williams, A. L., McLeod, S., & McCauley, R. J. (2010). *Interventions for speech sound disorders in children*. Communication and Language Intervention Series. Baltimore, MD: Paul H. Brookes.

World Health Organization. (2010, 2011). *International classification of impairments, disabilities, and handicaps.* Geneva, Switzerland: Author.

Yorkston, K. M., & Karlan, G. (1986). Assessment procedures. In S. W. Blackstone & D. M. Bruskin (Eds.), *Augmentative communication: An introduction* (pp. 163–196). Rockville, MD: American Speech-Language-Hearing Association.

Index

G

I

R

S